LIVER METABOLISM AND FATTY LIVER DISEASE

OXIDATIVE STRESS AND DISEASE

Series Editors

LESTER PACKER, PhD
ENRIQUE CADENAS, MD, PhD

UNIVERSITY OF SOUTHERN CALIFORNIA SCHOOL OF PHARMACY
LOS ANGELES, CALIFORNIA

LIVER METABOLISM AND FATTY LIVER DISEASE

EDITED BY
OREN TIROSH

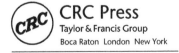

CRC Press
Taylor & Francis Group
Boca Raton London New York

CRC Press is an imprint of the
Taylor & Francis Group, an **informa** business

CRC Press
Taylor & Francis Group
6000 Broken Sound Parkway NW, Suite 300
Boca Raton, FL 33487-2742

First issued in paperback 2020

© 2015 by Taylor & Francis Group, LLC
CRC Press is an imprint of Taylor & Francis Group, an Informa business

No claim to original U.S. Government works

ISBN-13: 978-1-4822-1245-7 (hbk)
ISBN-13: 978-0-367-65908-0 (pbk)

Library of Congress Cataloging-in-Publication Data

Liver metabolism and fatty liver disease / editor, Oren Tirosh.
  p. ; cm.
  Includes bibliographical references and index.
  ISBN 978-1-4822-1245-7 (hardcover : alk. paper)
  I. Tirosh, Oren, editor.
  [DNLM: 1. Fatty Liver--metabolism. 2. Fatty Liver--etiology. 3. Fatty Liver--therapy. 4. Liver--metabolism. WI 700]

  QP185
  612.3'5--dc23   2014022997

Visit the Taylor & Francis Web site at
http://www.taylorandfrancis.com

and the CRC Press Web site at
http://www.crcpress.com

Contents

SECTION I Introduction to Fatty Liver Disease and Consequences

SECTION II Fatty Liver Disease and Consequences

SECTION III   Nutrition Role in Liver Protection and Damage

Series Preface

OXYGEN BIOLOGY AND MEDICINE

Through evolution, oxygen—itself a free radical—was chosen as the terminal electron acceptor for respiration. The two unpaired electrons of oxygen spin in the same direction; thus, oxygen is a biradical. Other oxygen-derived free radicals, such as superoxide anion or hydroxyl radicals, formed during metabolism or by ionizing radiation are stronger oxidants, i.e., endowed with a higher chemical reactivity. Oxygen-derived free radicals are generated during metabolism and energy production in the body and are involved in regulation of signal transduction and gene expression, activation of receptors and nuclear transcription factors, oxidative damage to cell components, the antimicrobial and cytotoxic action of immune system cells as well as in aging and age-related degenerative diseases. Conversely, the cell conserves antioxidant mechanisms to counteract the effect of oxidants; these antioxidants may remove oxidants either in a highly specific manner (e.g., by superoxide dismutases) or in a less specific manner (e.g., small molecules such as vitamin E, vitamin C, and glutathione). Oxidative stress as classically defined is an imbalance between oxidants and antioxidants. Overwhelming evidence indicates that oxidative stress can lead to cell and tissue injury. However, the same free radicals that are generated during oxidative stress are produced during normal metabolism and, as a corollary, are involved in both human health and disease.

UNDERSTANDING OXIDATIVE STRESS

In recent years, research disciplines interested in oxidative stress have grown and enormously increased our knowledge of the importance of the cell redox status and the recognition of oxidative stress as a process with implications for many pathophysiological states. From this multidisciplinary and interdisciplinary interest in oxidative stress emerges a concept that attests to the vast consequences of the complex and dynamic interplay of oxidants and antioxidants in the cellular and tissue settings. Consequently, our view of oxidative stress is growing in scope and new future directions. Likewise, the term "reactive oxygen species"—adopted at some stage to highlight nonradical oxidants such as H_2O_2 and $^1O_2$—fails to reflect the rich variety of other reactive species in free radical biology and medicine, i.e., encompassing nitrogen-, sulfur-, oxygen-, and carbon-centered radicals. With the discovery of nitric oxide, nitrogen-centered radicals gathered momentum and has matured into an area of enormous importance in biology and medicine. Nitric oxide or nitrogen monoxide (NO), a free radical generated in a variety of cell types by nitric oxide synthases (NOS), is involved in a wide array of physiological and pathophysiological phenomena, such as vasodilation, neuronal signaling, and inflammation. Of great importance is the radical–radical reaction of nitric oxide with superoxide anion: this is among the most rapid nonenzymatic reactions in biology (well over the diffusion-controlled limits) and yields the potent nonradical oxidant, peroxynitrite. The involvement of this species in tissue injury through oxidation and nitration reactions is well documented.

Virtually all diseases thus far examined involve free radicals. In most cases, free radicals are secondary to the disease process, but in some instances, causality established by free radicals themselves is known. Thus, there is a delicate balance between oxidants and antioxidants in health and disease. Their proper balance is essential for ensuring healthy aging.

Both reactive oxygen and nitrogen species are involved in the redox regulation of cell functions. Oxidative stress is increasingly viewed as a major upstream component in the signaling cascade involved in inflammatory responses, stimulation of cell adhesion molecules, and chemoattractant production and as an early component in age-related neurodegenerative disorders, such as Alzheimer disease, Parkinson disease, Huntington disease, and amyotrophic lateral sclerosis. Hydrogen peroxide is probably the most important redox signaling molecule that, among others, can activate NF-κB, Nrf2, and other universal transcription factors. Increasing steady-state levels of hydrogen peroxide has been linked to the cell's redox status, with clear involvement in adaptation, proliferation, differentiation, apoptosis, and necrosis. The identification of oxidants in regulation of redox cell signaling and gene expression was a significant breakthrough in the field of oxidative stress: the classical definition of oxidative stress as an *imbalance between the production of oxidants and the occurrence of cell antioxidant defenses* proposed by Sies in 1985 now seems to provide a limited concept of oxidative stress, but it emphasizes the significance of the cell's redox status. Because individual signaling and control events occur through discreet redox pathways rather than through global balances, a new definition of oxidative stress was advanced by Dean P. Jones (*Antioxidants and Redox Signaling*, 2006) as a disruption of redox signaling and control that recognizes the occurrence of compartmentalized cellular redox circuits. Recognition of discreet thiol redox circuits led D. P. Jones provide this new definition of oxidative stress. Measurements of GSH/GSSG or cysteine/cystine, $thioredoxin_{reduced}/thioredoxin_{oxidized}$ provide a quantitative definition of oxidative stress. The redox status is thus dependent on the degree to which tissue-specific cell components are in the oxidized state. In general, the reducing environment inside cells helps to prevent oxidative damage. In this reducing environment, disulfide bonds (S–S) do not spontaneously form because sulfhydryl groups are maintained in the reduced state (SH), thus preventing protein misfolding or aggregation. The reducing environment is maintained by metabolism and by the enzymes involved in maintenance of thiol/disulfide balance and substances, such as glutathione, thioredoxin, vitamins E and C, and enzymes such as superoxide dismutases, catalase, and the selenium-dependent glutathione reductase and glutathione, and thioredoxin-dependent hydroperoxidases (periredoxins), which serve to remove reactive oxygen species (hydroperoxides). Also of importance is the recognition of the existence of many tissue- and cell-compartment–specific isoforms of antioxidant enzymes and proteins.

Compelling support for the involvement of free radicals in disease development originates from epidemiological studies showing that an enhanced antioxidant status is associated with reduced risk of several diseases. Of high significance is the role that micronutrients play in modulation of redox cell signaling: this establishes a strong link between diet and health and disease, and centered on the ability of micronutrients to regulate redox cell signaling and modify gene expression.

These concepts are anticipated notions to serve as a platform for development of tissue-specific therapeutics tailored to discreet, compartmentalized redox circuits. This, in essence, dictates principles of drug development by guided by knowledge of mechanisms of oxidative stress. Hence, successful interventions will take advantage of new knowledge of compartmentalized redox control and free radical scanvenging.

OXIDATIVE STRESS IN HEALTH AND DISEASE

Oxidative stress is an underlying factor in health and disease. In this series of books, the importance of oxidative stress and disease associated with organ systems of the body is highlighted by exploring the scientific evidence and the clinical applications of this knowledge. This series is intended for researchers in the basic biomedical sciences and clinicians. The potential of such knowledge for healthy aging and disease prevention warrants further knowledge about how oxidants and antioxidants modulate cell and tissue function.

Liver Metabolism and Fatty Liver Disease, edited by Oren Tirosh of the Hebrew University of Jerusalem, covers several of the current areas of investigation into this widespread human disorder. The nonalcoholic form of fatty liver disease (NAFLD), known as steatohepatitis, is characterized by massive accumulation of lipid droplets in hepatic tissue, leading to pathology associated with disease progression.

The reported mechanisms that initiate NAFLD include oxidative stress, dietary lipids, obesity, insulin resistance, and inflammation; these mechanisms are integrated into the steps inherent in disease progression. The chapters in this volume address the role of cell organelles and metabolism involved in NAFLD.

Oren Tirosh and other internationally recognized leaders have contributed authoritative information on the mechanism of disease progression; they are to be congratulated for producing this excellent and timely book in an emerging field of health sciences research.

Lester Packer
Enrique Cadenas

Preface

LIVER METABOLISM AND FATTY LIVER DISEASE

Nonalcoholic fatty liver disease (NAFLD) comprises a spectrum of hepatic pathology, ranging from simple steatosis (SS), in which there is an increase of fat accumulation in hepatocytes, to nonalcoholic steatohepatitis (NASH), to cirrhosis. Primary NAFLD is associated with obesity, insulin resistance and metabolic syndrome, diabetes, and dyslipidemia. Secondary NAFLD is associated with all forms of liver damage including viral infections, autoimmune and hereditary diseases, drugs, toxins, and nutrition (parenteral nutrition, vitamin B12/folic acid deficiency, etc.). NASH is a progressive lesion in which steatosis is accompanied by hepatocyte injury and death as well as by hepatic infiltration of inflammatory cells. NASH-related liver damage often triggers liver fibrosis. In severe cases, NASH may progress to cirrhosis and possibly to hepatocellular carcinoma. NAFLD is one of the most common liver diseases worldwide affecting all racial, ethnic, and age groups without sex predilection. The prevalence of NAFLD is between 15% and 45% of the general population, whereas NASH affects about 3% of the lean population (those weighing no more than 110% of their ideal body weight), 19% of the obese population, and almost half of morbidly obese people.

It has become evident that progression from SS to NASH is not just a consequence of free fatty acid (FFA)–derived triglyceride (TG) accumulation in hepatocytes but, rather, the inadequate adaptation of the cells to toxic lipid–derived metabolites. Those may include unsaturated FFA, lipid peroxidation products, and others, which may induce multiple inflammatory pathways, mitochondrial dysfunction, oxidative stress, and endoplasmic reticulum stress—all leading eventually to cellular damage and apoptosis.

Oren Tirosh
The Hebrew University of Jerusalem

Editor

Oren Tirosh received his PhD from the School of Pharmacy, Faculty of Medicine, The Hebrew University of Jerusalem in 1997. He has done his postdoctoral fellowship with Lester Packer at the University of California Berkeley. Since 2001, he has been a staff member of the School of Nutrition Science, Institute of Biochemistry, Food Science and Nutrition, Faculty of Agriculture, Food and Environment, The Hebrew University of Jerusalem. In 2011, he was appointed the head of the School of Nutrition and received an academic rank of associate professor. Dr. Tirosh holds lifetime honorary membership in the Oxygen Club of California. He is active in the board of the Israel Society of Free Radical and Oxygen Research. His research interests include nitric oxide and redox biology, oxidative stress and liver pathology, and lipid metabolism in the liver under disease conditions.

Contributors

Michal Aharoni-Simon
Institute of Biochemistry, Food Science
and Nutrition
The Hebrew University of Jerusalem
Rehovot, Israel

and

Child and Family Research Institute
(CFRI)
Department of Surgery
University of British Columbia
Vancouver, British Columbia, Canada

Duah Alkam
Institute for Drug Research
The Hebrew University
Jerusalem, Israel

Anna Aronis
Institute of Biochemistry, Food Science
and Nutrition
The Hebrew University of Jerusalem
Rehovot, Israel

Jaime Bosch
Barcelona Hepatic Hemodynamic
Laboratory
Institut d'Investigacions Biomèdiques
August Pi i Sunyer (IDIBAPS)
Barcelona, Spain

Noga Budick-Harmelin
Institute of Biochemistry, Food Science
and Nutrition
The Hebrew University of Jerusalem
Rehovot, Israel

Dionysios V. Chartoumpekis
Department of Pharmacology and
Chemical Biology
University of Pittsburgh
Pittsburgh, Pennsylvania

Christopher M. Depner
The Linus Pauling Institute
Oregon State University
Corvallis, Oregon

Rabindra Dhital
Institute of Biochemistry, Food Science
and Nutrition
The Hebrew University of Jerusalem
Rehovot, Israel

Juan Carlos García-Pagán
Barcelona Hepatic Hemodynamic
Laboratory
Institut d'Investigacions Biomèdiques
August Pi i Sunyer (IDIBAPS)
Barcelona, Spain

Jordi Gracia-Sancho
Barcelona Hepatic Hemodynamic
Laboratory
Institut d'Investigacions Biomèdiques
August Pi i Sunyer (IDIBAPS)
Barcelona, Spain

Derick Han
Department of Biopharmaceutical
Sciences
Keck Graduate Institute
Claremont, California

A. Ruth He
Lombardi Comprehensive Cancer
    Center
Georgetown University
Washington, DC

Donald B. Jump
The Linus Pauling Institute
Oregon State University
Corvallis, Oregon

Thomas W. Kensler
Department of Pharmacology and
    Chemical Biology
University of Pittsburgh
Pittsburgh, Pennsylvania

and

Department of Environmental Health
    Sciences
The Johns Hopkins University
Baltimore, Maryland

Ho Leung
Department of Biopharmaceutical
    Sciences
Keck Graduate Institute
Claremont, California

Shelly C. Lu
Division of Gastroenterology and
    Liver Diseases
University of Southern California
Los Angeles, California

Kelli A. Lytle
The Linus Pauling Institute
Oregon State University
Corvallis, Oregon

Zecharia Madar
Institute of Biochemistry, Food Science
    and Nutrition
The Hebrew University of Jerusalem
Rehovot, Israel

Ihtzaz Ahmed Malik
Department of Internal Medicine
Georg-August-University
Göttingen, Germany

Noa Mashav
Department of Gastroenterology
Tel-Aviv Medical Center and Tel-Aviv
    University Sackler School of Medicine
Tel-Aviv, Israel

Lopa Mishra
The University of Texas
MD Anderson Cancer Center
Houston, Texas

Tommy Pacana
Department of Internal Medicine
Virginia Commonwealth University
Richmond, Virginia

Guiliano Ramadori
Department of Internal Medicine
Georg-August-University
Göttingen, Germany

Komal Ramani
Division of Gastroenterology and
    Liver Diseases
University of Southern California
Los Angeles, California

Nicole Rubin
Department of Biopharmaceutical
    Sciences
Keck Graduate Institute
Claremont, California

Arun J. Sanyal
Department of Internal Medicine
Virginia Commonwealth University
Richmond, Virginia

Oren Shibolet
Department of Gastroenterology
Tel-Aviv Medical Center and Tel-Aviv
    University Sackler School of Medicine
Tel-Aviv, Israel

Boaz Tirosh
Institute for Drug Research
The Hebrew University
Jerusalem, Israel

Oren Tirosh
Institute of Biochemistry, Food Science
    and Nutrition
The Hebrew University of Jerusalem
Rehovot, Israel

Sasmita Tripathy
The Linus Pauling Institute
Oregon State University
Corvallis, Oregon

Dotan Uzi
Institute for Drug Research
The Hebrew University
Jerusalem, Israel

Jacob E. Valk
Department of Biopharmaceutical
    Sciences
Keck Graduate Institute
Claremont, California

Stephen M. Wertheimer
Department of Biopharmaceutical
    Sciences
Keck Graduate Institute
Claremont, California

Shira Zelber-Sagi
Department of Gastroenterology
Tel-Aviv Medical Center
Tel-Aviv, Israel

and

School of Public Health
University of Haifa
Haifa, Israel

Section I

Introduction to Fatty Liver Disease and Consequences

1 Clinical Aspects of Nonalcoholic Fatty Liver Disease

Noa Mashav and Oren Shibolet

CONTENTS

INTRODUCTION

Nonalcoholic fatty liver disease (NAFLD) is characterized by accumulation of fat, mostly in the form of triglycerides, in the cytoplasm of hepatocytes, exceeding 5% to 10% by weight, as demonstrated by histology or imaging. It requires exclusion of other causes of steatosis, such as excessive alcohol consumption, drugs, or genetic diseases [1,2]. About 20% to 30% of adults with NAFLD will develop nonalcoholic steatohepatitis (NASH), a chronic hepatic inflammatory condition, which is the more severe form of the disease. In NASH, sustained liver injury can lead to progressive fibrosis and cirrhosis, liver-related morbidity, and hepatocellular carcinoma (HCC).

EPIDEMIOLOGY

With the increasing prevalence of obesity and diabetes mellitus (DM) worldwide, there is a significant increase in the incidence and prevalence of NAFLD [3,4].

INCIDENCE

Few studies investigated the incidence of NAFLD in the general population. In a recent study from Japan, the incidence of nonalcoholic hypertransaminasemia was 31 per 1000 person-years [5] and was higher in the younger than in the older age group (14.7% and 8.1%, respectively). Zelber-Sagi et al. published a prospective follow-up on a cohort of 147 healthy subjects that did not have NAFLD at baseline, of whom 28 (19%) developed NAFLD over a 7-year follow-up [6].

PREVALENCE

Prevalence of NAFLD varies greatly depending on definitions, populations studied, and the diagnostic methods (liver enzymes, imaging, histology, or their combinations) and is estimated at 20%–30% of the general population [7].

Autopsy studies allow for the diagnosis of NAFLD and NASH histologically and are considered accurate tools to estimate disease prevalence in the general population. In a recent study from Greece, liver biopsy material from a total of about 500 autopsies demonstrated a high prevalence of NAFLD and NASH: 31.3% and 39.8%, respectively [8]. In another study, autopsy NASH and fibrosis was found in 18.5% and 13.8% and 2.7% and 6.6% of markedly obese and lean patients, respectively [9]. In autopsies in children aged between 2 and 19 years old who died accidentally, NAFLD was present in 13% of subjects, steatohepatitis in 23% of those with fatty liver (3% of total study population), and severe fibrosis or cirrhosis in 9% of those with steatohepatitis. Fatty liver prevalence increased with age, ranging from 0.7% for ages 2 to 4 up to 17.3% for ages 15 to 19 years. The highest rate of fatty liver was seen in obese children (38%) [10].

The gold standard for the diagnosis of NAFLD is liver biopsy. The prevalence of NAFLD in potential liver transplant donors that underwent liver biopsy was 20% and 51% in American and Korean studies, respectively [11,12].

Imaging methods to diagnose NAFLD rely mostly on abdominal ultrasound (US). The prevalence of NAFLD by US was 17% to 46%, depending on the population studied [7]. Lazo et al. analyzed data from 12,454 adults who participated in the Third National Health and Nutrition Examination Survey (NHANES-III), conducted in the United States from 1988 to 1994. NAFLD was found in 19% of subjects, as diagnosed by US [13]. Magnetic resonance (MR) spectroscopy is a new imaging modality and is considered the most accurate imaging method to assess liver fat content. When MR spectroscopy was used in a nonselected population, the prevalence of NAFLD was 31% [11].

The most common method to diagnose NAFLD/NASH is by serum liver enzymes. The prevalence of NAFLD as assessed by increased liver enzyme levels, without imaging or histology, ranges from 7% to 11% in the general population. It should be noted that enzymes levels can be normal in patients with NAFLD, resulting in substantial underdiagnosis [7]. According to the NHANES-III database, the prevalence of elevated alanine aminotransferase (ALT) was 6.0%, in the studied population, and among these subjects, 41% had NAFLD. The prevalence of elevated aspartate aminotransferase (AST) was 5.6%, and 33.8% of these subjects had NAFLD [13].

The above-mentioned data suggest that the prevalence of NAFLD ranges from 2% to 35% in the general population, but can be markedly higher in patients with risk factors. Several factors were shown to be associated with increased prevalence of NAFLD.

AGE AND GENDER

NAFLD is a male dominant disease, and this predominance is more evident in Caucasian populations [14]. In an Asian population survey, NAFLD was diagnosed in 24% of the participants using abdominal US; the prevalence of NAFLD in men (31%) was significantly higher than that in women (16%) [15]. In a study with a predominantly Caucasian population, in which NAFLD was diagnosed by US and biopsy, 59% of subjects with NAFLD were men [16].

The underlying mechanisms leading to gender differences in NAFLD are unknown, but may be related to a protective effect of estrogen against the development of steatosis. This hypothesis is backed by an increased prevalence of NAFLD in postmenopausal women, higher rates of NAFLD in woman with polycystic ovary syndrome [17], and a reduction in liver enzymes in postmenopausal women taking hormone replacement therapy [18].

Another explanation for the higher rates of NAFLD in males is the excess abdominal adipose tissue compared with females with equal body mass index (BMI) [19]. The association between fat distribution and increased risk for NAFLD as part of the metabolic syndrome is well established [20,21].

The prevalence of NAFLD and NASH increases with age, as shown in multiple studies conducted in various countries and ethnic populations [14,22–24]. Frith et al. reviewed the data of 351 patients with biopsy-proven NAFLD in three age groups. NAFLD was significantly more prevalent in middle-aged and elderly subjects [25]. Age is not only an independent risk factor for the development of NAFLD but also for advanced fibrosis, HCC, and mortality [11,22,26].

ETHNICITY

Several studies have investigated the contribution of race and ethnicity to the prevalence of NAFLD and NASH in the general population. In the U.S. population, NAFLD is most prevalent in Hispanic subjects, followed by Caucasians and African Americans [7,14,27,28].

Higher rates of obesity and insulin resistance (IR) in patients of Hispanic origin can partly explain the ethnic differences in NAFLD prevalence. Yet, high rates of metabolic disturbances are also observed in African-Americans, which have the lowest NAFLD prevalence. The conflicting data led to the hypothesis that patients of Hispanic and African-American origin have different metabolic responses to obesity and IR. Indeed, studies that compared body fat distribution in the three major U.S. ethnic groups using various imaging methods showed that controlling for intraperitoneal fat content almost entirely eliminated ethnic differences in levels of steatosis [27,29]. These studies suggest that African-Americans appear to be more resistant to both the accretion of triglyceride in the abdominal adipose tissue and to hypertriglyceridemia induced by IR.

Genetic variability can also account for the ethnic differences in NAFLD prevalence. The adiponutrin (PNPLA3) rs738409 polymorphism has been associated with susceptibility to NAFLD [30,31]. The PNPLA3 allele is most common in Hispanic subjects, in correlation to the higher prevalence of hepatic steatosis [32]. Furthermore, a different single-nucleoside polymorphism (SNP) of PNPLA3 (rs6006460) was associated with lower hepatic fat content in African Americans, the group at lowest risk of NAFLD, implying that variation in PNPLA3 contributes to the ethnic susceptibility to NAFLD.

METABOLIC RISK FACTORS

The metabolic syndrome (MS) is the coexistence of multiple risk factors for subsequent development of cardiovascular disease (CVD) and DM, including obesity, glucose intolerance, hypertension, and hyperlipidemia. Both IR and visceral obesity play a predominant role in its development. The role of these metabolic derangements and obesity in the pathogenesis of NAFLD are discussed in Chapters 5, 8, 9, 11, 12, and 13 of this book.

ENVIRONMENTAL AND OTHER FACTORS

Environmental factors are also thought to play a role in the development of NAFLD. Caffeine consumption was found to have a possible protective effect against steatosis [33], whereas active and passive smoking increased the risk for NAFLD [34]. Incretin hormones, bile acids, selenium, taurine, and numerous other compounds were shown to influence the development NAFLD, yet their exact role requires further research and validation [35–38].

CLINICAL FEATURES

Most patients with NAFLD are asymptomatic [39], yet some may experience non-specific fatigue and malaise, nausea, and right upper abdominal pain or discomfort. Often, the diagnosis of NAFLD is made following an incidental finding of increased liver enzymes or abnormal imaging results.

NAFLD patients have been shown to experience a significant decrease in quality of life (QoL), most prominently in physical health, but also in mental health scores, in comparison with the general U.S. population [40]. Decreased QoL was evident even in patients with limited hepatic injury, and further decreased with increased fibrosis. Subjects with NAFLD-induced cirrhosis had significantly lower QoL scores compared with patients with chronic viral hepatitis B or hepatitis C infection [41].

Recent studies suggest that NAFLD is specifically associated with depression and also with generalized anxiety disorder and attention deficit/hyperactivity disorders [42–44]. It was recently suggested that NAFLD may even be an independent modifiable risk factor for depression [45].

There are several clinical manifestations that are associated with obesity, DM, and hypertension that are common in patients with NAFLD, but are associated with the metabolic syndrome and are not directly related to hepatic steatosis. Similarly, once cirrhosis has developed, its clinical manifestation is not directly related to the underlying liver disease.

DIAGNOSIS

NAFLD and NASH are diagnosed by imaging studies and/or histology, when other causes of steatosis or chronic liver disease have been ruled out.

Other common underlying causes of hepatic steatosis are excessive alcohol consumption (defined by consumption of more than 21 weekly doses of alcohol for men and more than 14 doses for women during the 2 years preceding the histological evidence of steatosis [46]), HCV infection (especially with genotype 3), medications (Table 1.1, Refs. [47–63]), total parenteral nutrition, malnutrition, and genetic syndromes.

It is important to distinguish "primary" NAFLD from other etiologies, as some underlying etiologies are treatable and treatment can resolve or improve steatosis [64]. Routine workup of patients with disturbed liver functions and steatosis include testing for viral hepatitis, autoimmune liver disease, hemochromatosis, thyroid disorders, celiac disease, and metabolic/genetic liver disease (Wilson disease, α-1-antitrypsin deficiency, and cystic fibrosis).

TABLE 1.1
Medications that Cause Hepatic Steatosis

Chronic steatosis	L-Asparaginase	Fibrosis and cirrhosis	Amiodarone
	Valproate		Methotrexate
	Perhexiline maleate		Methyldopa
	Amiodarone		Floxuridine
	Tetracycline		Azathioprine
			Mercaptopurine
Steatohepatitis	Amiodarone		Oral contraceptives
	Diethylaminoethoxyhexestrol		Inorganic arsenic
	Irinotecan		Copper sulphate
	Perhexiline maleate		Vinyl chloride
	Tamoxifen		Vitamin A
(rarely cause, but	5-fluorouracil		
may exacerbate)	Cisplatin	Phospholipidosis	Amiodarone
	Chloroform		Amitriptyline
	Diethylstilbestrol		Chloroquine
	Ethanol		Perhexiline maleate
	Glucocorticoids		Chlorpheniramine
	Gold		Chlorpromazine
	Griseofulvin		Thioridazine
	Methotrexate		
	Mercury		
	Nifedipine		
	Nitrofurantoin		
	NSAIDs		

Sources: Simon, J.B. et al., *N Engl J Med*, 1984; 311:167–72; Pessayre, D. et al., *Gastroenterology*, 1979; 76:170–7; Fromenty, B. and D. Pessayre, *Pharmacol Ther*, 1995; 67:101–54; Agozzino, F. et al., *Ital Heart J*, 2002; 3:686–8; Rigas, B., *Hepatology*, 1989; 10:116–7; Gehenot, M. et al., *J Hepatol*, 1994; 20:842; Lewis, J.H. et al., *Hepatology*, 1989; 9:679–85; Poucell, S. et al., *Gastroenterology*, 1984; 86:926–36; Ramachandran, R. and S. Kakar, *J Clin Pathol*, 2009; 62:481–92; Zorzi, D. et al., *Br J Surg*, 2007; 94:274–86; Pawlik, T.M. et al., *J Gastrointest Surg*, 2007; 11:860–8; Lee, W.M., *N Engl J Med*, 1995; 333:1118–27; Newman, M. et al., *Arch Dermatol*, 1989; 125:1218–24; Lee, W.M. and W.T. Denton, *J S C Med Assoc*, 1989; 85:75–9; Beyeler, C. et al., *Br J Rheumatol*, 1997; 36:338–44; Geubel, A.P. et al., *Gastroenterology*, 1991; 100:1701–9; Letteron, P. et al., *J Hepatol*, 1996; 24:200–8.

BIOPSY AND HISTOLOGY

To this date, liver biopsy remains the gold standard for the diagnosis of NAFLD and for differentiating it from NASH as well as from other etiologies of liver fibrosis. However, biopsy is costly, invasive, and has complications requiring hospitalization in 1%–3% of the cases and a procedural mortality of 0.001%. Furthermore, liver biopsy suffers from intraobserver and interobserver variability and from sample inadequacy or variability due to uneven disease distribution, which leads to missing a diagnosis of NASH in up to 27% of cases [65]. Even in the case of fibrosis that is considered uniform, results may vary from one part of the liver to another [66,67].

Histology may reveal a fatty change that is predominantly macrovesicular. The amount of steatosis is determined by the proportion of hepatocytes containing fat droplets (<10% mild, 10%–30% moderate, >30% severe). Features of steatohepatitis include hepatocyte ballooning sometimes associated with the formation of Mallory's hyaline (Mallory's bodies) and mega-mitochondria occurring mainly in zone 3 of the liver lobule.

The most distinct feature distinguishing NASH from NAFLD is the presence of parenchymal inflammation consisting of a mixed population of cells including mainly neutrophils, lymphocytes, macrophages/Kupffer cells, and some natural killer cells. Isolated biliary changes, siderosis, and mild portal and lobular changes mimicking chronic hepatitis may also occur. The fibrosis in NAFLD typically has a perisinusoidal and pericellular distribution and can lead to cirrhosis [68–72].

A quantitative scoring system of the following histological features: steatosis (0–3), lobular inflammation (0–2), and hepatocellular ballooning with the addition of fibrosis (0–4) has been validated and termed the NAFLD activity score (NAS) [73].

A NAS greater than or equal to 5 corresponds to NASH, a score of 0–2 is more likely to correspond with NAFLD, and a score of 3 or 4 is indeterminate [74].

Currently, liver biopsy is not routinely performed in patients with suspected NAFLD because of the perceived risk and because of the negligible effect of the results in determining therapeutic options due to lack of effective drug treatment [75].

Therefore, diagnosis of NAFLD relies on clinical skills, laboratory tests, imaging studies, and different scoring systems. None of these methods distinguishes between NAFLD and NASH, and many do not give an accurate assessment of the degree of fibrosis [76].

NONINVASIVE DIAGNOSTIC METHODS FOR NAFLD

IMAGING

Abdominal Ultrasound

Abdominal US is the most widely used imaging method for the diagnosis of hepatic steatosis with liver fat manifesting as increased echogenicity. The sensitivity and specificity of US for detecting hepatic steatosis ranges from 60% to 94% and from 88% to 95%, respectively. The sensitivity decreases with lower degrees of steatosis, reaching 55% when hepatic fat content is below 20% [77]. Several other factors affect the accuracy of US in diagnosing steatosis, including BMI and fibrosis [78]. The hepatorenal index (HRI) refers to the ratio of echogenicity of the liver parenchyma and the adjacent renal cortex. Its validity has been compared with liver biopsies and is a valuable tool in diagnosing even a small amount of hepatic fat [79].

Computed Tomography

Although computed tomography (CT) is considered a reliable technique to assess steatosis, its use is limited because of radiation exposure and complexity of technique (requiring precise contrast injection algorithms). In addition, it is less sensitive than US and MR imaging (MRI) [80]. On CT scan, hepatic steatosis has a low attenuation and appears darker than the spleen. The sensitivity and specificity of CT for detecting hepatic fat ranges from 50% to 86% and from 75% to 87%, respectively [80,81]. Accuracy is affected by fibrosis and by infiltration of the liver by iron or copper. Similar to US, CT is not sensitive in detecting low amounts of fatty infiltration [82].

Magnetic Resonance Imaging

Both MRI and MR spectroscopy are reliable at detecting and quantifying steatosis and have a higher diagnostic accuracy than US or CT. However, their use is limited by cost and lack of availability. Furthermore, similar to all imaging modalities it cannot distinguish NAFLD from NASH. The sensitivity and specificity of MRI in detecting steatosis is 85% and 100%, respectively [83]. MRI is currently the most accurate imaging modality to detect small amounts of fatty infiltration as low as 3% [84]. MR spectroscopy is a new MR modality that provides information about the chemical composition of the liver (e.g., hepatic triglyceride content). The values obtained with spectroscopy were validated compared with liver biopsy, and its use is expanding [85].

Transient Elastography (Fibroscan®)

A noninvasive technique used to assess liver stiffness (measured in kilopascal and correlated to fibrosis), and is currently FDA approved for the evaluation of liver fibrosis in NAFLD. A recent meta-analysis showed high sensitivity and specificity for Fibroscan® in identifying fibrosis in NAFLD, with the exception of patients with high BMI [86,87].

Two other noninvasive technologies for assessing tissue stiffness have recently been introduced. Acoustic radiation force impulse (ARFI) shear wave imaging and real-time elastography (RTE). ARFI technology estimates liver stiffness by measuring tissue deformation produced by the mechanical excitation of tissue with short duration acoustic pulses that produce shear wave propagation. RTE measures echo signals before and under slight compression to show the physical property of liver tissue. Both methods are used to assess fibrosis in NAFLD patients with good correlation to liver biopsies [88,89].

A major limitation of the methods described above is that they have been studied mainly in cross-sectional studies; thus, their efficiency in monitoring response to treatment and progression is not well established. None of the available noninvasive diagnostic tools can distinguish simple steatosis from NASH.

GENETICS

Patatin-Like Phospholipase 3 (PNPL3)

The *PNPL3* gene is located on the long arm of chromosome 22 at position 13.31. It encodes a triacylglycerol lipase protein that mediates triacylglycerol hydrolysis in adipocytes. In 2008, Romeo et al. revealed a strong association between variations in *PNPL3* alleles and differences in hepatic fat content and susceptibility to NAFLD; homozygotes carriers of the single-nucleotide polymorphism rs738409[G] in the *PNPL3* gene showed significantly higher and rs6006460[T] carriers showed lower levels of hepatic fat in comparison to noncarriers [32]. These results were similar in Japanese, American, and Italian populations [90–92].

Apolipoprotein C-III (*APOC-III*)

The *APOC3* gene is located on the long arm of chromosome 11 at position 23.3, encoding for the apolipoprotein C-III protein, a component of very-low-density lipoprotein (VLDL) and a primary cause of hypertriglyceridemia [93]. Although several SNPs in the *APOC-III* gene were shown to be associated with increased prevalence of NAFLD and IR, this association is still controversial and requires further validation [94–96].

Human Hemochromatosis (*HFE*)

The *HFE* gene is located on the short arm of chromosome 6 at location 6p21.3, regulates iron absorption and is associated with hereditary hemochromatosis. It has been suggested that the *HFE* gene is involved in NAFLD pathogenesis but its role is still unknown [97–99].

Other Genes

Other genes potentially involved in the pathogenesis of NAFLD include *NCAN*, *GCKR*, *LYPLAL1*, *PPP1R3B*, and *TNFR1* [31]. The contributory role of these genes to NAFLD is currently under intense research.

BIOMARKERS

Cytokeratin 18

Cytokeratin 18 (CK18) is the major intermediate filament protein in the liver, and during apoptosis, it is cleaved by caspases and released into the bloodstream.

Hepatocyte apoptosis plays an important role in liver injury in NASH [100] and NAFLD [101], making caspase-cleaved CK18 measurements a potential effective noninvasive biomarker in their diagnosis and monitoring [102,103]. Joka et al. measured levels of capase-cleaved CK18 (M30 and M65). Both assays could distinguish patients with different stages of fibrosis from healthy controls, but the M65 assay was shown to be able to differentiate low and higher grades of steatosis [104].

NAFLD Fibrosis Scoring Systems

Because of the difficulty in diagnosing NAFLD, differentiating it from NASH, and predicting outcome, several scoring systems using a myriad of assays, parameters, and methods have emerged. These systems are discussed here in brief.

NAFLD Fibrosis Score

The most extensively validated scoring system, comprised of six parameters (age, BMI, presence of IFG/DM, platelets, albumin, and AST/ALT ratio). It generates a score that can predict the presence or absence of advanced fibrosis in NAFLD and possibly reduce the need for liver biopsy in some patients. NAFLD fibrosis score

(NFS) was investigated and validated worldwide, with negative predictive value of 89%–93%, positive predictive value of 72%–91%, and sensitivity and specificity of 90% and 97%, respectively.

FibroTest

A six-parameter score (α-2-macroglobulin, haptoglobin, apolipoprotein A1, γ-gluta-myltranspeptidase (GGT), total bilirubin, and ALT), corrected for age and gender. It was evaluated and validated compared with liver biopsy in HCV [105], HBV [106], alcoholic liver disease [107], and NAFLD. A large meta-analysis demonstrated a mean standardized area under the ROC curves (AUROCs) of 0.84 for the diagnosis of NAFLD [108].

AST-to-Platelet Ratio Index

The AST-to-platelet ratio index (APRI) was initially developed for predicting significant fibrosis and cirrhosis in patients with HCV [109]. It is calculated using the formula (AST/ULN)/platelets × 100. The APRI score is a simple and noninvasive tool for identifying advanced fibrosis. Different studies estimated its sensitivity and specificity from 75% and 86% to 60% and 73%, respectively [110,111] and an average AUROC of 0.85 [112] to predict long-term outcomes of patients with NAFLD [113].

Enhanced Liver Fibrosis Panel

Enhanced liver fibrosis panel (ELF) combines measurements of three matrix turn-over proteins: hyaluronic acid (HA), amino-terminal propeptide of type III procollagen (PIIINP), and tissue inhibitor of metalloproteinase 1 (TIMP-1) adjusted to age. The ELF test was found to be accurate in determining the degree of fibrosis in NAFLD patients [114,115]. It has an area under the curve (AUC) of 0.90 for distinguishing severe fibrosis, 0.82 for moderate fibrosis, and 0.76 for no fibrosis. Simplification of the algorithm by removing age did not alter diagnostic performance [114].

SteatoTest

A combination of the FibroTest (Biopredictive, Paris, France) and the Acti-Test (Biopredictive, Paris, France) [107,116] with body mass index, serum cholesterol, triglycerides, and glucose adjusted for age and gender as a marker of fibrosis and steatosis.

Fatty Liver Index

A formula assembled of four parameters: BMI, waist circumference, triglycerides, and GGT levels. In a recent validation study, fatty liver index identified subjects with NAFLD with an AUROC curve of 0.813 [117].

Various other scores used for the identification of NAFLD and for predicting fibrosis and progression exist, including lipid accumulation product (LAP), NASHtest, Acetotest, Visceral Adiposity Index (VAI), and others. These methods require further validation.

TREATMENT

Fatty liver disease is essentially the hepatic manifestation of metabolic syndrome; therefore, treatment should focus on combating the separate components and risk factors for this disorder, such as obesity, hyperlipidemia, and diabetes.

NAFLD patients without signs of liver damage and fibrosis have limited disease progression. Therefore, pharmacological therapy should be considered only in patients with NASH [118].

LIFESTYLE INTERVENTION

Dietary changes in combination with physical exercise can induce substantial improvement in hepatic steatosis, inflammation, and fibrosis.

A meta-analysis of studies conducted from 1967 to 2000 using a variety of diet regiments with different caloric restrictions and nutrient composition clearly showed that weight reduction improved hepatic outcomes. However, the authors cautioned that studies in the meta-analysis were small and very few used histological evidence to support their findings [119].

Another meta-analysis compared aerobic exercise and/or progressive resistance training versus nonexercise controls. The authors show clear evidence for a benefit of exercise therapy on liver fat, but not ALT levels. This benefit was apparent even with minimal or no weight loss and at low exercise levels [120].

In a randomized controlled trial (RCT) by Promrat et al., participants with biopsy proven NASH were assigned to an aggressive weight loss and exercise program versus structured education alone. After 1-year follow-up, the treatment group showed a 9% weight reduction versus only 0.2% in the controls. Participants who reduced over 7% of their body weight showed significant improvement in NAS [121].

Based on these data, weight reduction and exercise are currently recommended treatments for NAFLD/NASH.

BARIATRIC SURGERY

Obese patients (BMI > 30 kg/m^2) are at greater risk of developing NAFLD and NASH [122]. The risk for hepatitis increases significantly if they also share other features of the metabolic syndrome such as IR, DM, hypertension, and dyslipidemia [123,124]. Bariatric surgery using either restrictive or malabsorptive techniques is rapidly becoming the best available treatment for obesity and type 2 DM.

Unfortunately, no RCTs are available regarding the different bariatric surgery techniques and their therapeutic effect on NAFLD or NASH, as most studies are observational or retrospective [125]. Nevertheless, histological changes in liver morphology in patients who underwent bariatric surgery were documented, especially in the first year following surgery. A large meta-analysis of observational studies regarding the outcome of bariatric surgery in patients with NAFLD/NASH showed considerable improvement in steatosis, steatohepatitis, and fibrosis [126].

Adverse effects of bariatric surgery include fulminant hepatitis and worsening fibrosis, particularly in patients with extreme weight loss during the first postoperative year [127]. Although overweight patients with NAFLD/NASH may benefit from bariatric surgery, both in terms of improvement in liver steatosis and fibrosis, and of eliminating other metabolic syndrome risk factors, strong evidence to support surgery as an established treatment of isolated NAFLD without metabolic derangements is still lacking [118].

PHARMACOLOGICAL THERAPY

Currently, there is only limited evidence to support the use of pharmacotherapy in NAFLD patients. Medications assessed thus far include insulin-sensitizing agents, vitamin E, ursodeoxycholic acid, lipase inhibitors, and weight reduction medications. These agents target IR, oxidative stress, and weight gain. Most trials were small, open label, and did not assess histological outcomes. They utilize changes in serum ALT and imaging end points.

VITAMIN E

Vitamin E is an antioxidant and has been investigated in the treatment of NASH [46], yet the trials conducted are difficult to compare because of the large variability of vitamin E doses and formulations used, other drugs used, and the inability to estimate changes in liver histology. A recent RCT evaluated the effect of high-dose vitamin E (800 IU/day), pioglitazone, or placebo in nondiabetic patients with NASH assessing histological end points. The PIVEN study showed that use of vitamin E improved steatosis, inflammation, and ballooning and led to resolution of steatohepatitis in adults with NASH, with no effect on hepatic fibrosis [128]. Another double-blind RCT assessing similar end points in pediatric patients with NAFLD compared high-dose vitamin E (800 IU/day) to metformin or placebo. Neither vitamin E nor metformin were superior to placebo in attaining the primary end point [129].

Of note, studies suggest that treatment with high-dose vitamin E supplements (>400 IU per day) increase all-cause mortality, but this point is still controversial [130,131].

INSULIN-SENSITIZING AGENTS: METFORMIN AND THIAZOLIDINEDIONES

Several studies examined the effect of metformin, pioglitazone, and rosiglitazone on the serum aminotransferases and hepatic histology in patients with NASH. Metformin had no significant effect on liver histology and is not currently recommended as treatment for NASH [118,129,132,133]. Studies assessing the effect of thiazolidinediones yielded conflicting results. A recent meta-analysis showed that pioglitazone significantly improved steatosis but not fibrosis and in the PIVEN trial pioglitazone led to resolution of NASH in a significant number of patients compared with placebo [7,128]. Concerns have been raised about the long-term safety of thiazolidinediones and their effect on congestive heart failure, weight gain, and bladder cancer [134–136]. Their use is currently very restricted, and several are no longer marketed.

Ursodeoxycholic Acid

Despite early enthusiasm, a recent RCT did not show benefit to ursodeoxycholic acid (UDCA) in improving histological outcomes in NAFLD patients as compared with placebo. High-dose UDCA reduced aminotransferase levels and decreased markers of fibrosis and IR, but histological end points were not examined. Its use is not currently recommended for the treatment of NASH [137,138].

Miscellaneous Agents

ω-3 polyunsaturated fatty acid (PUFA) has shown benefit in NAFLD, but the optimal dose is currently unknown [139]. Orlistat, a reversible inhibitor of gastric and pancreatic lipase, was shown to induce limited weight loss in selected patients, but side effects such as diarrhea and bloating make it less desirable. Although initially shown to improve liver outcomes [140], it was later shown that orlistat does not induce weight loss or improve histological NAFLD scores.

Recently, the FDA approved two new medications for weight loss. Lorcaserin is serotonergic and an anorectic drug that was shown together with behavioral modification to induce mild weight loss over a 1-year follow-up period [141]. Another drug, a combination of phentermine and topiramate, was also shown to induce weight loss over a 2-year follow-up [142]. The effect of these drugs on NAFLD has not been evaluated, and their long-term safety remains to be seen. There are multiple other medications under investigation for the treatment of NAFLD/NASH. Their detailed evaluation is beyond the scope of this chapter.

PREVENTION

The most common cause of death in patients with NAFLD or NASH is CVD; thus, identification of cardiovascular risk factors, and adjusting treatment accordingly, is an inseparable part of overall management.

Statins

Statins are the cornerstone of CVD treatment, and their use in patients with NAFLD has been widely advocated and has been associated with improvements in liver biochemistry and histology [143–146]. Despite their beneficial effect, their use is limited because of a conceived risk of hepatic injury. There are ample data to suggest that these fears are unfounded, and statins can be safely used in NAFLD and NASH patients [147–149].

Alcohol

Heavy alcohol consumption should be discouraged in NAFLD patients. No recommendation can be made regarding low-dose alcohol consumption in this population [118].

NATURAL HISTORY AND PROGRESSION

Studies have failed to provide sufficient evidence as to the changes in histological characteristics in patients with NAFLD and NASH over time. However, it is currently suggested that patients with simple steatosis show modest progression to cirrhosis and liver failure [7,150]. In contrast, 20% of patients with NASH are at risk of developing liver cirrhosis over the course of their lifetime [151].

Overall mortality in NAFLD patients is higher in comparison to the general population, with CVD being the leading cause of death. Patients with advanced disease who progress to NASH have higher mortality rates from complications of liver disease with a further increase in mortality rates in cirrhotics [22,152,153].

Surprisingly, analysis of all-cause mortality over an 18-year span of subjects from the NHANES III study did not find access mortality in patients with NAFLD compared with participants without steatosis [154].

Several studies have compared the natural history of patients with NASH cirrhosis to that of patients with HCV-induced cirrhosis. One study demonstrated lower rates of decompensation and mortality in patients with NASH cirrhosis compared with cirrhosis due to HCV [155]. Another large prospective multicenter cohort study showed that patients with NAFLD and advanced fibrosis or cirrhosis have lower rates of liver-related complications and HCC than corresponding patients with HCV infection, with similar overall mortality [156]. In contrast, however, recent analyses showed 10 years' survival to be similar among NAFLD patients and controls.

The risk for HCC was higher in NAFLD patients than controls, but limited to those with advanced fibrosis or cirrhosis and was lower than the risk for HCV cirrhotics [157–161]. Several studies suggested that the risk for HCC is not limited to NASH cirrhosis and that tumors can occur in nonfibrotic livers [155,162]. A recent meta-analysis questioned these findings claiming that the absolute risk for HCC in noncirrhotic NASH patients is only minimally elevated [163].

SCREENING

Routine screening for NAFLD is debatable, in terms of both method and efficacy. Laboratory finding alone are insufficient since liver enzymes may not always be disturbed in patients with NAFLD or NASH [7].

Alternatively, ultrasonographic studies are more expensive, less available, and subjected to user interpretation, making it inconvenient [46]. To date, performing routine screening tests for NAFLD is not recommended, even among high-risk populations, as long-term benefit and cost effectiveness is still unclear [46]. For similar reasons, screening of diagnosed NAFLD patients' family members is not recommended, despite the genetic link in NAFLD [46].

In some cases, imaging studies performed for various reasons other than elevated liver enzymes or suggestive clinical features reveal findings characteristic of liver steatosis. Once symptoms related to liver dysfunction or abnormal laboratory values are evident, evaluation for suspected NAFLD should be performed, otherwise, screening for metabolic risk factors (obesity, IFG, dyslipidemia), and other potential etiologies for liver damage, such as excessive consumption of alcohol or drugs, is warranted. A liver biopsy is not advised for diagnosis in cases of incidental findings.

SUMMARY

NAFLD is rapidly becoming the major cause of liver disease in the world. The disease can progress to NASH and lead to fibrosis and cirrhosis causing liver-related morbidity and mortality. Patients with NAFLD have a decreased QoL both physically and psychologically and the disease increases the risk for metabolic complications and CVDs.

Currently, treatment is lifestyle modifications with limited surgical and pharmacological therapy available. It is thus of extreme importance to understand the molecular mechanisms at the basis of the disease to guide our therapies and possibly identify modifiable risk factors and drug targets.

REFERENCES

1. Angulo, P. and K.D. Lindor, Non-alcoholic fatty liver disease. *J Gastroenterol Hepatol,* 2002; 17:S186–90.
2. Neuschwander-Tetri, B.A. and S.H. Caldwell, Nonalcoholic steatohepatitis: Summary of an AASLD single topic conference. *Hepatology,* 2003; 37:1202–19.
3. Bjornsson, E. and P. Angulo, Non-alcoholic fatty liver disease. *Scand J Gastroenterol,* 2007; 42:1023–30.
4. Flegal, K.M. et al., Prevalence and trends in obesity among US adults, 1999–2000. *JAMA,* 2002; 288:1723–1727.
5. Suzuki, A. et al., Chronological development of elevated aminotransferases in a nonalcoholic population. *Hepatology,* 2005; 41:64–71.
6. Zelber-Sagi, S. et al., Predictors for incidence and remission of NAFLD in the general population during a seven-year prospective follow-up. *J Hepatol,* 2012; 56:1145–51.
7. Vernon, G., A. Baranova, and Z.M. Younossi, Systematic review: The epidemiology and natural history of non-alcoholic fatty liver disease and non-alcoholic steatohepatitis in adults. *Aliment Pharmacol Ther,* 2011; 34:274–85.
8. Zois, C.D. et al., Steatosis and steatohepatitis in postmortem material from Northwestern Greece. *World J Gastroenterol,* 2010; 16:3944–9.
9. Wanless, I.R. and J.S. Lentz, Fatty liver hepatitis (steatohepatitis) and obesity: An autopsy study with analysis of risk factors. *Hepatology,* 1990; 12:1106–10.
10. Schwimmer, J.B. et al., Prevalence of fatty liver in children and adolescents. *Pediatrics,* 2006; 118:1388–93.
11. Lee, J.Y. et al., Prevalence and risk factors of non-alcoholic fatty liver disease in potential living liver donors in Korea: A review of 589 consecutive liver biopsies in a single center. *J Hepatol,* 2007; 47:239–44.
12. Marcos, A. et al., Selection and outcome of living donors for adult to adult right lobe transplantation. *Transplantation,* 2000; 69:2410–5.
13. Lazo, M. et al., Prevalence of Nonalcoholic Fatty Liver Disease in the United States: The Third National Health and Nutrition Examination Survey, 1988–1994. *Am J Epidemiol,* 2013; 178(1):38–45.
14. Browning, J.D. et al., Prevalence of hepatic steatosis in an urban population in the United States: Impact of ethnicity. *Hepatology,* 2004; 40:1387–95.

15. Chen, Z.W. et al., Relationship between alanine aminotransferase levels and metabolic syndrome in nonalcoholic fatty liver disease. *J Zhejiang Univ Sci B*, 2008; 9:616–22.
16. Williams, C.D. et al., Prevalence of nonalcoholic fatty liver disease and nonalcoholic steatohepatitis among a largely middle-aged population utilizing ultrasound and liver biopsy: A prospective study. *Gastroenterology*, 2011; 140:124–31.
17. Gutierrez-Grobe, Y. et al., Prevalence of non alcoholic fatty liver disease in premenopausal, posmenopausal and polycystic ovary syndrome women. The role of estrogens. *Ann Hepatol*, 2010; 9:402–9.
18. McKenzie, J. et al., Effects of HRT on liver enzyme levels in women with type 2 diabetes: A randomized placebo-controlled trial. *Clin Endocrinol (Oxf)*, 2006; 65:40–4.
19. Lemieux, S. et al., Sex differences in the relation of visceral adipose tissue accumulation to total body fatness. *Am J Clin Nutr*, 1993; 58:463–7.
20. Marchesini, G. et al., Nonalcoholic fatty liver, steatohepatitis, and the metabolic syndrome. *Hepatology*, 2003; 37:917–23.
21. Stefan, N., K. Kantartzis, and H.U. Haring, Causes and metabolic consequences of fatty liver. *Endocr Rev*, 2008; 29:939–60.
22. Adams, L.A. et al., The natural history of nonalcoholic fatty liver disease: A population-based cohort study. *Gastroenterology*, 2005; 129:113–21.
23. Chen, C.H. et al., Prevalence and etiology of elevated serum alanine aminotransferase level in an adult population in Taiwan. *J Gastroenterol Hepatol*, 2007; 22:1482–9.
24. Park, S.H. et al., Prevalence and risk factors of non-alcoholic fatty liver disease among Korean adults. *J Gastroenterol Hepatol*, 2006; 21:138–43.
25. Frith, J. et al., Non-alcoholic fatty liver disease in older people. *Gerontology*, 2009; 55:607–13.
26. Hu, X. et al., Prevalence and factors associated with nonalcoholic fatty liver disease in Shanghai work-units. *BMC Gastroenterol*, 2012; 12:123.
27. Lomonaco, R. et al., Role of ethnicity in overweight and obese patients with nonalcoholic steatohepatitis. *Hepatology*, 2011; 54:837–45.
28. Bambha, K. et al., Ethnicity and nonalcoholic fatty liver disease. *Hepatology*, 2012; 55:769–80.
29. Guerrero, R. et al., Ethnic differences in hepatic steatosis: An insulin resistance paradox? *Hepatology*, 2009; 49:791–801.
30. Zain, S.M. et al., A multi-ethnic study of a PNPLA3 gene variant and its association with disease severity in non-alcoholic fatty liver disease. *Hum Genet*, 2012; 131:1145–52.
31. Speliotes, E.K. et al., Genome-wide association analysis identifies variants associated with nonalcoholic fatty liver disease that have distinct effects on metabolic traits. *PLoS Genet*, 2011; 7:e1001324.
32. Romeo, S. et al., Genetic variation in PNPLA3 confers susceptibility to nonalcoholic fatty liver disease. *Nat Genet*, 2008; 40:1461–5.
33. Birerdinc, A. et al., Caffeine is protective in patients with non-alcoholic fatty liver disease. *Aliment Pharmacol Ther*, 2012; 35:76–82.
34. Liu, Y. et al., Active smoking, passive smoking, and risk of nonalcoholic fatty liver disease (NAFLD): A population-based study in China. *J Epidemiol*, 2013; 23:115–21.
35. Clarke, C. et al., Selenium supplementation attenuates procollagen-1 and interleukin-8 production in fat-loaded human C3A hepatoblastoma cells treated with TGFbeta1. *Biochim Biophys Acta*, 2010; 1800:611–8.
36. Zarrinpar, A. and R. Loomba, Review article: The emerging interplay among the gastrointestinal tract, bile acids and incretins in the pathogenesis of diabetes and non-alcoholic fatty liver disease. *Alimen Pharmacol Ther*, 2012; 36:909–921.
37. Gentile, C.L. et al., Experimental evidence for therapeutic potential of taurine in the treatment of nonalcoholic fatty liver disease. *Am J Physiol Regul Integr Comp Physiol*, 2011; 301:R1710–22.

38. Warskulat, U. et al., Chronic liver disease is triggered by taurine transporter knockout in the mouse. *FASEB J*, 2006; 20:574–6.
39. Lewis, J.R. and S.R. Mohanty, Nonalcoholic fatty liver disease: A review and update. *Dig Dis Sci*, 2010; 55:560–78.
40. David, K. et al., Quality of life in adults with nonalcoholic fatty liver disease: Baseline data from the nonalcoholic steatohepatitis clinical research network. *Hepatology*, 2009; 49:1904–12.
41. Dan, A.A. et al., Health-related quality of life in patients with non-alcoholic fatty liver disease. *Aliment Pharmacol Ther*, 2007; 26:815–20.
42. Suzuki, A., M. Binks, and A. Wachholtz, and A.M. Diehl, Relationship of psychological issues and sleep disturbance to liver function in obese patients at a residential weight loss program. *Gastroenterology*, 2007; 132:A–811.
43. Sayuk, G.S., E.d.S., J.E. Elwing, P. Lustman, M. Lisker-Melman, J.S. Crippin, R.E. Clouse, Severity of depression symptoms and transaminase levels are related in non-alcoholic steatohepatitis (NASH) and chronic hepatitis C. *Gastroenterology*, 2007; 132:A–813..
44. Lee, C.K. and M.M. Jonas, High prevalence of psychiatric and attention-deficit/hyperactivity disorders in children with NAFLD at children's hospital Boston 1995–2005: A retrospective study. *Gastroenterology*, 2007; 132:A–738–A739.
45. Zelber-Sagi, S. et al., Elevated alanine aminotransferase independently predicts new onset of depression in employees undergoing health screening examinations. *Psychol Med*, 2013; 1–11.
46. Fan, J.G. et al., Prevalence of and risk factors for fatty liver in a general population of Shanghai, China. *J Hepatol*, 2005; 43:508–14.
47. Simon, J.B. et al., Amiodarone hepatotoxicity simulating alcoholic liver disease. *N Engl J Med*, 1984; 311:167–72.
48. Pessayre, D. et al., Perhexiline maleate-induced cirrhosis. *Gastroenterology*, 1979; 76:170–7.
49. Fromenty, B. and D. Pessayre, Inhibition of mitochondrial beta-oxidation as a mechanism of hepatotoxicity. *Pharmacol Ther*, 1995; 67:101–54.
50. Agozzino, F., M. Picca, and G. Pelosi, Acute hepatitis complicating intravenous amiodarone treatment. *Ital Heart J*, 2002; 3:686–8.
51. Rigas, B., The evolving spectrum of amiodarone hepatotoxicity. *Hepatology*, 1989; 10:116–7.
52. Gehenot, M. et al., Subfulminant hepatitis requiring liver transplantation after benzarone administration. *J Hepatol*, 1994; 20:842.
53. Lewis, J.H. et al., Amiodarone hepatotoxicity: Prevalence and clinicopathologic correlations among 104 patients. *Hepatology*, 1989; 9:679–85.
54. Poucell, S. et al., Amiodarone-associated phospholipidosis and fibrosis of the liver. Light, immunohistochemical, and electron microscopic studies. *Gastroenterology*, 1984; 86:926–36.
55. Ramachandran, R. and S. Kakar, Histological patterns in drug-induced liver disease. *J Clin Pathol*, 2009; 62:481–92.
56. Zorzi, D. et al., Chemotherapy-associated hepatotoxicity and surgery for colorectal liver metastases. *Br J Surg*, 2007; 94:274–86.
57. Pawlik, T.M. et al., Preoperative chemotherapy for colorectal liver metastases: Impact on hepatic histology and postoperative outcome. *J Gastrointest Surg*, 2007; 11:860–8.
58. Lee, W.M., Drug-induced hepatotoxicity. *N Engl J Med*, 1995; 333:1118–27.
59. Newman, M. et al., The role of liver biopsies in psoriatic patients receiving long-term methotrexate treatment. Improvement in liver abnormalities after cessation of treatment. *Arch Dermatol*, 1989; 125:1218–24.
60. Lee, W.M. and W.T. Denton, Chronic hepatitis and indolent cirrhosis due to methyldopa: The bottom of the iceberg? *J S C Med Assoc*, 1989; 85:75–9.

61. Beyeler, C. et al., Quantitative liver function in patients with rheumatoid arthritis treated with low-dose methotrexate: A longitudinal study. *Br J Rheumatol*, 1997; 36:338–44.
62. Geubel, A.P. et al., Liver damage caused by therapeutic vitamin A administration: Estimate of dose-related toxicity in 41 cases. *Gastroenterology*, 1991; 100:1701–9.
63. Letteron, P. et al., Acute and chronic hepatic steatosis lead to in vivo lipid peroxidation in mice. *J Hepatol*, 1996; 24:200–8.
64. Poynard, T. et al., Effect of treatment with peginterferon or interferon alfa-2b and ribavirin on steatosis in patients infected with hepatitis C. *Hepatology*, 2003; 38:75–85.
65. Ratziu, V. et al., Sampling variability of liver biopsy in nonalcoholic fatty liver disease. *Gastroenterology*, 2005; 128:1898–906.
66. Poynard, T. et al., Prospective analysis of discordant results between biochemical markers and biopsy in patients with chronic hepatitis C. *Clin Chem*, 2004; 50:1344–55.
67. Arun, J. et al., Influence of liver biopsy heterogeneity and diagnosis of nonalcoholic steatohepatitis in subjects undergoing gastric bypass. *Obes Surg*, 2007; 17:155–161.
68. Brunt, E.M. and D.G. Tiniakos, Histopathology of nonalcoholic fatty liver disease. *World J Gastroenterol*, 2010; 16:5286–96.
69. Hubscher, S.G., Histological assessment of non-alcoholic fatty liver disease. *Histopathology*, 2006; 49:450–65.
70. Matteoni, C.A. et al., Nonalcoholic fatty liver disease: A spectrum of clinical and pathological severity. *Gastroenterology*, 1999; 116:1413–9.
71. Yeh, M.M. and E.M. Brunt, Pathology of nonalcoholic fatty liver disease. *Am J Clin Pathol*, 2007; 128:837–47.
72. Mofrad, P. et al., Clinical and histologic spectrum of nonalcoholic fatty liver disease associated with normal ALT values. *Hepatology*, 2003; 37:1286–92.
73. Kleiner, D.E. et al., Design and validation of a histological scoring system for nonalcoholic fatty liver disease. *Hepatology*, 2005; 41:1313–21.
74. Brunt, E.M. et al., Nonalcoholic fatty liver disease (NAFLD) activity score and the histopathologic diagnosis in NAFLD: Distinct clinicopathologic meanings. *Hepatology*, 2011; 53:810–20.
75. Rockey, D.C. et al., Liver biopsy. *Hepatology*, 2009; 49:1017–1044.
76. Wieckowska, A. and A.E. Feldstein, Diagnosis of nonalcoholic fatty liver disease: Invasive versus noninvasive. *Semin Liver Dis*, 2008; 28:386–95.
77. Ryan, C.K. et al., One hundred consecutive hepatic biopsies in the workup of living donors for right lobe liver transplantation. *Liver Transplant*, 2002; 8:1114–22.
78. Mottin, C.C. et al., The role of ultrasound in the diagnosis of hepatic steatosis in morbidly obese patients. *Obes Surg*, 2004; 14:635–7.
79. Webb, M. et al., Diagnostic value of a computerized hepatorenal index for sonographic quantification of liver steatosis. *AJR Am J Roentgenol*, 2009; 192:909–14.
80. Jacobs, J.E. et al., Diagnostic criteria for fatty infiltration of the liver on contrast-enhanced helical CT. *AJR Am J Roentgenol*, 1998; 171:659–64.
81. Grandison, G.A. and P. Angulo, Can NASH be diagnosed, graded, and staged noninvasively? *Clin Liver Dis*, 2012; 16:567–585.
82. Saadeh, S. et al., The utility of radiological imaging in nonalcoholic fatty liver disease. *Gastroenterology*, 2002; 123:745–50.
83. Fishbein, M. et al., Hepatic MRI for fat quantitation: Its relationship to fat morphology, diagnosis, and ultrasound. *J Clin Gastroenterol*, 2005; 39:619–25.
84. Qayyum, A. et al., Accuracy of liver fat quantification at MR imaging: Comparison of out-of-phase gradient-echo and fat-saturated fast spin-echo techniques—initial experience. *Radiology*, 2005; 237:507–11.
85. Szczepaniak, L.S. et al., Magnetic resonance spectroscopy to measure hepatic triglyceride content: Prevalence of hepatic steatosis in the general population. *Am J Physiol Endocrinol Metab*, 2005; 288:E462–8.

86. Angulo, P. et al., The NAFLD fibrosis score: A noninvasive system that identifies liver fibrosis in patients with NAFLD. *Hepatology*, 2007; 45:846–54.
87. Musso, G. et al., Meta-analysis: Natural history of non-alcoholic fatty liver disease (NAFLD) and diagnostic accuracy of non-invasive tests for liver disease severity. *Ann Med*, 2011; 43:617–49.
88. Palmeri, M.L. et al., Noninvasive evaluation of hepatic fibrosis using acoustic radiation force-based shear stiffness in patients with nonalcoholic fatty liver disease. *Journal of Hepatology*, 2011; 55:666–672.
89. Ochi, H. et al., Real-time tissue elastography for evaluation of hepatic fibrosis and portal hypertension in nonalcoholic fatty liver diseases. *Hepatology*, 2012; 56:1271–1278.
90. Dunn, W. et al., The interaction of rs738409, obesity, and alcohol: A population-based autopsy study. *Am J Gastroenterol*, 2012; 107:1668–74.
91. Hotta, K. et al., Association of the rs738409 polymorphism in PNPLA3 with liver damage and the development of nonalcoholic fatty liver disease. *BMC Med Genet*, 2010; 11:172.
92. Valenti, L. et al., Patatin-like phospholipase domain-containing 3 I148M polymorphism, steatosis, and liver damage in chronic hepatitis C. *Hepatology*, 2011; 53:791–9.
93. Ito, Y. et al., Hypertriglyceridemia as a result of human apo CIII gene expression in transgenic mice. *Science*, 1990; 249:790–3.
94. Hyysalo, J. et al., Genetic variation in PNPLA3 but not APOC3 influences liver fat in non-alcoholic fatty liver disease. *J Gastroenterol Hepatol*, 2012; 27:951–6.
95. Petersen, K.F. et al., Apolipoprotein C3 gene variants in nonalcoholic fatty liver disease. *N Engl J Med*, 2010; 362:1082–9.
96. Valenti, L. et al., The APOC3 T-455C and C-482T promoter region polymorphisms are not associated with the severity of liver damage independently of PNPLA3 I148M genotype in patients with nonalcoholic fatty liver. *J Hepatol*, 2011; 55:1409–14.
97. Valenti, L. et al., Increased susceptibility to nonalcoholic fatty liver disease in heterozygotes for the mutation responsible for hereditary hemochromatosis. *Dig Liver Dis*, 2003; 35:172–8.
98. Valenti, L. et al., HFE genotype, parenchymal iron accumulation, and liver fibrosis in patients with nonalcoholic fatty liver disease. *Gastroenterology*, 2010; 138:905–12.
99. Raszeja-Wyszomirska, J. et al., Nonalcoholic fatty liver disease and HFE gene mutations: A Polish study. *World J Gastroenterol*, 2010; 16:2531–6.
100. Feldstein, A.E. et al., Hepatocyte apoptosis and fas expression are prominent features of human nonalcoholic steatohepatitis. *Gastroenterology*, 2003; 125:437–43.
101. Feldstein, A.E. and G.J. Gores, Apoptosis in alcoholic and nonalcoholic steatohepatitis. *Front Biosci*, 2005; 10:3093–9.
102. Feldstein, A.E. et al., Cytokeratin-18 fragment levels as noninvasive biomarkers for nonalcoholic steatohepatitis: A multicenter validation study. *Hepatology*, 2009; 50:1072–8.
103. Shen, J. et al., Non-invasive diagnosis of non-alcoholic steatohepatitis by combined serum biomarkers. *J Hepatol*, 2012; 56:1363–70.
104. Joka, D. et al., Prospective biopsy-controlled evaluation of cell death biomarkers for prediction of liver fibrosis and nonalcoholic steatohepatitis. *Hepatology*, 2012; 55:455–64.
105. Ngo, Y. et al., A prospective analysis of the prognostic value of biomarkers (FibroTest) in patients with chronic hepatitis C. *Clin Chem*, 2006; 52:1887–96.
106. Halfon, P., M. Munteanu, and T. Poynard, FibroTest-ActiTest as a non-invasive marker of liver fibrosis. *Gastroenterol Clin Biol*, 2008; 32:22–39.
107. Naveau, S. et al., Biomarkers for the prediction of liver fibrosis in patients with chronic alcoholic liver disease. *Clin Gastroenterol Hepatol*, 2005; 3:167–74.
108. Poynard, T. et al., Meta-analyses of FibroTest diagnostic value in chronic liver disease. *BMC Gastroenterol*, 2007; 7:40.

109. Wai, C.T. et al., A simple noninvasive index can predict both significant fibrosis and cirrhosis in patients with chronic hepatitis C. *Hepatology*, 2003; 38:518–26.
110. Kruger, F.C. et al., APRI: A simple bedside marker for advanced fibrosis that can avoid liver biopsy in patients with NAFLD/NASH. *S Afr Med J*, 2011; 101:477–80.
111. Yilmaz, Y. et al., Noninvasive assessment of liver fibrosis with the aspartate transaminase to platelet ratio index (APRI): Usefulness in patients with chronic liver disease: APRI in chronic liver disease. *Hepat Mon*, 2011; 11:103–6.
112. Cales, P. et al., Comparison of blood tests for liver fibrosis specific or not to NAFLD. *J Hepatol*, 2009; 50:165–73.
113. Angulo, P. et al., Simple noninvasive systems predict long-term outcomes of patients with nonalcoholic fatty liver disease. *Gastroenterology*, 2013; 145:782–9.e4.
114. Guha, I.N. et al., Noninvasive markers of fibrosis in nonalcoholic fatty liver disease: Validating the European Liver Fibrosis Panel and exploring simple markers. *Hepatology*, 2008; 47:455–60.
115. Rosenberg, W.M. et al., Serum markers detect the presence of liver fibrosis: A cohort study. *Gastroenterology*, 2004; 127:1704–13.
116. Myers, R.P. et al., Prediction of liver histological lesions with biochemical markers in patients with chronic hepatitis B. *J Hepatol*, 2003; 39:222–30.
117. Koehler, E.M. et al., External validation of the fatty liver index for identifying nonalcoholic fatty liver disease in a population-based study. *Clin Gastroenterol Hepatol*, 2013; 11:1201–4.
118. Chalasani, N. et al., The diagnosis and management of non-alcoholic fatty liver disease: Practice guideline by the American Association for the Study of Liver Diseases, American College of Gastroenterology, and the American Gastroenterological Association. *Am J Gastroenterol*, 2012; 107:811–26.
119. Wang, R.T., R.L. Koretz, and H.F. Yee, Jr., Is weight reduction an effective therapy for nonalcoholic fatty liver? A systematic review. *Am J Med*, 2003; 115:554–9.
120. Keating, S.E. et al., Exercise and non-alcoholic fatty liver disease: A systematic review and meta-analysis. *J Hepatol*, 2012; 57:157–66.
121. Promrat, K. et al., Randomized controlled trial testing the effects of weight loss on nonalcoholic steatohepatitis. *Hepatology*, 2010; 51:121–9.
122. Ong, J.P. et al., Predictors of nonalcoholic steatohepatitis and advanced fibrosis in morbidly obese patients. *Obes Surg*, 2005; 15:310–5.
123. Younossi, Z.M. et al., Nonalcoholic fatty liver disease in patients with type 2 diabetes. *Clin Gastroenterol Hepatol*, 2004; 2:262–5.
124. Dixon, J.B., P.S. Bhathal, and P.E. O'Brien, Nonalcoholic fatty liver disease: Predictors of nonalcoholic steatohepatitis and liver fibrosis in the severely obese. *Gastroenterology*, 2001; 121:91–100.
125. Chavez-Tapia, N.C. et al., Bariatric surgery for non-alcoholic steatohepatitis in obese patients. *Cochrane Database Syst Rev*, 2010; CD007340.
126. Mummadi, R.R. et al., Effect of bariatric surgery on nonalcoholic fatty liver disease: Systematic review and meta-analysis. *Clin Gastroenterol Hepatol*, 2008; 6:1396–402.
127. Mathurin, P. et al., Prospective study of the long-term effects of bariatric surgery on liver injury in patients without advanced disease. *Gastroenterology*, 2009; 137:532–40.
128. Sanyal, A.J. et al., Pioglitazone, vitamin E, or placebo for nonalcoholic steatohepatitis. *N Engl J Med*, 2010; 362:1675–85.
129. Lavine, J.E. et al., Effect of vitamin E or metformin for treatment of nonalcoholic fatty liver disease in children and adolescents: The TONIC randomized controlled trial. *JAMA*, 2011; 305:1659–68.
130. Miller, E.R. 3rd et al., Meta-analysis: High-dosage vitamin E supplementation may increase all-cause mortality. *Ann Intern Med*, 2005; 142:37–46.

131. Abner, E.L. et al., Vitamin E and all-cause mortality: A meta-analysis. *Curr Aging Sci*, 2011; 4:158–70.
132. Torres, D.M. et al., Rosiglitazone versus rosiglitazone and metformin versus rosiglitazone and losartan in the treatment of nonalcoholic steatohepatitis in humans: A 12-month randomized, prospective, open-label trial. *Hepatology*, 2011; 54:1631–9.
133. Musso, G. et al., A meta-analysis of randomized trials for the treatment of nonalcoholic fatty liver disease. *Hepatology*, 2010; 52:79–104.
134. Nesto, R.W. et al., Thiazolidinedione use, fluid retention, and congestive heart failure: A consensus statement from the American Heart Association and American Diabetes Association. October 7, 2003. *Circulation*, 2003; 108:2941–8.
135. Mamtani, R. et al., Association between longer therapy with thiazolidinediones and risk of bladder cancer: A cohort study. *J Natl Cancer Inst*, 2012; 104:1411–21.
136. Boettcher, E. et al., Meta-analysis: Pioglitazone improves liver histology and fibrosis in patients with non-alcoholic steatohepatitis. *Aliment Pharmacol Ther*, 2012; 35:66–75.
137. Lindor, K.D. et al., Ursodeoxycholic acid for treatment of nonalcoholic steatohepatitis: Results of a randomized trial. *Hepatology*, 2004; 39:770–8.
138. Ratziu, V. et al., A randomized controlled trial of high-dose ursodesoxycholic acid for nonalcoholic steatohepatitis. *J Hepatol*, 2011; 54:1011–9.
139. Parker, H.M. et al., Omega-3 supplementation and non-alcoholic fatty liver disease: A systematic review and meta-analysis. *J Hepatol*, 2012; 56:944–951.
140. Zelber-Sagi, S. et al., A double-blind randomized placebo-controlled trial of orlistat for the treatment of nonalcoholic fatty liver disease. *Clin Gastroenterol Hepatol*, 2006; 4:639–44.
141. Smith, S.R. et al., Multicenter, placebo-controlled trial of lorcaserin for weight management. *N Engl J Med*, 2010; 363:245–56.
142. Gadde, K.M. et al., Effects of low-dose, controlled-release, phentermine plus topiramate combination on weight and associated comorbidities in overweight and obese adults (CONQUER): A randomised, placebo-controlled, phase 3 trial. *Lancet*, 2011; 377:1341–52.
143. Foster, T. et al., Atorvastatin and antioxidants for the treatment of nonalcoholic fatty liver disease: The St Francis Heart Study randomized clinical trial. *Am J Gastroenterol*, 2011; 106:71–7.
144. Gomez-Dominguez, E. et al., A pilot study of atorvastatin treatment in dyslipemid, non-alcoholic fatty liver patients. *Aliment Pharmacol Ther*, 2006; 23:1643–7.
145. Hyogo, H. et al., Efficacy of atorvastatin for the treatment of nonalcoholic steatohepatitis with dyslipidemia. *Metabolism*, 2008; 57:1711–8.
146. Rallidis, L.S., C.K. Drakoulis, and A.S. Parasi, Pravastatin in patients with nonalcoholic steatohepatitis: Results of a pilot study. *Atherosclerosis*, 2004; 174:193–6.
147. Lewis, J.H. et al., Efficacy and safety of high-dose pravastatin in hypercholesterolemic patients with well-compensated chronic liver disease: Results of a prospective, randomized, double-blind, placebo-controlled, multicenter trial. *Hepatology*, 2007; 46:1453–63.
148. Athyros, V.G. et al., Safety and efficacy of long-term statin treatment for cardiovascular events in patients with coronary heart disease and abnormal liver tests in the Greek Atorvastatin and Coronary Heart Disease Evaluation (GREACE) Study: A post-hoc analysis. *Lancet*, 2010; 376:1916–22.
149. Onofrei, M.D. et al., Safety of statin therapy in patients with preexisting liver disease. *Pharmacotherapy*, 2008; 28:522–9.
150. Gupte, P. et al., Non-alcoholic steatohepatitis in type 2 diabetes mellitus. *J Gastroenterol Hepatol*, 2004; 19:854–8.
151. Edmison, J. and A.J. McCullough, Pathogenesis of non-alcoholic steatohepatitis: Human data. *Clin Liver Dis*, 2007; 11:75–104, ix.
152. Soderberg, C. et al., Decreased survival of subjects with elevated liver function tests during a 28-year follow-up. *Hepatology*, 2010; 51:595–602.

153. Hui, J.M. et al., Long-term outcomes of cirrhosis in nonalcoholic steatohepatitis compared with hepatitis C. *Hepatology*, 2003; 38:420–7.
154. Lazo, M. et al., Non-alcoholic fatty liver disease and mortality among US adults: Prospective cohort study. *BMJ*, 2011; 343:d6891.
155. Sanyal, A.J. et al., Similarities and differences in outcomes of cirrhosis due to nonalcoholic steatohepatitis and hepatitis C. *Hepatology*, 2006; 43:682–9.
156. Bhala, N. et al., The natural history of nonalcoholic fatty liver disease with advanced fibrosis or cirrhosis: An international collaborative study. *Hepatology*, 2011; 54:1208–16.
157. Leite, N.C. et al., Prevalence and associated factors of non-alcoholic fatty liver disease in patients with type-2 diabetes mellitus. *Liver Int*, 2009; 29:113–9.
158. Bugianesi, E. et al., Expanding the natural history of nonalcoholic steatohepatitis: From cryptogenic cirrhosis to hepatocellular carcinoma. *Gastroenterology*, 2002; 123:134–40.
159. Hashimoto, E. et al., Hepatocellular carcinoma in patients with nonalcoholic steatohepatitis. *J Gastroenterol*, 2009; 44:89–95.
160. Smedile, A. and E. Bugianesi, Steatosis and hepatocellular carcinoma risk. *Eur Rev Med Pharmacol Sci*, 2005; 9:291–3.
161. Ascha, M.S. et al., The incidence and risk factors of hepatocellular carcinoma in patients with nonalcoholic steatohepatitis. *Hepatology*, 2010; 51:1972–8.
162. Yatsuji, S. et al., Clinical features and outcomes of cirrhosis due to non-alcoholic steatohepatitis compared with cirrhosis caused by chronic hepatitis C. *J Gastroenterol Hepatol*, 2009; 24:248–54.
163. White, D.L., F. Kanwal, and H.B. El-Serag, Association between nonalcoholic fatty liver disease and risk for hepatocellular cancer, based on systematic review. *Clin Gastroenterol Hepatol*, 2012; 10:1342–1359.e2.

Section II

Fatty Liver Disease and Consequences

2 Fatty Liver Vulnerability to Hypoxic and Inflammatory Stress

Rabindra Dhital and Oren Tirosh

CONTENTS

INTRODUCTION

Fatty liver is one of the most important causes responsible for liver cirrhosis and liver damage in developed as well as developing countries. Fatty liver is the result of the accumulation of various types of lipids (Postic and Girard, 2008), but mostly there is infiltration of triglycerides (TGs) into the liver cells more than 5% of its total weight. Traditionally, fatty liver has been considered a benign and reversible condition, and it usually causes the expression of a nonspecific response of the liver to metabolic stress of different origin (Day and Yeaman, 1994; Teli et al., 1995).

There are a number of articles suggesting the significant association between fatty liver and metabolic syndrome. Marceau et al. (1999) studied 551 severely obese patients undergoing antiobesety surgery. Steatosis was found in 86%, fibrosis in 74%, mild inflammation or steatohepatitis in 24%, and unexpected cirrhosis in 2% (n = 11) of the patients.

Terminologies of Fatty Liver Disease

The term nonalcoholic steatohepatitis (NASH) was coined by Ludwig et al. in 1980 to describe the morphologic pattern of liver injury in 20 patients evaluated at the Mayo Clinic over a 10-year period. These patients had histological evidence suggestive of alcoholic hepatitis on liver biopsy (i.e., steatosis and lobular inflammation) but no history of alcohol abuse. These patients were mostly female (60%) and the majority were obese (90%). Several other terms have been used to refer to this entity, including pseudo-alcoholic liver disease, alcohol-like hepatitis, diabetic hepatitis, nonalcoholic Laennec disease, and steatonecrosis (Sheth et al., 1997). However, seeing that the disease represents a spectrum of pathology, the umbrella term "nonalcoholic fatty liver disease" (NAFLD), first introduced in 1986, became the preferred one (Schaffner and Thaler, 1986).

Fatty liver encompass a wide spectrum of liver injury, ranging from steatosis to steatohepatitis, fibrosis, and cirrhosis (Reid, 2001). Insulin resistance, disrupted fatty acid metabolism, mitochondrial dysfunction, oxidative stress, and dysregulation of adipocytokine networks are proposed to be critical factors in the development of steatohepatitis from the steatosis. In steatohepatitis, fat accumulation is associated with liver cell inflammation and different degrees of deterioration. Steatohepatitis is rather a serious condition that may lead to severe liver cirrhosis. Cirrhosis is characterized by replacement of liver tissue by fibrosis, scar tissue and regenerative nodules ultimately causing liver dysfunction. In serious conditions, patients who develop cirrhosis may eventually require a liver transplant.

Broadly, fatty liver can be categorized into following terms on the basis of alcohol consumption:

1. Alcoholic fatty liver disease: The primary cause of this type of fatty liver is heavy consumption of alcohol. Fatty liver develops after chronic alteration of lipid metabolism due to prolonged alcoholic ingestion. Researchers have shown that prolonged alteration of lipid metabolism is responsible for the accumulation of triacylglycerol in the hepatocytes.
2. Nonalcoholic fatty liver disease: The nonalcoholic fatty liver resembles the pathological condition related to the alcoholic fatty liver but it develops in the people who are no heavy drinker. It is one of the most common causes of chronic liver disease worldwide. It is generally associated with dyslipidemia and decreased insulin sensitivity.

Fatty liver is the most common liver disease in Western countries. The prevalence of FLD in the general population ranges from 10% to 24% in various countries (Angulo, 2002). However, the condition is observed in up to 75% of obese people, 35% of whom will progress to NAFLD (Hamaguchi et al., 2005), despite no evidence of excessive alcohol consumption. FLD is the most common cause of abnormal liver function tests in the United States (Angulo, 2002). Fatty livers occur in 33% of European Americans, 45% of Hispanic Americans, and 24% of African Americans.

MECHANISM BEHIND THE DEVELOPMENT OF FATTY LIVER

Several mechanisms may lead to a fatty liver (Fabbrini et al., 2008):

1. Increased free fatty acids supply due to increased lipolysis from both visceral/subcutaneous adipose tissue and/or increased intake of dietary fat;
2. Decreased free fatty acid oxidation;
3. Increased de novo hepatic lipogenesis (DNL);
4. Decreased hepatic very-low-density lipoprotein–TG secretion.

Almost two thirds of the total free fatty acids are transported from the diet. Elevated free fatty acid and de novo lipogenesis significantly contribute to the formation of fatty liver. Besides this sterol response element-binding protein (SREBP) or carbohydrate response element-binding protein (ChREBP), an X-box-binding protein 1 (XBP1), known as a key regulator of the unfolded protein response (UPR) secondary to ER stress, is characterized as a regulator of hepatic lipogenesis (Lee et al., 2008).

Mechanism of Alcoholic Fatty Liver Formation

Fatty liver in alcoholism is a malnutrition-related disorder related to the hepatotoxic effect of ethanol (Lieber, 2004). Ethanol metabolism leads the synthesis of alcohol dehydrogenase and cytochrome P4502E1 (CYP2E1) in the MEOS synthesizing toxic acetaldehyde (Lieber and DeCarli, 1970). In addition, ALD-mediated ethanol metabolism leads to generation of reduced form of nicotinamide adenine dinucleotide (NADH), which promotes synthesis of fatty acid as well as oppose β-oxidation resulting steatosis in the liver.

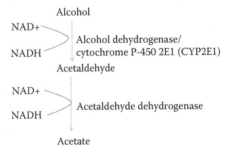

Sketch showing metabolism of alcohol.

The induction of CYP2E1 has been shown to play a key role in the pathogenesis of alcoholic liver injury, including alcoholic steatohepatitis, because of the oxidative stress it generates (Lieber, 1997). In addition, CYP2E1 is invariably elevated in the liver of patients with NASH (Weltman et al., 1998) because fatty acids (which increase in obesity) and ketones (which increase in diabetes) are also substrates for CYP2E1; their excess upregulates CYP2E1. Additionally, CYP2E1 activity is increased not only by its substrate ethanol but also by fatty acids (Cederbaum et al., 2001).

Excess dietary lipids has been found to promote steatosis, whereas medium-chain TG replacement attenuates the process. Reduction of pyruvate causes elevation of NADH, which also increases lactate, stimulating collagen synthesis in myofibroblasts (Savolainen et al., 1984). The excess activity of MEOS-induced CYP2E1 leads to the formation of free radicals, which cause oxidative stress resulting lipid peroxidation, which causes cell membrane damage as well as altered enzyme activities. Products of lipid peroxidation such as 4-hydroxynonenal stimulate collagen generation and fibrosis, which are also increased by reduced negative feedback of collagen synthesis because of adduct formation by acetaldehyde with procollagen in hepatic stellate cells (HSCs) (Ma et al., 1997). Acetaldehyde is very toxic to the mitochondria and worsens oxidative stress by binding with glutathione and promoting its leakage.

Oxidative stress and associated cell injury lead to the inflammatory response to the cell, which promotes the synthesis of different types of cytokines such as TNF-α in the Kupffer cells (KCs), which worsens the situation. These are activated by induction of their CYP2E1 as well as by endotoxin. The endotoxin-stimulated TNF-α release is decreased by dilinoleoylphosphatidylcholine, the active phosphatidylcholine (PC) species of polyenylphosphatidylcholine (PPC).

Mechanism of Nonalcoholic Fatty Liver Formation

Increased hepatic fatty acid oxidation can produce reactive oxygen radicals (ROS) that may aid mitochondrial dysfunction, lipid peroxidation, and/or cytokine secretion (Feher and Lengyel, 2003). A two-hit model has been proposed (Day and James, 1998) involving a cellular chain of events that, in steatotic liver, promote(s) inflammation, fibrosis, cell death, and cirrhosis. It is accepted that hepatic fat accumulation is linked to insulin resistance (IR) (Marchesini et al., 1999), which is associated with NAFLD, but the exact mechanism is unclear (Cheung and Sanyal, 2010). However, hepatic steatosis (i.e., TG accumulation) is dissociated from IR in patients with familial hypobetalipoproteinemia, providing further evidence that increased intrahepatic TG content might be more a marker rather than a cause of IR (Amaro et al., 2010). It is still a matter of debate as to whether IR causes NAFLD or whether excessive accumulation of TG or precursors on the synthetic pathway precedes and then causes IR (Postic and Girard, 2008). Regardless of which comes first, it is likely that hepatic insulin sensitivity deteriorates with increasing hepatic fat accumulation, resulting in increased hepatic gluconeogenesis and increased hepatic glucose output. Insulin resistance in NAFLD is characterized by reduced whole-body, hepatic, and adipose tissue insulin sensitivity. The mechanism(s) underlying the accumulation of fat in the liver may include excess dietary fat, increased delivery of free fatty acids to the liver, inadequate fatty acid oxidation, and increased de novo lipogenesis (Bugianesi et al., 2005) (Figure 2.1).

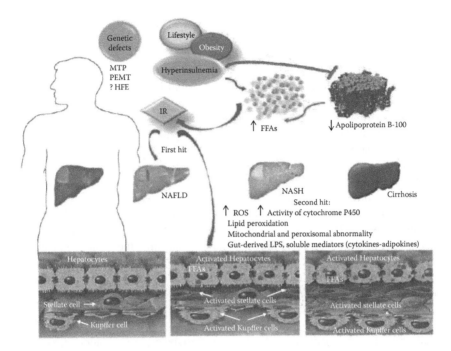

FIGURE 2.1 Sketch showing mechanism of NAFLD development. (From Malaguarnera, M. et al., *J Mol Med (Berl)*. 2009, 87, 679–695. With permission.)

Another proposed mechanism is that when there is an increase in delivery of fatty acids to muscle or a decrease in intracellular metabolism of fatty acids leads to an increase in intracellular fatty acid metabolites such as diacylglycerol (Schmitz-Peiffer and Biden, 2008), fatty acyl CoA, and ceramides. These metabolites activate a serine/threonine kinase cascade (possibly initiated by protein kinase Cθ), leading to the phosphorylation of serine/threonine sites on insulin receptor substrates (IRS-1 and IRS-2), which in turn reduces the ability of the insulin receptor substrates to activate PI3 kinase. Intracellular diacylglycerols (DAGs) is responsible for inhibition of insulin signaling by activation of novel PKC isoforms (Samuel et al., 2004), which ultimately block insulin receptor kinase phosphorylation of insulin receptor substrates 1 and 2. Intracellular ceramides are also thought to prevent Akt2 activation (Schmitz-Peiffer, 2010; Summers, 2006). Activation of endoplasmic reticulum (ER) stress pathways, Inflammation, and increase of hepatocellular lipids have all been suggested to cause IR in animal models of NAFLD (Samuel et al., 2010; Savage and Semple, 2010; Shulman, 2000) Second, adipocytokines (e.g., TNF-α, interleukin [IL] 1β, IL-6) interfere with insulin signaling through activation of the JNK or inhibitor of IκB kinase β pathways (Hotamisligil, 2010; Solinas and Karin, 2010; Tilg and Moschen, 2008). Finally, the unfolded protein response or ER stress pathways are also implicated in the pathogenesis of IR (Ozcan et al., 2004). As a consequence, glucose transport activity and other events downstream of insulin receptor signaling are diminished.

PATHOGENESIS OF FATTY LIVER DISEASE

Two-Hit Theory

Although the pathogenesis of NAFLD and NASH has not yet been fully elucidated, a popular mechanism is the "two-hit" theory (Day and James, 1998; Garcia-Monzon, 2001), in which the first hit is the accumulation of fatty acids, by several causes (e.g., obesity), in the liver, and the second hit is the peroxidation of these fatty acids because of the oxidative stress produced by different factors such as CYP2E1 induction (Angulo and Lindor, 2001).

The first hit of steatosis is caused by excess free fatty acids (FFA) in the liver, which are sterified to TGs, giving rise to the first lesions, (Charlton et al., 2002; Sanyal et al., 2001). These initial lesions make the liver vulnerable to aggressive factors of the second hit, which is caused by the oxidative stress and proinflammatory cytokines (TNF-α, TGF-β, IL-6, IL-8). This leads to the occurrence of lesions in the hepatocytes, inflammation, and fibrosis, and consequently, the evolution of hepatic steatosis to steatohepatitits. Some poorly understood genetic factors may explain whether steatosis evolves to steatohepatitis or not (Chitturi and Farrell, 2001; Day and James, 1998; Harrison et al., 2002).

First Hit

Insulin resistance is a feature of obesity, type 2 diabetes, hyperlipidemia, and metabolic syndrome X (Chitturi and Farrell, 2001; Pagano et al., 2002). Adipocyte insensitivity to insulin, inhibits the regulation of the lipase in the adipose tissue, and a large amount of free fatty acids (FFAs) is released (Fabbrini et al., 2008; Oneta and Dufour, 2002). Oversupply of FFAs to the liver is the main mechanism that leads to steatosis in these patients. However, there are also other mechanisms. One of these is an increase in insulinemia, whether or not caused by IR, which inhibits the carnitine palmitoyltransferase enzyme and reduces the mytochondria β-oxidation of FFAs (Fong et al., 2000; Mannaerts et al., 2000; Reddy and Hashimoto, 2001; Reddy and Rao, 2006). Hyperinsulinism also decreases the synthesis of apolipoprotein B-100 in the liver, which causes a decrease in the secretion of very-low-density lipoproteins (VLDL) (Charlton et al., 2002; Valenti et al., 2002). Finally, excess production of exogenous and endogenous glucose (in obesity and diabetes, respectively), together with hyperinsulinemia, increases the synthesis of FFAs in the liver. The final result is a positive FFA balance, from oversupply and/or failure in lipid beta oxidation, leading to accumulation in the liver. It is not well understood why not all patients with risk factors (obesity, type 2 diabetes mellitus, hyperlipidemia) develop NAFLD. It has also been demonstrated that patients with NAFLD have an increased prevalence of polymorphism in TNF-α 238 (TNFA allele), inducing an overexpression of TNF-α in adipose tissue, and this, in turn, disrupts insulin receptors, causing resistance to insulin (Crespo et al., 2001; Fernandez-Real et al., 2002; Valenti et al., 2002). The transcription factor HNF3α (hepatocyte nuclear factor) is an important target for research. Its presence is related to the inhibition of the accumulation of fatty acids. If overexpressed, this transcription factor triggers a reduction in the synthesis of fatty acids, that is, it has an opposite effect to steatosis (Hughes et al., 2003; Li and Klaassen, 2004; Morral et al., 2007).

Second Hit

FFAs cause an increase in the expression of cytochrome P450 2E1 (CYP 2E1). This is a microsomal enzyme that takes part in the β-oxidation of long- and very-long-chain FFAs, causing the production of reactive oxygen metabolites (Weltman et al., 1998). Meanwhile, some long-chain FFAs are metabolized by peroxisomal β-oxidation. This oxidation generates hydrogen peroxide, which produces hydroxyl radicals in the presence of iron, both being reactive oxygen metabolites (Rao and Reddy, 2001). The excess of reactive oxygen metabolites depletes natural antioxidants such as glutathione and vitamin E in the liver, causing oxidative stress resulting in lipid peroxidation (Garcia-Monzon et al., 2000; Neuschwander-Tetri and Caldwell, 2003; Sanyal et al., 2001). In turn, this causes damage in the hepatocyte organelles and membranes, leading to degeneration and hepatocellular necrosis (Garcia-Monzon et al., 2000). The damage caused by lipid peroxidation in mitochondria, apart from changing their morphology (megamitochondria), distorts the transfer of electrons in the respiratory chain, and this results in more production of reactive oxygen metabolites, closing the cycle by causing more oxidative stress (Browning and Horton, 2004; Harrison et al., 2002; Solis Herruzo et al., 2006).

Oxidative stress activates the Fas ligand and nuclear factor κB (NF-κB), in which activated Fas ligand causes degeneration and hepatocyte death, whereas NF-κB stimulates the synthesis of proinflammatory cytokines (TNF-α, TGF-β, IL-8) (Angulo, 2002). In addition, the final products of lipid peroxidation, malonaldehyde, and 4-hydroxynonenal have chemotactic properties, activating proinflammatory cytokines (TNF-α, TGF-β, IL-6, IL-8), and stimulating hepatic collagen-producing stellate cells. The end result is a mixed lesion, known as steatohepatitis, characterized by degeneration and hepatocyte necrosis, inflammatory infiltrate, and fibrosis as well as steatosis (Angulo, 2002). Malonaldehyde and 4-hydroxynonenal are also covalently bound to proteins and produce protein clusters with antigenic properties. Secondarily, antibodies that are able to cause immune-mediated hepatocellular injury (autoimmune hepatitis) may appear. One of these protein inclusions corresponds to Mallory's hyaline (Pessayre et al., 2001). Ongoing oxidative stress and lipid peroxidation result in the continued production of collagen leading to fibrosis reaching the stage of hepatic cirrhosis (Chitturi and Farrell, 2001).

The passage of endotoxins from the intestine to the splenic circulation causes portal endotoxemia. Endotoxins stimulate the synthesis of proinflammatory cytokines in the liver (Chitturi and Farrell, 2001). This mechanism is essential in the development of steatohepatitis associated with intestinal bypass, since this type of surgery encourages bacterial overgrowth and endotoxemia from the dysfunctionalized loop (Chitturi and Farrell, 2001). Obese patients have intense intrahepatic expression of the enzyme nitric oxide synthase (Garcia-Monzon et al., 2000), which is induced by endotoxins and TNF-α; furthermore, obese mice have been found to experience hepatic hypersensitivity, which causes them to develop more severe degrees of steatohepatitis (Garcia-Monzon, 2001).

ROLES OF DIFFERENT FACTORS IN THE DEVELOPMENT OF FATTY LIVER

In this complex context, the roles of several molecules are involved.

1. Leptin is a hormone secreted from adipocytes (fat cells) and functions to suppress appetite and increase energy expenditure (Singh et al., 2009; Zhang et al., 1994). Leptin levels are elevated in obesity (Tsochatzis et al., 2009). It is believed that leptin has a lipostatic function: when the quantity of fat stored in the adipocytes increases, leptin is released into the bloodstream. This constitutes a negative feedback signal to the hypothalamus, informing the hippocampus that the body has enough food and the appetite should be reduced. When the adipose tissue mass increases a certain level beyond equilibrium, there is an increase of the synthesis and secretion of leptin, triggering several compensating effects in the hypothalamus: a decrease in appetite by the production of anorexigenic peptides (inducing loss of appetite) and the suppression of orexigenic peptides; an increase in energy expenditure by increasing of the basal metabolism and body temperature; and also a change in the equilibrium levels of hormones to reduce lipogenesis (production of fats) and to increase lipolysis (use of the body fat stored to produce energy) in the adipose tissue. The regulation of the secretion of leptin takes place on long timescales, mainly due to variations in body mass and stimulating effects of insulin. It has been found to prevent the occurrence of NAFLD, indirectly though the central neural pathway, and directly through the activation of adenosine monophosphate-activated protein kinase AMPK (Andreelli et al., 2006; Marra and Bertolani, 2009; Rabe et al., 2008). In patients with NAFLD it has been observed that leptin levels are directly correlated to the severity of the disease. Leptin deficient *ob/ob* mice show markedly reduced levels of energy expenditure and become obese even when pair fed compared with littermate controls. The marked steatosis observed in this group indicates that leptin prevents fatty liver, both indirectly, through central neural pathways, and directly via hepatic activation of AMPK. In NAFLD patients, the analysis of circulating levels of leptin, has provided results more conflicting. Leptin levels found to be increased in NASH, independently of BMI, with higher in patients with advanced disease (Uygun et al., 2000). In another study, leptin levels directly correlated with the severity of steatosis but not with inflammation or fibrosis (Chitturi et al., 2002). However, the strong evidence for leptin as a fibrogenic agent in animal models is not clearly paralleled by evidence on circulating levels in patients (Marra and Bertolani, 2009).

2. Adiponectin is a type of adipocytes secreted hormone with a wide range of beneficial effects on obesity-related medical complications. Numerous epidemiological investigations in diverse ethnic groups have identified a lower adiponectin level as an independent risk factor for NAFLDs and liver dysfunctions. It is considered as an anti-inflammatory adipokine (Tsochatzis et al., 2009). It takes part in the metabolism of glucose and fatty acids. In

general, adiponectin reduces inflammation, stimulating secretion of anti-inflammatory cytokines (e.g., IL-10), blocking nuclear factor κB activation, and inhibiting release of TNF-α, IL-6, and chemokines (Tilg and Moschen, 2006). Adiponectin concentrations inversely correlated with fat mass and are downregulated in obesity and type 2 diabetes. Adiponectin exerts insulin-sensitizing effects in the liver, skeletal muscle, and adipose tissue. Like leptin, adiponectin regulates whole-body lipid partitioning and has hepato-protective and anti-fibrogenic effect in condition of liver injury (Tsochatzis et al., 2009). Adiponectin possesses potent protective effects against alcoholic fatty liver disease, NAFLD, and steatohepatitis (Xu et al., 2003). In both ethanol-fed and *oblob* obese mice, chronic treatment with recombinant adiponectin markedly attenuated hepatomegaly and steatosis and significantly decreased hepatic inflammation and serum alanine aminotransferase (ALT) levels.

In experimental alcoholic and nonalcoholic models, the administration of adiponectin, improved the necro-inflammation, and steatosis, partly via inhibition of TNF-α (Xu et al., 2003). In obese mice, the administration of adiponectin improved liver injury, increased PPAR-α, and reduced TNF-α (Masaki et al., 2004). In patients with NASH, adiponectin levels were reduced in comparison with control and simple steatosis patients (Hui et al., 2004). Bugianesi et al. (2005) found that adiponectin levels correlate with suppression of endogenous glucose production and predict the presence of the metabolic syndrome. However, adiponectin levels was inversely associated only with intrahepatic fat but not with inflammation and fibrosis. In patients with diabetes, levels of adiponectin are inversely correlated to hepatic fat content and to endogenous glucose production. This hit suggests, that adiponectin may represent a link between hepatic fat and IR (Bajaj et al., 2004). Also, genetic factors produce alterations in the adiponectin levels. Polymorphisms of the adiponectin gene have been associated with higher risk of type 2 diabetes and cardiovascular disease (Qi et al., 2006).

3. IL-6 has a pleiotropic action, and in animals models it has been associated with protection against steatosis (Marra and Bertolani, 2009). It is associated with hyperinsulinemia and IR. IL-6 is overexpressed in the adipose tissue of obese patients (Marra and Bertolani, 2009). Increased hepatic IL-6 production may play an important role in NASH development, as well as in systemic IR and diabetes (Wieckowska et al., 2008). Chronically elevated IL-6 levels lead to inappropriate hyperinsulinemia, reduced body weight, impaired insulin-stimulated glucose uptake by the skeletal muscles, and marked inflammation in the liver. Thus, the pleiotrophic effects of chronically elevated IL-6 levels preclude any obvious usefulness in treating obesity or its associated metabolic complications in man, despite the fact that weight reduction may be expected (Franckhauser et al., 2008).

4. Farnesoid X receptor (FXR) and its downstream targets play a key role in the control of hepatic de novo lipogenesis, very-low-density lipoprotein–TG export, and plasma TG turnover. Bile acid supplementation in normal or hypertriglyceridemic patients results in the lowering of serum TG

(Claudel et al., 2005). FXR-deficient (FXR$^{-/-}$) mice develop hepatic steatosis and hypertriglyceridemia, reflecting the central role of FXR in the
regulation of hepatic lipid metabolism in some studies (Houten et al., 2006;
Thomas et al., 2008).

5. Insulin resistance is often associated with chronic low-grade inflammation,
and numerous mediators released from immune cells and adipocytes may
contribute to liver damage and liver disease progression.

FATTY LIVER VULNERABILITY TO HYPOXIA

ROLE OF HYPOXIA IN FLD

The liver has a unique vascular and metabolic system that relatively protects against
hypoxic injury. Cardiac output contributes about 20%–25% of its blood supply to the
liver, in which 30% is received through the hepatic artery, whereas 70% is received
through the portal vein. Because of its dual supply of blood, the liver is generally
protected from ischemic injury (Ebert, 2006).

Livers of well-nourished individuals also contain up to 7% glycogen by weight.
This glycogen supports adenosine triphosphate (ATP) generation by anaerobic glycolysis. During anoxia and ischemia, glycolytic ATP formation replaces, in part,
the ATP lost from oxidative phosphorylation and delays anoxic hepatocellular cell
death by hours compared with glycogen-depleted livers. Even with the protection
of a dual blood supply and the anaerobic metabolism of glycogen, hypoxic liver
damage is quite common in systemic hypoxemia and cardiogenic, hemorrhagic, and
septic shock. Due to the intralobular oxygen gradient, hypoxic injury in low-flow
states occurs first in the pericentral (zone 3) region of hepatic lobules, where there
is low amount of oxygen supply. If severe enough, pericentral liver hypoxia leads to
a syndrome of ischemic hepatitis characterized by a sharp increase in serum transaminase activities in the absence of other causes of hepatic necrosis, such as viral
or drug-induced hepatitis (Naschitz et al., 2000). The liver, unlike other tissues, has
enormous regenerative capacity. Thus, virtually complete restoration of normal liver
structure and function can occur after hypoxic injury when normal hepatic perfusion
is restored. Repeated cycles of hypoxic injury, however, may lead to chronic liver
injury. In alcoholic liver disease, cycles of hypoxic injury are postulated to contribute to hepatic fibrosis and alcoholic cirrhosis (Arteel et al., 1997). Savransky et al.
(2007) found that chronic intermittent hypoxia in combination with a high-fat diet
(HFD) induces inflammation and lipid peroxidation in mice, with increased steatosis
observed in the hypoxia exposure group.

Hypoxic liver injury may arise with the obstruction of either the portal vein or
the hepatic artery, depending on several factors: blood flow in the other vessel, collateral vessel formation, and the ability of the liver to increase oxygen extraction to
compensate for the decrease in perfusion.

Interaction of Hypoxia and Fatty Liver

There is strong interaction between hypoxia and its effect on liver and more specifically on fatty liver. The study by Chin et al. (2003) found that the continuous

positive airway pressure decreases the aminotransferase level in 35% who have obstructive sleep apnea hypopnea syndrome (OSAHS). OSAHS is defined as a sleep disorder that involves cessation or significant decrease in airflow in the presence of breathing effort leading to a drop in oxygen saturation in the arterial blood, increased respiratory muscle work, arousals, and sleep fragmentation (Guilleminault et al., 1976).

Another study by Jouet et al. (2007) also showed that morbidly obese people who have OSAHS have elevated liver enzyme compared with those with no OSAHS. The study by Kallwitz et al. (2007) supports the above conclusion. However, obesity appears to be a strong predisposing factor of the fatty liver disease. There was no significance difference between levels of blood liver enzyme in nonobese people with and without OSASH (Tatsumi and Saibara, 2005).

Feng et al. (2011) have studied the dynamic process of the influence that chronic intermittent hypoxia in rat on levels of liver enzyme in the blood, hepatic histology, and ultrastructure based on lipid disorders (Figure 2.2). A total of 72 male Wistar rats were randomly divided into three groups. The control group was fed with a regular chow diet, with a HFD, and HFD plus intermittent-hypoxia group. It was concluded that under the conditions of high fat and intermittent hypoxia, the injury to the liver function, hepatic histology, and ultrastructure is more severe than that of the high-fat group and the normal group. The injury mainly was characterized by NAFLD and becomes more severe with increased exposure time. Oxidative stress plays an important role in the mechanism.

Similar types of results were obtained in various other studies. Anavi et al. (2012) showed marked lipid accumulation within the hypoxic cells compared with normoxic control cells treated with fatty acid mix.

Ip et al. (2002) suggested that hypoxic patient were significantly associated with IR parameter. For every unit increase in the apnea hypopnea index, the level of insulin increases by about 0.5% and the same correlation also exist in nonobese patient. The exact mechanism is unknown, but it is surmised that the mechanism might be related to central obesity. Oxidative stress induced by intermittent hypoxia, sleep deprivation, participation of inflammatory cytokines, fat factor, etc. (Carneiro et al., 2007; Zhang, 2008). A study by Li et al. (2005) has also shown that chronic intermittent hypoxia upregulates genes of lipid biosynthesis in obese mice.

Chronic hypoxia has been associated as a contributing factor in liver injury in response to obstructive sleep apnea (Tanne et al., 2005), which has also been linked to the cardiometabolic syndrome and NASH (Jouet et al., 2007). Piguet et al. (2009) have investigated the effect of hypoxia on NAFLD. Piguet et al. used 8-week-old female PTEN-deficient mice, exposed to hypoxia for 7 days with matched control without hypoxia. They showed that there was a 10% increase in hematocrit to prove the animals were hypoxic. Affected animals were more insulin resistant, lighter in weight, hypertriglyceridemic, glucose intolerant, and had a marked increase in Kleiner score, a histopathogical scoring system used to quantitative severity of NAFLD (8.3 versus 2.3, $p < 0.01$), in keeping with NASH. In investigating the pathogenesis of hypoxia-induced NASH, they also show that expression of key genes in the hepatic lipogenesis pathway were increased, whereas expression of a marker of

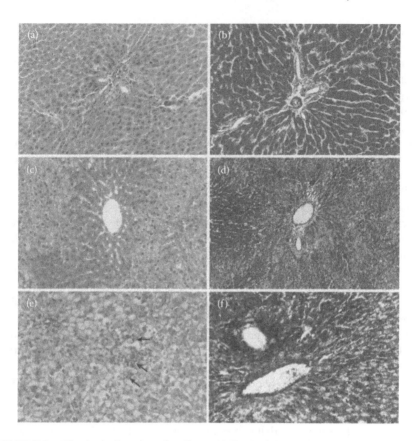

FIGURE 2.2   Histological section of rat livers. (a) Group A (control group), 6 weeks, rat normal liver cell (H&E, magnification ×200). (b) Group A (control group), 9 weeks, rat normal liver cell (Masson's trichrome, magnification ×200). (c) Group B (high-fat group), 6 weeks, steatosis of liver cells, cell swelling (H&E, magnification ×200). (d) Group B (high-fat group), 9 weeks, mild hyperplasia in periportal collagen fibers (Masson's trichrome, magnification ×100). (e) Group C (high-fat-plus-intermittent-hypoxia group), 9 weeks, steatosis of liver cells, cell swelling, inflammatory cell infiltration, focal necrosis (arrow) (H&E, magnification ×200). (f) Group C (the high-fat-plus-intermittent-hypoxia group), 9 weeks, hyperplasia in periportal collagen fibers (Masson's trichrome, magnification ×200). (From Feng, S.Z. et al., *Sleep Breath*, 15, 493–502, 2011. With permission.)

β-oxidation (carnitine palmitoyltransferase I) was decreased. They concluded that hypoxia may worsen the case of NAFLD to NASH.

Vascular endothelial growth factor (VEGF) is a signal protein produced by cells that stimulates vasculogenesis and angiogenesis. It is part of the system that restores the oxygen supply to tissues when blood circulation is inadequate. The normal function of VEGF is to create new blood vessels during embryonic development, new blood vessels after injury, muscle following exercise, and new vessels (collateral circulation) to bypass blocked vessels. VEGF is required for normal growth and survival in early life, whereas for angiogenesis later in life (Gerber et al., 1999). Redaelli et al. (2004) have studied the effects of VEGF on functional recovery after hepatectomy in lean and obese mice. They come into a conclusion that hepatic resection elicits an angiogenic response in the remnant liver, which is impaired in case of steatosis. It also clearly shows that the fatty liver is more vulnerable to the hypoxic stress due to impairment of VEGF signaling.

Hypoxia-Inducible Factor (HIF) and Fatty Liver

HIFs are transcription factors that mediate cellular adaptations to oxygen deprivation. Over 100 direct HIF target genes have been identified that regulate a number of cellular processes, including glucose metabolism, angiogenesis, erythropoiesis, proliferation, and invasion. HIF can also indirectly regulate cellular processes such as proliferation and differentiation through interactions with other signaling proteins such as C-Myc and Notch. There are multiple mechanisms by which HIF can become activated and promote tumor progression.

During low O_2 (hypoxic) conditions, cells activate a number of adaptive responses to match O_2 supply with metabolic, bioenergetics, and redox demands. Cells temporarily arrest in the cell cycle, reduce energy consumption, and secrete survival and proangiogenic factors. These events are coordinated by various cellular pathways, including the unfolded protein response (UPR), mTOR signaling, and gene regulation by hypoxia-inducible factors (HIFs). Initially identified as a regulator of erythropoietin (EPO) production, HIF is recognized as a key modulator of the transcriptional response to hypoxic stress. Hypoxia-inducible factors (HIFs) are essential mediators of the cellular oxygen signaling pathway. They are heterodimeric transcription factors consisting of an oxygen-sensitive α subunit (HIF-1α) and a constitutive β-subunit (HIF-β) that facilitate both oxygen delivery and adaptation to oxygen deprivation by regulating the expression of genes that control glucose uptake, metabolism, angiogenesis, erythropoiesis, cell proliferation, and apoptosis.

Evidence indicates the crucial roles of HIF-1α in the regulation of glucose metabolism through activating glycolysis (Semenza, 2009) and the inhibiting entry of pyruvate into TCA cycle (Rankin et al., 2009).

Studies indicate that mitochondrial reactive oxygen species (ROS) plays an important role in regulating HIF protein levels under hypoxia. Multiple studies have observed that genetic and chemical inhibition of the mitochondrial electron transport chain and ROS production results in decreased or increased HIF stability under hypoxic conditions (Brunelle et al., 2005; Chandel et al., 1998; Guzy et al., 2005; Mansfield et al., 2005).

HIF-1α is found to have a protective role against alcoholic fatty liver disease. Nishiyama et al. (2012) address the question of the role of HIF-1α in the metabolic and histological changes associated with alcoholic liver disease. They employ a technique of hepatocyte specific HIF-1α deletion and demonstrate that in a model of alcohol-induced liver disease in mice, there is an upregulation of HIF-1α in a central venous distribution, and in the absence of hepatocyte HIF-1α, there is greater pathology with increased liver weight, steatosis, and increased liver and serum TGs. This is strong evidence that the alcohol-induced increase in hepatic HIF-1α is adaptive and protective.

However, in a previous study, Nath et al. (2011) also found that an alcohol-rich diet upregulates HIF-1α in mice, but subsequently demonstrated that HIF-1α, rather than inducing adaptive and protective changes from the development of steatosis and that this is a key step in the development of steatosis and hypertriglyceridemia (Mehal, 2012). This study used two genetic manipulations, one in which there was constitutively active HIF-1α in hepatocytes, and a second that used the same hepatocyte specific HIF-1α deletion approach. Both genetic manipulations gave concordant results, with mice expressing constitutively active HIF-1α in hepatocytes developing increased liver steatosis and hypertriglyceridemia and mice lacking HIF-1α in hepatocytes having reduced liver steatosis and hypertriglyceridemia (Nath et al., 2011).

Role of Mitochondrial Bioenergetics and Microcirculation and Kupffer Cell Activation in Fatty Liver Exposed to Hypoxia

An uncoupling protein (UCP) is a mitochondrial inner membrane protein that can dissipate the proton gradient before it can be used to provide the energy for oxidative phosphorylation (Nedergaard et al., 2005). Although the precise physiological function of UCP2 is still unclear, a body of evidence has suggested that UCP2 functions as a negative regulator of mitochondria-derived ROS production. Therefore, the activation and/or increased expression of UCP2 may represent an alternative adaptive response to mitochondria-derived ROS generation in the cell. It has been previously reported that UCP2 expression in fatty liver is increased (Chavin et al., 1999). This finding can be attributed to an overabundance of substrate and an insufficient concentration of the terminal electron acceptor, O_2, resulting in diminished hepatic ATP stores in *ob/ob* livers rendering the steatotic hepatocytes vulnerable to ischemic damage (Chavin et al., 1999).

The Effect of Impaired Microcirculation

The microcirculation of the liver has important roles in maintenance of liver function. It guarantees the supply of the parenchymal tissue with oxygen and nutrients, serves as the gate for leukocyte entrance in hepatic inflammation, and is responsible for the clearance of toxic materials and foreign bodies from the bloodstream. Fatty liver contribute to the substantial changes in blood flow to the hepatocytes due to macrovescicular and microvesicular lipid deposition (Ijaz et al., 2003). The changes in hepatic microcirculation in the fatty liver may have a subsequent effect on cellular morphology and function, as reduced blood flow within sinusoids potentially may lead to exposure of the cells under the environment of chronic hypoxia (Hayashi et al., 1993). Reduced sinusoidal perfusion in fatty human liver compared with healthy human liver has been detected (Seifalian et al., 1998), and this reduction is perfusion is also correlated with the severity of fat deposition in parenchymal cells (Seifalian et al., 1998). The severity of the steatosis contributes to the severity of impaired microcirculation. Several macrophages also play role in progression of impaired microcirculation. They intensified the impairment either by mechanically trapping in the narrowed sinusoids or by adhering as a result of hepatic microvascular inflammatory response. Activation of KCs and other hepatic macrophages with the release of proinflammatory cytokines as well as free radicals are the contributing factors for inflammatory responses. Together, they contribute to the hepatic inflammatory response in steatohepatitis, stimulate stellate cells to produce collagen, and exacerbate the oxidative stress in the liver, which progressively increases during the course of fatty liver disease (Farrell et al., 2008). In addition, these microcirculatory and cellular changes in the fatty liver sensitize the organ the effects of ischemia–reperfusion injury, toxins, and drugs leading to an exacerbated response to liver damage (Farrell et al., 2008).

The Effect of Hypoxia on KC Activation

The concept that hypoxia may play a critical role in the etiology of liver diseases is well established in other pathologies associated with steatosis. For example, Arteel et al. (1996, 1997) demonstrated that due to increase demand of O_2 supply for the alcohol metabolism, chronic and acute alcohol exposure causes hypoxia in the pericentral region of the liver presumably and through the release of vasoconstrictive eicosanoids from KCs. Levels of plasma endotoxin, intercellular adhesion molecule 1, free radical production, infiltrating neutrophils, and nuclear factor κB are increased in hypoxia, which are found to promote KC activation (Thurman, 1998) and excessive liver damage in hypoxic fatty livers.

ROLE OF INFLAMMATORY STRESS IN FLD

Inflammation is part of the complex biological response of vascular tissues to harmful stimuli, such as pathogens, damaged cells, or irritants (Ferrero-Miliani et al., 2007). Inflammation is a protective attempt by the organism to remove the injurious stimuli and to initiate the healing process. Upon various kinds of infections and injuries, the liver tends to stimulate inflammatory reactions to maintain its normal metabolic states.

There are various types of process and molecules liver tends to maintain its normal physiological properties. When liver accumulates fats, then the normal inflammatory processes are altered. Some of the inflammatory agents and their abnormalities are discussed here.

Kupffer Cells

KCs are liver-resident macrophages that provide important protection against the emergence of endotoxins and harmful exogenous particles from the portal vein to the systemic circulation (Fox et al., 1990). The pathogenesis of NASH is incompletely understood, but may encompass hyperendotoxemia (Creely et al., 2007) secondary to impaired phagocytotic function of KCs (Loffreda et al., 1998) and consequent KC overproduction of, and increased sensitivity, to cytokines such as TNF-α and IL-1β (Diehl, 2002). Impaired phagocytotic function of KCs may therefore lead to higher endotoxin levels in the systemic circulation, as has been observed in patients with NASH and in animal models of NASH (Solga and Diehl, 2003). In addition, aggregates of enlarged KCs exist in perivenular regions of the livers of patients with NASH compared with the diffuse distribution seen in simple steatosis (Park et al., 2007). Absent KCs or impaired KC function may be associated with harmful effects. Resultant impaired clearance of bacterial products, lipopolysaccharides (LPS), endotoxins, and other dangerous molecules may accelerate pathogenesis of liver diseases. Activation of cellular defense programs, in particular, activation of KCs, offers additional stress stimuli and may influence the fate of hepatocytes from survival toward apoptosis by altering lipid oxidation and the intracellular redox state. Activated KCs produce inflammatory mediators, which in turn activate HSCs to synthesize collagen whose overproduction leads to hepatic fibrosis and cirrhosis.

Given that overproduction and increased sensitivity to cytokines such as TNF-α and IL-1b from KCs (Diehl, 2002; Solga and Diehl, 2003) are also implicated in the pathogenesis of NASH, failure of KCs to clear endotoxins and LPS because of defective phagocytotic function may further drive the production of these proinflammatory cytokines by KCs. Meanwhile, it is also considered that KCs that produce cytokines may differ from KCs with phagocytotic activity, and LPS-responsive KCs (CD14-positive KCs) are potential sources of proinflammatory and profibrogenic cytokine release. Cytokines such IL-1, IL-6, and TNF-α are released from CD14-positive KCs by stimulation of LPS (Su, 2002). CD14-transgenic mice that overexpress CD14 on monocytes have increased sensitivity to LPS (Ferrero et al., 1993). In contrast, CD14-deficient mice are completely unable to release cytokine when exposed to LPS (Haziot et al., 1996). Even when the CD14 expression on KCs is low, CD14 is still critical for LPS activation. In addition, isolated KCs respond to low concentrations of LPS with production of proinflammatory cytokines. Although the expression of CD14-positive KCs is low in normal livers (Ikejima et al., 1999), these cells increase in many types of liver disease by progression of hepatic fibrosis, advanced stage, and stimulation of LPS (Leicester et al., 2006).

Tonan et al. (2012) clearly showed that the number of CD14-positive KCs in the livers of patients with NASH increased compared with those in patients with steatosis, although the number of CD68-positive KCs was not different. This result may indicate that the sensitivity for LPS and endotoxin might increase in the livers of patients with NASH compared with steatosis, and hypersensitivity for LPS may be an important pathogenic factor for progression of NASH. Activation of CD14-positive KCs and elevation of the LPS concentration promote the activation of proinflammatory cytokine release, which leads to the development of NASH. Therefore, as they showed, the number of CD14-positive KCs might be correlated to the degree of necroinflammation and severity of fibrosis in the livers of patients with NASH. CD14-positive KCs were reportedly physiologically associated with septal myofibroblasts expressing a-smooth muscle actin. This finding raises the possibility that LPS- and CD14-positive KCs may be involved in fibrosis across a broad spectrum of liver diseases. As already noted, impaired phagocytotic function of KCs may cause elevation of the circulating LPS concentration. They also showed that the degree of impaired phagocytic function of KCs was correlated to the degree of necroinflammation and severity of fibrosis in the livers of patients with NASH, although it was previously reported that severity of NASH, grading, and staging were not related to the impairment of KC phagocytic function. The mechanism underlying the observed impaired phagocytic function of KCs also remains unclear. However, impaired phagocytotic function of KCs may influence the increased expression of CD14-positive KCs and sensitivity for LPS and leads to hyperrelease of proinflammatory cytokines and progression of NASH.

These results indicate that impaired phagocytotic function of KCs may also be an important pathogenic factor for progression of NASH. In conclusion, impaired

KC function is significant in the pathogenesis of NASH, a contention that receives further support by these elegant imaging studies by Tonan and colleagues. Further mechanistic studies are indicated to clarify the pathogenic mechanisms of KC function impairment in NASH.

Ma et al. (2008) investigated the inflammatory stress in hepatic cells and fatty livers of apolipoprotein E knockout mice. They have showed that inflammatory stress increased cholesterol accumulation in hepatic cells and in the livers. They come to a conclusion that stress exacerbates lipid accumulation in liver by upregulating LDL-mediated cholesterol influx and downregulates ABCA1-mediated cholesterol efflux in vivo and in vitro. These findings demonstrated that inflammatory stress disrupted cholesterol trafficking in the liver by reducing cholesterol efflux and increasing cholesterol influx. As NAFLD progresses, a subsequent or persistent inflammatory stimulus, the second hit, will worsen cholesterol trafficking. This, together with dysregulation of TGs and free fatty acids, will result in increased lipid accumulation and progression of NAFLD.

It also became clear that the presence of chronic inflammatory diseases, such as rheumatoid arthritis or hepatitis, significantly increases the risk of development of IR, thus providing an additional and important link between chronic inflammatory states and impaired insulin action in humans, subsequently leading to progression of fatty liver.

Study by Koskinas et al. (2008) investigated liver biopsies obtained immediately after the death of the 15 patients with sepsis. Steatosis was observed in 11 (73.3%) of 15 patients affecting 5%–80% of liver parenchyma. Among the histological features, the presence of portal inflammation in liver biopsy was associated with increased hospitalization in the ICU prior death ($p = 0.026$). These findings also suggest that people with fatty liver is more vulnerable to sepsis and inflammatory responses.

Fatty Liver and Cardiovascular Disease

Fatty liver also play a role in the development of atherosclerosis. In studies, NAFLD has been shown as a risk factor for atherosclerosis. The initial event in atherogenesis is the increased transcytosis of low density lipoprotein, and its subsequent deposition, retention, and modification in the subendothelium. It is followed by the infiltration of activated inflammatory cells from the coronary circulation into the arterial wall. There they secrete ROS and produce oxidized lipoproteins capable of inducing endothelial cell apoptosis, and thereby plaque erosion. Activated T lymphocytes, macrophages, and mast cells accumulate in the eroded plaque where they secrete a variety of proteases capable of inducing degradation of extracellular proteins, thereby rendering the plaques more prone to rupture. Population studies showed a strong correlation between proinflammatory biomarkers (such as C-reactive protein, IL-6, and TNF-α) and perturbations in glucose homeostasis, obesity, and atherosclerosis (Duncan et al., 2003; Pradhan et al., 2001). Another emerging risk factor is oxidized low-density lipoprotein (ox-LDL) that activates circulating monocytes, thereby increasing their ability to infiltrate the vascular wall. This increased infiltration is a key event in atherogenesis.

Akabame et al. (2008) investigated 298 consecutive patients who were receiving multislice computed tomography (MSCT) to diagnose coronary artery disease. They found that NAFLD is related to the remodeling lesions of the coronary artery and lipid core plaques and they come into conclusion that NAFLD is the risk factor for developing vulnerable plaques.

Huang and colleagues (Huang et al., 2012) investigated atherosclerosis in middle aged and elderly Chinese. They measured NAFLD by ultrasonography. Carotid intima–media thickness (CIMT) and brachial–ankle pulse wave velocity (ba-PWV) in each participant. They come into a conclusion that NAFLD was associated with elevated CIMT and ba-PWV, independent of conventional CVD risk factors and the presence of metabolic syndrome. The study added more evidence to the notion that the risk of CVD increased in patients with NAFLD. The study by Kim et al. (2009) also demonstrated that that NAFLD is independently associated with carotid atherosclerosis only in people who have multiple metabolic abnormalities. The study by Salvi et al. (2010) has also shown independent role of NAFLD in determining arterial stiffness.

The study by Colak et al. (2012) evaluated the endothelial functions in patients with NAFLD. In this observational case–control study, a total of 51 patients with NAFLD in study group and a total of 21 with age- and sex-matched individuals in control group were enrolled. In both patients and control groups, levels of asymmetric dimethylarginine (ADMA), systemic endothelial function (brachial artery flow-mediated dilation) (FMD), and carotid artery intima–media thickness (C-IMT) were measured. C-IMT was significantly higher in patients with NAFLD group than control group (0.67 ± 0.09 versus 0.52 ± 0.11 mm, $p < 0.001$). Measurement of brachial artery FMD was significantly lower in patients with NAFLD group compared with control group (7.3 ± 4.8 versus $12.5 \pm 7.1\%$, $p < 0.001$). The increase in C-IMT and decrease in FMD was independent from metabolic syndrome, and it was also more evident in patients with simple steatosis and NASH compared with the control group. From these data, they concluded that NAFLD is associated with endothelial dysfunction and increased earlier in patients with atherosclerosis compared with control subjects.

Thakur et al. (2012) studied the association of subclinical atherosclerosis and endothelial dysfunction with NAFLD in Asian Indians. They included 40 nondiabetic subjects with NAFLD and 40 matched controls without NAFLD with similar age, gender, and BMI. They concluded in their paper that in Indians NAFLD is significantly associated with subclinical atherosclerosis and endothelial dysfunction independent of obesity and metabolic syndrome.

CONCLUSION

Fatty liver disease is one of the most significant health problems in the developing as well as developed world. Different factors contribute to the deterioration of fatty liver, and NAFLD has become a significant public health problem mostly in westernized countries. Fatty liver is one of the most important clinical conditions associated with many complications. Mainly associated with IR and metabolic syndrome and cardiovascular risks, the fatty liver developed to severe steatohepatitis and cirrhotic form by multiple mechanisms leading to serious liver injuries. Stress factors such as hypoxic stress and inflammatory stress are found to accentuating the progression of fatty liver. Excess production of cytokines and ROS and shortage of glutathione, adiponectin, and superoxide dismutase are some factors that play key role in pathogenesis of both NAFLD and ALD. Defective immune system are associated with fatty liver leading to the progression of the disease such as anti-inflammatory cytokines and antioxidants are unable to overcome inflammation and fibrosis in progressive liver injury. Fatty liver has vulnerability to various other factors associated with hypoxic and inflammatory stresses. These stresses contribute the severity and worsen the liver damage and deterioration.

REFERENCES

Akabame, S., M. Hamaguchi, K. Tomiyasu, M. Tanaka, Y. Kobayashi-Takenaka, K. Nakano, Y. Oda, and T. Yoshikawa. 2008. Evaluation of vulnerable coronary plaques and non-alcoholic fatty liver disease (NAFLD) by 64-detector multislice computed tomography (MSCT). *Circ J.* 72:618–625.

Amaro, A., E. Fabbrini, M. Kars, P. Yue, K. Schechtman, G. Schonfeld, and S. Klein. 2010. Dissociation between intrahepatic triglyceride content and insulin resistance in familial hypobetalipoproteinemia. *Gastroenterology.* 139:149–153.

Anavi, S., N.B. Harmelin, Z. Madar, and O. Tirosh. 2012. Oxidative stress impairs HIF1alpha activation: A novel mechanism for increased vulnerability of steatotic hepatocytes to hypoxic stress. *Free Radic Biol Med.* 52:1531–1542.

Andreelli, F., M. Foretz, C. Knauf, P.D. Cani, C. Perrin, M.A. Iglesias, B. Pillot, A. Bado, F. Tronche, G. Mithieux, S. Vaulont, R. Burcelin, and B. Viollet. 2006. Liver adenosine monophosphate-activated kinase-alpha2 catalytic subunit is a key target for the control of hepatic glucose production by adiponectin and leptin but not insulin. *Endocrinology.* 147:2432–2441.

Angulo, P. 2002. Nonalcoholic fatty liver disease. *N Engl J Med.* 346:1221–1231.

Angulo, P., and K.D. Lindor. 2001. Insulin resistance and mitochondrial abnormalities in NASH: A cool look into a burning issue. *Gastroenterology.* 120:1281–1285.

Arteel, G.E., Y. Iimuro, M. Yin, J.A. Raleigh, and R.G. Thurman. 1997. Chronic enteral ethanol treatment causes hypoxia in rat liver tissue in vivo. *Hepatology.* 25:920–926.

Arteel, G.E., J.A. Raleigh, B.U. Bradford, and R.G. Thurman. 1996. Acute alcohol produces hypoxia directly in rat liver tissue in vivo: Role of Kupffer cells. *Am J Physiol.* 271:G494–500.

Bajaj, M., S. Suraamornkul, P. Piper, L.J. Hardies, L. Glass, E. Cersosimo, T. Pratipanawatr, Y. Miyazaki, and R.A. DeFronzo. 2004. Decreased plasma adiponectin concentrations are closely related to hepatic fat content and hepatic insulin resistance in pioglitazone-treated type 2 diabetic patients. *J Clin Endocrinol Metab.* 89:200–206.

Browning, J.D., and J.D. Horton. 2004. Molecular mediators of hepatic steatosis and liver injury. *J Clin Invest.* 114:147–152.

Brunelle, J.K., E.L. Bell, N.M. Quesada, K. Vercauteren, V. Tiranti, M. Zeviani, R.C. Scarpulla, and N.S. Chandel. 2005. Oxygen sensing requires mitochondrial ROS but not oxidative phosphorylation. *Cell Metab.* 1:409–414.

Bugianesi, E., A.J. McCullough, and G. Marchesini. 2005. Insulin resistance: A metabolic pathway to chronic liver disease. *Hepatology.* 42:987–1000.

Carneiro, G., F.F. Ribeiro Filho, S.M. Togeiro, S. Tufik, and M.T. Zanella. 2007. [Interactions between obstructive sleep apnea syndrome and insulin resistance]. *Arq Bras Endocrinol Metabol.* 51:1035–1040.

Cederbaum, A.I., D. Wu, M. Mari, and J. Bai. 2001. CYP2E1-dependent toxicity and oxidative stress in HepG2 cells. *Free Radic Biol Med.* 31:1539–1543.

Chandel, N.S., E. Maltepe, E. Goldwasser, C.E. Mathieu, M.C. Simon, and P.T. Schumacker. 1998. Mitochondrial reactive oxygen species trigger hypoxia-induced transcription. *Proc Natl Acad Sci USA*. 95:11715–11720.

Charlton, M., R. Sreekumar, D. Rasmussen, K. Lindor, and K.S. Nair. 2002. Apolipoprotein synthesis in nonalcoholic steatohepatitis. *Hepatology*. 35:898–904.

Chavin, K.D., S. Yang, H.Z. Lin, J. Chatham, V.P. Chacko, J.B. Hoek, E. Walajtys-Rode, A. Rashid, C.H. Chen, C.C. Huang, T.C. Wu, M.D. Lane, and A.M. Diehl. 1999. Obesity induces expression of uncoupling protein-2 in hepatocytes and promotes liver ATP depletion. *J Biol Chem*. 274:5692–5700.

Cheung, O., and A.J. Sanyal. 2010. Recent advances in nonalcoholic fatty liver disease. *Curr Opin Gastroenterol*. 26:202–208.

Chin, K., T. Nakamura, K. Takahashi, K. Sumi, Y. Ogawa, H. Masuzaki, S. Muro, N. Hattori, H. Matsumoto, A. Niimi, T. Chiba, K. Nakao, M. Mishima, and M. Ohi. 2003. Effects of obstructive sleep apnea syndrome on serum aminotransferase levels in obese patients. *Am J Med*. 114:370–376.

Chitturi, S., G. Farrell, L. Frost, A. Kriketos, R. Lin, C. Fung, C. Liddle, D. Samarasinghe, and J. George. 2002. Serum leptin in NASH correlates with hepatic steatosis but not fibrosis: A manifestation of lipotoxicity? *Hepatology*. 36:403–409.

Chitturi, S., and G.C. Farrell. 2001. Etiopathogenesis of nonalcoholic steatohepatitis. *Semin Liver Dis*. 21:27–41.

Claudel, T., B. Staels, and F. Kuipers. 2005. The Farnesoid X receptor: A molecular link between bile acid and lipid and glucose metabolism. *Arterioscler Thromb Vasc Biol*. 25:2020–2030.

Colak, Y., E. Senates, A. Yesil, Y. Yilmaz, O. Ozturk, L. Doganay, E. Coskunpinar, O.T. Kahraman, B. Mesci, C. Ulasoglu, and I. Tuncer. 2012. Assessment of endothelial function in patients with nonalcoholic fatty liver disease. *Endocrine*.

Creely, S.J., P.G. McTernan, C.M. Kusminski, M. Fisher, N.F. Da Silva, M. Khanolkar, M. Evans, A.L. Harte, and S. Kumar. 2007. Lipopolysaccharide activates an innate immune system response in human adipose tissue in obesity and type 2 diabetes. *Am J Physiol Endocrinol Metab*. 292:E740–E747.

Crespo, J., A. Cayon, P. Fernandez-Gil, M. Hernandez-Guerra, M. Mayorga, A. Dominguez-Diez, J.C. Fernandez-Escalante, and F. Pons-Romero. 2001. Gene expression of tumor necrosis factor alpha and TNF-receptors, p55 and p75, in nonalcoholic steatohepatitis patients. *Hepatology*. 34:1158–1163.

Day, C.P., and O.F. James. 1998. Steatohepatitis: A tale of two "hits"? *Gastroenterology*. 114:842–845.

Day, C.P., and S.J. Yeaman. 1994. The biochemistry of alcohol-induced fatty liver. *Biochim Biophys Acta*. 1215:33–48.

Diehl, A.M. 2002. Nonalcoholic steatosis and steatohepatitis IV. Nonalcoholic fatty liver disease abnormalities in macrophage function and cytokines. *Am J Physiol Gastrointest Liver Physiol*. 282:G1–G5.

Duncan, B.B., M.I. Schmidt, J.S. Pankow, C.M. Ballantyne, D. Couper, A. Vigo, R. Hoogeveen, A.R. Folsom, and G. Heiss. 2003. Low-grade systemic inflammation and the development of type 2 diabetes: The atherosclerosis risk in communities study. *Diabetes*. 52:1799–1805.

Ebert, E.C. 2006. Hypoxic liver injury. *Mayo Clin Proc*. 81:1232–1236.

Fabbrini, E., B.S. Mohammed, F. Magkos, K.M. Korenblat, B.W. Patterson, and S. Klein. 2008. Alterations in adipose tissue and hepatic lipid kinetics in obese men and women with nonalcoholic fatty liver disease. *Gastroenterology*. 134:424–431.

Farrell, G.C., N.C. Teoh, and R.S. McCuskey. 2008. Hepatic microcirculation in fatty liver disease. *Anat Rec (Hoboken)*. 291:684–692.

Feher, J., and G. Lengyel. 2003. A new approach to drug therapy in non-alcoholic steatohepatitis (NASH). *J Int Med Res*. 31:537–551.

Feng, S.Z., J.L. Tian, Q. Zhang, H. Wang, N. Sun, Y. Zhang, and B.Y. Chen. 2011. An experimental research on chronic intermittent hypoxia leading to liver injury. *Sleep Breath.* 15:493–502.

Fernandez-Real, J.M., M. Broch, J. Vendrell, and W. Ricart. 2002. To: T. Skoog et al. (2001) Tumour necrosis factor-alpha(TNF-alpha) polymorphisms –857C/A and –863C/A are associated with TNF-alpha secretion from human adipose tissue. *Diabetologia* 44: 654–655. *Diabetologia.* 45:149–150.

Ferrero-Miliani, L., O.H. Nielsen, P.S. Andersen, and S.E. Girardin. 2007. Chronic inflammation: Importance of NOD2 and NALP3 in interleukin-1beta generation. *Clin Exp Immunol.* 147:227–235.

Ferrero, E., D. Jiao, B.Z. Tsuberi, L. Tesio, G.W. Rong, A. Haziot, and S.M. Goyert. 1993. Transgenic mice expressing human CD14 are hypersensitive to lipopolysaccharide. *Proc Natl Acad Sci USA.* 90:2380–2384.

Fong, D.G., V. Nehra, K.D. Lindor, and A.L. Buchman. 2000. Metabolic and nutritional considerations in nonalcoholic fatty liver. *Hepatology.* 32:3–10.

Fox, E.S., S.A. Broitman, and P. Thomas. 1990. Bacterial endotoxins and the liver. *Lab Invest.* 63:733–741.

Franckhauser, S., I. Elias, V. Rotter Sopasakis, T. Ferre, I. Nagaev, C.X. Andersson, J. Agudo, J. Ruberte, F. Bosch, and U. Smith. 2008. Overexpression of Il6 leads to hyperinsulinaemia, liver inflammation and reduced body weight in mice. *Diabetologia.* 51:1306–1316.

Garcia-Monzon, C. 2001. [Non-alcoholic steatohepatitis]. *Gastroenterol Hepatol.* 24:395–402.

Garcia-Monzon, C., E. Martin-Perez, O.L. Iacono, M. Fernandez-Bermejo, P.L. Majano, A. Apolinario, E. Larranaga, and R. Moreno-Otero. 2000. Characterization of pathogenic and prognostic factors of nonalcoholic steatohepatitis associated with obesity. *J Hepatol.* 33:716–724.

Gerber, H.P., K.J. Hillan, A.M. Ryan, J. Kowalski, G.A. Keller, L. Rangell, B.D. Wright, F. Radtke, M. Aguet, and N. Ferrara. 1999. VEGF is required for growth and survival in neonatal mice. *Development.* 126:1149–1159.

Guilleminault, C., A. Tilkian, and W.C. Dement. 1976. The sleep apnea syndromes. *Annu Rev Med.* 27:465–484.

Guzy, R.D., B. Hoyos, E. Robin, H. Chen, L. Liu, K.D. Mansfield, M.C. Simon, U. Hammerling, and P.T. Schumacker. 2005. Mitochondrial complex III is required for hypoxia-induced ROS production and cellular oxygen sensing. *Cell Metab.* 1:401–408.

Hamaguchi, M., T. Kojima, N. Takeda, T. Nakagawa, H. Taniguchi, K. Fujii, T. Omatsu, T. Nakajima, H. Sarui, M. Shimazaki, T. Kato, J. Okuda, and K. Ida. 2005. The metabolic syndrome as a predictor of nonalcoholic fatty liver disease. *Ann Intern Med.* 143:722–728.

Harrison, S.A., S. Kadakia, K.A. Lang, and S. Schenker. 2002. Nonalcoholic steatohepatitis: What we know in the new millennium. *Am J Gastroenterol.* 97:2714–2724.

Hayashi, M., Y. Tokunaga, T. Fujita, K. Tanaka, Y. Yamaoka, and K. Ozawa. 1993. The effects of cold preservation on steatotic graft viability in rat liver transplantation. *Transplantation.* 56:282–287.

Haziot, A., E. Ferrero, F. Kontgen, N. Hijiya, S. Yamamoto, J. Silver, C.L. Stewart, and S.M. Goyert. 1996. Resistance to endotoxin shock and reduced dissemination of Gram-negative bacteria in CD14-deficient mice. *Immunity.* 4:407–414.

Hotamisligil, G.S. 2010. Endoplasmic reticulum stress and the inflammatory basis of metabolic disease. *Cell.* 140:900–917.

Houten, S.M., M. Watanabe, and J. Auwerx. 2006. Endocrine functions of bile acids. *EMBO J.* 25:1419–1425.

Huang, Y., Y. Bi, M. Xu, Z. Ma, Y. Xu, T. Wang, M. Li, Y. Liu, J. Lu, Y. Chen, F. Huang, B. Xu, J. Zhang, W. Wang, X. Li, and G. Ning. 2012. Nonalcoholic fatty liver disease is associated with atherosclerosis in middle-aged and elderly Chinese. *Arterioscler Thromb Vasc Biol.* 32:2321–2326.

Hughes, D.E., D.B. Stolz, S. Yu, Y. Tan, J.K. Reddy, S.C. Watkins, A.M. Diehl, and R.H. Costa. 2003. Elevated hepatocyte levels of the Forkhead box A2 (HNF-3beta) transcription factor cause postnatal steatosis and mitochondrial damage. *Hepatology.* 37:1414–1424.

Hui, J.M., A. Hodge, G.C. Farrell, J.G. Kench, A. Kriketos, and J. George. 2004. Beyond insulin resistance in NASH: TNF-alpha or adiponectin? *Hepatology.* 40:46–54.

Ijaz, S., W. Yang, M.C. Winslet, and A.M. Seifalian. 2003. Impairment of hepatic microcirculation in fatty liver. *Microcirculation.* 10:447–456.

Ikejima, K., N. Enomoto, V. Seabra, A. Ikejima, D.A. Brenner, and R.G. Thurman. 1999. Pronase destroys the lipopolysaccharide receptor CD14 on Kupffer cells. *Am J Physiol.* 276:G591–598.

Ip, M.S., B. Lam, M.M. Ng, W.K. Lam, K.W. Tsang, and K.S. Lam. 2002. Obstructive sleep apnea is independently associated with insulin resistance. *Am J Respir Crit Care Med.* 165:670–676.

Jouet, P., J.M. Sabate, D. Maillard, S. Msika, C. Mechler, S. Ledoux, F. Harnois, and B. Coffin. 2007. Relationship between obstructive sleep apnea and liver abnormalities in morbidly obese patients: A prospective study. *Obes Surg.* 17:478–485.

Kallwitz, E.R., J. Herdegen, J. Madura, S. Jakate, and S.J. Cotler. 2007. Liver enzymes and histology in obese patients with obstructive sleep apnea. *J Clin Gastroenterol.* 41:918–921.

Kim, H.C., D.J. Kim, and K.B. Huh. 2009. Association between nonalcoholic fatty liver disease and carotid intima-media thickness according to the presence of metabolic syndrome. *Atherosclerosis.* 204:521–525.

Koskinas, J., I.P. Gomatos, D.G. Tiniakos, N. Memos, M. Boutsikou, A. Garatzioti, A. Archimandritis, and A. Betrosian. 2008. Liver histology in ICU patients dying from sepsis: A clinico-pathological study. *World J Gastroenterol.* 14:1389–1393.

Lee, A.H., E.F. Scapa, D.E. Cohen, and L.H. Glimcher. 2008. Regulation of hepatic lipogenesis by the transcription factor XBP1. *Science.* 320:1492–1496.

Leicester, K.L., J.K. Olynyk, E.M. Brunt, R.S. Britton, and B.R. Bacon. 2006. Differential findings for CD14-positive hepatic monocytes/macrophages in primary biliary cirrhosis, chronic hepatitis C and nonalcoholic steatohepatitis. *Liver Int.* 26:559–565.

Li, J., D.N. Grigoryev, S.Q. Ye, L. Thorne, A.R. Schwartz, P.L. Smith, C.P. O'Donnell, and V.Y. Polotsky. 2005. Chronic intermittent hypoxia upregulates genes of lipid biosynthesis in obese mice. *J Appl Physiol.* 99:1643–1648.

Li, N., and C.D. Klaassen. 2004. Role of liver-enriched transcription factors in the downregulation of organic anion transporting polypeptide 4 (oatp4; oatplb2; slc21a10) by lipopolysaccharide. *Mol Pharmacol.* 66:694–701.

Lieber, C.S. 1997. Cytochrome P-4502E1: Its physiological and pathological role. *Physiol Rev.* 77:517–544.

Lieber, C.S. 2004. Alcoholic fatty liver: Its pathogenesis and mechanism of progression to inflammation and fibrosis. *Alcohol.* 34:9–19.

Lieber, C.S., and L.M. DeCarli. 1970. Hepatic microsomal ethanol-oxidizing system. in vitro characteristics and adaptive properties in vivo. *J Biol Chem.* 245:2505–2512.

Loffreda, S., S.Q. Yang, H.Z. Lin, C.L. Karp, M.L. Brengman, D.J. Wang, A.S. Klein, G.B. Bulkley, C. Bao, P.W. Noble, M.D. Lane, and A.M. Diehl. 1998. Leptin regulates proinflammatory immune responses. *FASEB J.* 12:57–65.

Ma, K.L., X.Z. Ruan, S.H. Powis, Y. Chen, J.F. Moorhead, and Z. Varghese. 2008. Inflammatory stress exacerbates lipid accumulation in hepatic cells and fatty livers of apolipoprotein E knockout mice. *Hepatology.* 48:770–781.

Ma, X., G. Svegliati-Baroni, J. Poniachik, E. Baraona, and C.S. Lieber. 1997. Collagen synthesis by liver stellate cells is released from its normal feedback regulation by acetaldehyde-induced modification of the carboxyl-terminal propeptide of procollagen. *Alcohol Clin Exp Res.* 21:1204–1211.

Malaguarnera, M., M. Di Rosa, F. Nicoletti, and L. Malaguarnera. 2009. Molecular mechanisms involved in NAFLD progression. *J Mol Med (Berl)*. 87:679–695.

Mannaerts, G.P., P.P. Van Veldhoven, and M. Casteels. 2000. Peroxisomal lipid degradation via beta- and alpha-oxidation in mammals. *Cell Biochem Biophys*. 32 Spring:73–87.

Mansfield, K.D., R.D. Guzy, Y. Pan, R.M. Young, T.P. Cash, P.T. Schumacker, and M.C. Simon. 2005. Mitochondrial dysfunction resulting from loss of cytochrome c impairs cellular oxygen sensing and hypoxic HIF-alpha activation. *Cell Metab*. 1:393–399.

Marceau, P., S. Biron, F.S. Hould, S. Marceau, S. Simard, S.N. Thung, and J.G. Kral. 1999. Liver pathology and the metabolic syndrome X in severe obesity. *J Clin Endocrinol Metab*. 84:1513–1517.

Marchesini, G., M. Brizi, A.M. Morselli-Labate, G. Bianchi, E. Bugianesi, A.J. McCullough, G. Forlani, and N. Melchionda. 1999. Association of nonalcoholic fatty liver disease with insulin resistance. *Am J Med*. 107:450–455.

Marra, F., and C. Bertolani. 2009. Adipokines in liver diseases. *Hepatology*. 50:957–969.

Masaki, T., S. Chiba, H. Tatsukawa, T. Yasuda, H. Noguchi, M. Seike, and H. Yoshimatsu. 2004. Adiponectin protects LPS-induced liver injury through modulation of TNF-alpha in KK-Ay obese mice. *Hepatology*. 40:177–184.

Mehal, W.Z. 2012. HIF-1alpha is a major and complex player in alcohol induced liver diseases. *J Hepatol*. 56:311–312.

Morral, N., H.J. Edenberg, S.R. Witting, J. Altomonte, T. Chu, and M. Brown. 2007. Effects of glucose metabolism on the regulation of genes of fatty acid synthesis and triglyceride secretion in the liver. *J Lipid Res*. 48:1499–1510.

Naschitz, J.E., G. Slobodin, R.J. Lewis, E. Zuckerman, and D. Yeshurun. 2000. Heart diseases affecting the liver and liver diseases affecting the heart. *Am Heart J*. 140:111–120.

Nath, B., I. Levin, T. Csak, J. Petrasek, C. Mueller, K. Kodys, D. Catalano, P. Mandrekar, and G. Szabo. 2011. Hepatocyte-specific hypoxia-inducible factor-1alpha is a determinant of lipid accumulation and liver injury in alcohol-induced steatosis in mice. *Hepatology*. 53:1526–1537.

Nedergaard, J., D. Ricquier, and L.P. Kozak. 2005. Uncoupling proteins: Current status and therapeutic prospects. *EMBO Rep*. 6:917–921.

Neuschwander-Tetri, B.A., and S.H. Caldwell. 2003. Nonalcoholic steatohepatitis: Summary of an AASLD Single Topic Conference. *Hepatology*. 37:1202–1219.

Nishiyama, Y., N. Goda, M. Kanai, D. Niwa, K. Osanai, Y. Yamamoto, N. Senoo-Matsuda, R.S. Johnson, S. Miura, Y. Kabe, and M. Suematsu. 2012. HIF-1alpha induction suppresses excessive lipid accumulation in alcoholic fatty liver in mice. *J Hepatol*. 56:441–447.

Oneta, C.M., and J.F. Dufour. 2002. Non-alcoholic fatty liver disease: Treatment options based on pathogenic considerations. *Swiss Med Wkly*. 132:493–505.

Ozcan, U., Q. Cao, E. Yilmaz, A.H. Lee, N.N. Iwakoshi, E. Ozdelen, G. Tuncman, C. Gorgun, L.H. Glimcher, and G.S. Hotamisligil. 2004. Endoplasmic reticulum stress links obesity, insulin action, and type 2 diabetes. *Science*. 306:457–461.

Pagano, G., G. Pacini, G. Musso, R. Gambino, F. Mecca, N. Depetris, M. Cassader, E. David, P. Cavallo-Perin, and M. Rizzetto. 2002. Nonalcoholic steatohepatitis, insulin resistance, and metabolic syndrome: Further evidence for an etiologic association. *Hepatology*. 35:367–372.

Park, J.W., G. Jeong, S.J. Kim, M.K. Kim, and S.M. Park. 2007. Predictors reflecting the pathological severity of non-alcoholic fatty liver disease: Comprehensive study of clinical and immunohistochemical findings in younger Asian patients. *J Gastroenterol Hepatol*. 22:491–497.

Pessayre, D., A. Berson, B. Fromenty, and A. Mansouri. 2001. Mitochondria in steatohepatitis. *Semin Liver Dis*. 21:57–69.

Piguet, A.C., D. Stroka, A. Zimmermann, and J.F. Dufour. 2009. Hypoxia aggravates non-alcoholic steatohepatitis in mice lacking hepatocellular PTEN. *Clin Sci (Lond)*. 118:401–410.

Postic, C., and J. Girard. 2008. Contribution of de novo fatty acid synthesis to hepatic steatosis and insulin resistance: Lessons from genetically engineered mice. *J Clin Invest.* 118:829–838.

Pradhan, A.D., J.E. Manson, N. Rifai, J.E. Buring, and P.M. Ridker. 2001. C-reactive protein, interleukin 6, and risk of developing type 2 diabetes mellitus. *JAMA.* 286:327–334.

Qi, L., A. Doria, J.E. Manson, J.B. Meigs, D. Hunter, C.S. Mantzoros, and F.B. Hu. 2006. Adiponectin genetic variability, plasma adiponectin, and cardiovascular risk in patients with type 2 diabetes. *Diabetes.* 55:1512–1516.

Rabe, K., M. Lehrke, K.G. Parhofer, and U.C. Broedl. 2008. Adipokines and insulin resistance. *Mol Med.* 14:741–751.

Rankin, E.B., J. Rha, M.A. Selak, T.L. Unger, B. Keith, Q. Liu, and V.H. Haase. 2009. Hypoxia-inducible factor 2 regulates hepatic lipid metabolism. *Mol Cell Biol.* 29:4527–4538.

Rao, M.S., and J.K. Reddy. 2001. Peroxisomal beta-oxidation and steatohepatitis. *Semin Liver Dis.* 21:43–55.

Redaelli, C.A., D. Semela, F.E. Carrick, M. Ledermann, D. Candinas, B. Sauter, and J.F. Dufour. 2004. Effect of vascular endothelial growth factor on functional recovery after hepatectomy in lean and obese mice. *J Hepatol.* 40:305–312.

Reddy, J.K., and T. Hashimoto. 2001. Peroxisomal beta-oxidation and peroxisome proliferator-activated receptor alpha: An adaptive metabolic system. *Annu Rev Nutr.* 21:193–230.

Reddy, J.K., and M.S. Rao. 2006. Lipid metabolism and liver inflammation. II. Fatty liver disease and fatty acid oxidation. *Am J Physiol Gastrointest Liver Physiol.* 290:G852–858.

Reid, A.E. 2001. Nonalcoholic steatohepatitis. *Gastroenterology.* 121:710–723.

Salvi, P., R. Ruffini, D. Agnoletti, E. Magnani, G. Pagliarani, G. Comandini, A. Pratico, C. Borghi, A. Benetos, and P. Pazzi. 2010. Increased arterial stiffness in nonalcoholic fatty liver disease: The Cardio-GOOSE study. *J Hypertens.* 28:1699–1707.

Samuel, V.T., Z.X. Liu, X. Qu, B.D. Elder, S. Bilz, D. Befroy, A.J. Romanelli, and G.I. Shulman. 2004. Mechanism of hepatic insulin resistance in non-alcoholic fatty liver disease. *J Biol Chem.* 279:32345–32353.

Samuel, V.T., K.F. Petersen, and G.I. Shulman. 2010. Lipid-induced insulin resistance: Unravelling the mechanism. *Lancet.* 375:2267–2277.

Sanyal, A.J., C. Campbell-Sargent, F. Mirshahi, W.B. Rizzo, M.J. Contos, R.K. Sterling, V.A. Luketic, M.L. Shiffman, and J.N. Clore. 2001. Nonalcoholic steatohepatitis: Association of insulin resistance and mitochondrial abnormalities. *Gastroenterology.* 120:1183–1192.

Savage, D.B., and R.K. Semple. 2010. Recent insights into fatty liver, metabolic dyslipidaemia and their links to insulin resistance. *Curr Opin Lipidol.* 21:329–336.

Savolainen, E.R., M.A. Leo, R. Timpl, and C.S. Lieber. 1984. Acetaldehyde and lactate stimulate collagen synthesis of cultured baboon liver myofibroblasts. *Gastroenterology.* 87:777–787.

Savransky, V., S. Bevans, A. Nanayakkara, J. Li, P.L. Smith, M.S. Torbenson, and V.Y. Polotsky. 2007. Chronic intermittent hypoxia causes hepatitis in a mouse model of diet-induced fatty liver. *Am J Physiol Gastrointest Liver Physiol.* 293:G871–877.

Schaffner, F., and H. Thaler. 1986. Nonalcoholic fatty liver disease. *Prog Liver Dis.* 8:283–298.

Schmitz-Peiffer, C. 2010. Targeting ceramide synthesis to reverse insulin resistance. *Diabetes.* 59:2351–2353.

Schmitz-Peiffer, C., and T.J. Biden. 2008. Protein kinase C function in muscle, liver, and beta-cells and its therapeutic implications for type 2 diabetes. *Diabetes.* 57:1774–1783.

Seifalian, A.M., V. Chidambaram, K. Rolles, and B.R. Davidson. 1998. in vivo demonstration of impaired microcirculation in steatotic human liver grafts. *Liver Transpl Surg.* 4:71–77.

Semenza, G.L. 2009. Regulation of oxygen homeostasis by hypoxia-inducible factor 1. *Physiology (Bethesda).* 24:97–106.

Sheth, S.G., F.D. Gordon, and S. Chopra. 1997. Nonalcoholic steatohepatitis. *Ann Intern Med.* 126:137–145.

Shulman, G.I. 2000. Cellular mechanisms of insulin resistance. *J Clin Invest.* 106:171–176.

Singh, A., M. Wirtz, N. Parker, M. Hogan, J. Strahler, G. Michailidis, S. Schmidt, A. Vidal-Puig, S. Diano, P. Andrews, M.D. Brand, and J. Friedman. 2009. Leptin-mediated changes in hepatic mitochondrial metabolism, structure, and protein levels. *Proc Natl Acad Sci USA.* 106:13100–13105.

Solga, S.F., and A.M. Diehl. 2003. Non-alcoholic fatty liver disease: Lumen-liver interactions and possible role for probiotics. *J Hepatol.* 38:681–687.

Solinas, G., and M. Karin. 2010. JNK1 and IKKbeta: Molecular links between obesity and metabolic dysfunction. *FASEB J.* 24:2596–2611.

Solis Herruzo, J.A., I. Garcia Ruiz, M. Perez Carreras, and M.T. Munoz Yague. 2006. Non-alcoholic fatty liver disease. From insulin resistance to mitochondrial dysfunction. *Rev Esp Enferm Dig.* 98:844–874.

Su, G.L. 2002. Lipopolysaccharides in liver injury: Molecular mechanisms of Kupffer cell activation. *Am J Physiol Gastrointest Liver Physiol.* 283:G256–265.

Summers, S.A. 2006. Ceramides in insulin resistance and lipotoxicity. *Prog Lipid Res.* 45:42–72.

Tanne, F., F. Gagnadoux, O. Chazouilleres, B. Fleury, D. Wendum, E. Lasnier, B. Lebeau, R. Poupon, and L. Serfaty. 2005. Chronic liver injury during obstructive sleep apnea. *Hepatology.* 41:1290–1296.

Tatsumi, K., and T. Saibara. 2005. Effects of obstructive sleep apnea syndrome on hepatic steatosis and nonalcoholic steatohepatitis. *Hepatol Res.* 33:100–104.

Teli, M.R., O.F. James, A.D. Burt, M.K. Bennett, and C.P. Day. 1995. The natural history of nonalcoholic fatty liver: A follow-up study. *Hepatology.* 22:1714–1719.

Thakur, M.L., S. Sharma, A. Kumar, S.P. Bhatt, K. Luthra, R. Guleria, R.M. Pandey, and N.K. Vikram. 2012. Nonalcoholic fatty liver disease is associated with subclinical atherosclerosis independent of obesity and metabolic syndrome in Asian Indians. *Atherosclerosis.* 223:507–511.

Thomas, C., R. Pellicciari, M. Pruzanski, J. Auwerx, and K. Schoonjans. 2008. Targeting bile-acid signalling for metabolic diseases. *Nat Rev Drug Discov.* 7:678–693.

Thurman, R.G. 1998. II. Alcoholic liver injury involves activation of Kupffer cells by endotoxin. *Am J Physiol.* 275:G605–611.

Tilg, H., and A.R. Moschen. 2006. Adipocytokines: Mediators linking adipose tissue, inflammation and immunity. *Nat Rev Immunol.* 6:772–783.

Tilg, H., and A.R. Moschen. 2008. Inflammatory mechanisms in the regulation of insulin resistance. *Mol Med.* 14:222–231.

Tonan, T., K. Fujimoto, A. Qayyum, Y. Morita, O. Nakashima, N. Ono, A. Kawahara, M. Kage, N. Hayabuchi, and T. Ueno. 2012. CD14 expression and Kupffer cell dysfunction in non-alcoholic steatohepatitis: Superparamagnetic iron oxide-magnetic resonance image and pathologic correlation. *J Gastroenterol Hepatol.* 27:789–796.

Tsochatzis, E.A., G.V. Papatheodoridis, and A.J. Archimandritis. 2009. Adipokines in non-alcoholic steatohepatitis: From pathogenesis to implications in diagnosis and therapy. *Mediators Inflamm.* 2009:831670.

Uygun, A., A. Kadayifci, Z. Yesilova, A. Erdil, H. Yaman, M. Saka, M.S. Deveci, S. Bagci, M. Gulsen, N. Karaeren, and K. Dagalp. 2000. Serum leptin levels in patients with non-alcoholic steatohepatitis. *Am J Gastroenterol.* 95:3584–3589.

Valenti, L., A.L. Fracanzani, P. Dongiovanni, G. Santorelli, A. Branchi, E. Taioli, G. Fiorelli, and S. Fargion. 2002. Tumor necrosis factor alpha promoter polymorphisms and insulin resistance in nonalcoholic fatty liver disease. *Gastroenterology.* 122:274–280.

Weltman, M.D., G.C. Farrell, P. Hall, M. Ingelman-Sundberg, and C. Liddle. 1998. Hepatic cytochrome P450 2E1 is increased in patients with nonalcoholic steatohepatitis. *Hepatology.* 27:128–133.

Wieckowska, A., B.G. Papouchado, Z. Li, R. Lopez, N.N. Zein, and A.E. Feldstein. 2008. Increased hepatic and circulating interleukin-6 levels in human nonalcoholic steatohepatitis. *Am J Gastroenterol.* 103:1372–1379.

Xu, A., Y. Wang, H. Keshaw, L.Y. Xu, K.S. Lam, and G.J. Cooper. 2003. The fat-derived hormone adiponectin alleviates alcoholic and nonalcoholic fatty liver diseases in mice. *J Clin Invest.* 112:91–100.

Zhang, X.L. 2008. [Obstructive sleep apnea syndromes and insulin resistance]. *Zhonghua Jie He He Hu Xi Za Zhi.* 31:644–646.

Zhang, Y., R. Proenca, M. Maffei, M. Barone, L. Leopold, and J.M. Friedman. 1994. Positional cloning of the mouse obese gene and its human homologue. *Nature.* 372:425–432.

3 Development of Hepatocellular Carcinoma

A. Ruth He and Lopa Mishra

CONTENTS

INTRODUCTION

Primary liver cancer is one of the most common and deadly cancers worldwide. Globally, it represents the fifth most common cancer and the third most common cause of cancer death, behind only lung cancer and stomach cancer (Parkin, 2001; El-Serag and Rudolph, 2007; Gomaa et al., 2008; World Health Organization, 2010a).

Hepatocellular carcinoma (HCC) accounts for the majority of these primary cancers of the liver. The World Health Organization and the Centers for Disease Control and Prevention project that, annually, some 600,000 chronically infected people die from HCC and chronic liver disease (World Health Organization, 2010b; Colvin and Mitchell, 2010). HCC is a unique cancer, given its wide diversity in geographic distribution, risk factors, and altered signaling transduction pathways in carcinogenesis. In this chapter, we will first introduce briefly the epidemiology of HCC, followed by discussion of risks factor including the well-established risk factors, such as viral hepatitis, alcohol cirrhosis, and NASH—an emerging risk factor for HCC in Western country. We then will summarize the signaling pathways that are important for hepatocarcinogenesis including NASH induced HCC, which supported by animal models experiments. Furthermore, the implication of molecular tumorigenesis in the development of therapeutics against HCC is discussed.

EPIDEMIOLOGY OF HCC

More than 80% of HCC cases occur in less developed countries, particularly East Asia and sub-Saharan Africa, and these are typically associated with chronic hepatitis B and C, although the incidence in these countries is decreasing (Parkin, 2001; El-Serag and Rudolph, 2007). Interestingly, the incidence of HCC in developed countries including Japan, Australia, Europe, Canada, and the United States has been increasing over the last 20 years (El-Serag and Mason, 1999; Bosch et al., 2004). In the United States alone, the annual incidence of HCC has increased about 80% during the last two decades (Gomaa et al., 2008). The emergence of hepatitis C virus (HCV) in developed countries accounts for about half of this increase in HCC (El-Serag and Mason, 1999; Gomaa et al., 2008). The etiology of HCC in 15%–50% of new HCC cases in developed countries remains unclear, however, which suggests that other risk factors also account for the increase (Bugianesi, 2007). In particular, nonalcoholic steatohepatitis (NASH) that accounts for a large proportion of idiopathic or cryptogenic cirrhosis has emerged as an important risk factor for HCC.

RISK FACTORS FOR HCC

The dominant risk factors tend to vary in high- and low-risk HCC regions. In most high-risk countries of Asia and Africa, chronic hepatitis B virus (HBV) infection and aflatoxin B1 exposure are the major risk factors. In contrast, HCV infection, excessive alcohol consumption, obesity, and diabetes play more important roles in low-risk HCC areas.

HBV INFECTION

The lifetime risk of HCC among HBV carriers is estimated to be 10% to 25%. The World Health Organization and the Centers for Disease Control and Prevention project that between 35 million and 87 million of the 350 million prevalent global HBV carriers will die of HCC (World Health Organization, 2013). Prevention of chronic infection with HBV via vaccination drastically reduces the risk of subsequent HCC, although the vaccine is ineffective in 5% to 10% of individuals. On the population level, it is anticipated that the widespread neonatal vaccination in many countries that started in the mid-1980s will result in notable decreases in the incidence of HBV-related HCC. In Taiwan, 20 years after the initiation of universal newborn vaccination, seropositivity rates of hepatitis B surface antigen in persons younger than 20 years have fallen from 10% to 17% to 0.7% to 1.7% (Chang et al., 2009a). Currently, 92% of all countries have integrated newborn hepatitis B vaccination into their routine vaccination programs, and 70% are now delivering three immunization doses (World Health Organization, 2013). However, vaccination is not routine in all high-risk countries, particularly those in sub-Saharan Africa. In these areas, control of aflatoxin is critically important because there is a synergistic effect of aflatoxin consumption and HBV infection on the risk of HCC.

HCV Infection

The highest rates of chronic HCV infection in the world occur in northern Africa, particularly Egypt, where the rate has been estimated to be 18% (Bostan and Mahmood, 2010). In Asia, the chronic HCV infection rate is considerably higher in Mongolia (10%) than in Vietnam (6%), Cambodia (4%), China (3%–4%), or Japan (2%) (Chung et al., 2010). European rates (0.5% to 2.5%) are similar to that in the United States (1.8%) but higher than the Canadian rate (0.1% to 0.8%), which is one of the lowest in the world. In developed countries where the HCC rate is low, Japan and Egypt are two exceptions due to the increased incidence of HCV infection, which is the dominant risk factor for HCC in these two countries. The cumulative lifetime (age 30–75 years) incidence of HCC for men and women positive for those positive HCV antibody is 24% and 17%, respectively (Huang et al., 2011).

Aflatoxin Infection

Aflatoxin, a mycotoxin produced by the molds *Aspergillus flavus* and *Aspergillus parasiticus*, contaminates maize, groundnuts, and tree nuts in warm, humid environments and is a well-established hepatic carcinogen (International Agency for Research on Cancer [IARC], 2002). The synergistic effect of aflatoxin B1 and chronic HBV infection on HCC risk was revealed in short-term prospective studies in Shanghai, China. Compared with persons without aflatoxin or HBV exposure, the risk of HCC was 4-fold greater among persons with increased levels of aflatoxin metabolites in urine, 7-fold greater among persons chronically infected with HBV and 60-fold greater among individuals with both risk factors (Ross et al., 1992; Qian et al., 1994). Aflatoxin B1 contamination is more common in areas where HBV is the dominant virus.

High Alcohol Consumption

In 1988, the IARC concluded that there was a causal relationship between alcohol consumption and liver cancer (IARC, 1988). In 2007, the World Cancer Research

Fund and the American Institute for Cancer Research, in a review of diet and physical activity studies, concluded that alcohol consumption was probably a direct cause of liver cancer (World Cancer Research Fund, 2007). Both HBV and HCV, in conjunction with alcohol, have synergistic effects on HCC risk (Kuper et al., 2000; Donato et al., 2002; Yuan et al., 2004). The same studies found that alcohol consumption is significantly associated with HCC in the absence of viral infection (odds ratio 2.4–7.0), although higher levels of alcohol consumption are likely required to increase risk in the absence of viral infection.

Animal and human studies have provided little evidence that ethanol is a carcinogen (McKillop and Schrum, 2009). Some of the mechanisms by which alcohol might increase risk include the production of acetaldehyde and free radicals during alcohol metabolism, cytochrome P4502E1 induction, modulation of cell regeneration, promotion or exacerbation of nutritional deficiencies, and alterations of the immune system (Seitz et al., 1998). What is certain is that alcohol induces cirrhosis, which is a factor in 60%–90% of HCCs. Whether alcohol is related to HCC independently of cirrhosis is less clear.

OBESITY

Obesity has been established as a significant risk factor for the development of various malignancies, including liver cancer (Ozturk, 1991; Iida et al., 1999; Seeff et al., 2000; IARC, 2002). A large, prospective mortality study by the American Cancer Society (Bordeaux et al., 2006) demonstrated increased cancer mortality with increased body weight. The death rates from all types of cancers among the heaviest patients in the study cohort (patients with a body mass index [BMI] > 40 kg/m^2) were 52% higher for men and 62% higher for women compared with patients of normal index BMI (BMI 18.5–24.9 kg/m^2). These mortality rates included deaths from esophageal, stomach, colorectal, liver, gallbladder, pancreatic, prostate, and kidney cancer as well as leukemia, non-Hodgkin lymphoma, and multiple myeloma. Compared with patients with normal BMI, the relative risk of mortality from liver cancer was 1.68 times higher in women and 4.52 times higher in men with a BMI > 35 kg/m^2. These findings confirmed the results of another population-based study from Denmark of more than 40,000 obese patients, which showed that the relative risk of liver cancer 1.9 compared with the general population (Hsu et al., 1991).

A study from South Korea published in 2005 examined the relationship between BMI and various cancers in 781,283 men without a prior diagnosis of cancer (Oh et al., 2005). The patients were followed over a 10-year period. Korean men with a BMI > 30 kg/m^2 had a 26% increase in risk for all types of cancer compared with men with a normal BMI (Wild and Hall, 2000). A relative risk of 1.53 was demonstrated for HCC in obese males compared with normal controls, even after controlling for HBV infection, which is the most common cause of HCC in Korea (Wild and Hall, 2000; Plymoth et al., 2009). This risk that obesity imposes for the development of HCC is likely conferred by two factors: the increased risk for nonalcoholic fatty liver disease (NAFLD) with subsequent progression to NASH and the carcinogenic potential of obesity alone (Altekruse et al., 2009).

DIABETES

A significant relationship between diabetes and liver cancer was first reported in 1986 (Lawson et al., 1986). More recently, a case–control study in the United States showed that diabetes was associated with an increased risk for HCC, but only in patients with concomitant HCV-, HBV-, or alcohol-related cirrhosis (IARC, 1988). In a larger longitudinal study, the same group compared 173,643 patients with diabetes with 650,620 nondiabetic control subjects over 10–15 years (World Cancer Research Fund, 2007). The incidence of HCC was found to be more than 2-fold higher among the patients, and the increase was higher among those with longer duration of follow-up. The risk of HCC with diabetes remained elevated even after exclusion of patients who were subsequently diagnosed with HCV, HBV, alcohol use, and/or fatty liver disease at any time during the follow-up (World Cancer Research Fund, 2007).

Diabetes is a clearly established independent risk factor for HCC. Statins have been shown to significantly reduce the risk of HCC among patients with diabetes (El-Serag et al., 2009). In a nested, matched, case–control study, a total of 1303 cases and 5212 controls were compared in patients with diabetes with or without statin treatment for risk of the development of HCC. The study demonstrated that the risk dropped between 25% and 40% for the development of HCC among diabetic patients who were prescribed statins (El-Serag et al., 2009). This risk reduction persisted in analysis of patients with and without known liver disease, or cirrhosis (El-Serag et al., 2009). Future studies should be conducted to confirm these findings in diabetic patients as well as to evaluate the benefit of statins in NAFLD and NASH.

NASH/NAFLD AND CIRRHOSIS

The most common form of chronic liver disease in developed countries is NAFLD, which includes a clinicopathologic spectrum of disease ranging from isolated hepatic steatosis to NASH, the more aggressive form of fatty liver disease, which can progress to cirrhosis and its associated complications, including hepatic failure and HCC. Globally, the prevalence of NAFLD in the general population ranges from 9% to 37% (Hilden et al., 1977; Ground, 1982; Nomura et al., 1988; Nonomura et al., 1992; Lai et al., 2002; Omagari et al., 2002; Shen et al., 2003; Bedogni et al., 2005). In the United States, NAFLD affects an estimated 30% of the general population and as high as 90% of the morbidly obese (Torres and Harrison, 2008).

NASH has been estimated to affect 5%–7% of the general population and as many as 34%–40% of patients who have elevated liver enzymes in the setting of negative serologic markers for liver disease (Daniel et al., 1999; Skelly et al., 2001; Mccullough, 2007; Ong and Younossi, 2007). Obesity, diabetes mellitus, hyperlipidemia, metabolic syndrome, and insulin resistance have been established as risk factors for primary NAFLD (Ludwig et al., 1980; Cortez-Pinto et al., 1999; Chitturi et al., 2002; Pagano et al., 2002; Marchesini et al., 2003; Ong and Younossi, 2007). With the progressive epidemics of obesity and diabetes mellitus, particularly in developed countries, the prevalence of NAFLD and its associated complications is expected to increase (Ong and Younossi, 2007).

Severe fibrosis occurs in 15% to 50% of patients with NASH and cirrhosis in 7% to 25% (Bugianesi et al., 2002). Burned-out NASH may be the cause of many cases of cryptogenic cirrhosis because many of the same comorbid conditions are equally present in NASH and cryptogenic cirrhosis (Powell et al., 1990; Caldwell et al., 1999; Poonawala et al., 2000). An analysis of risk factors for HCC in the United States between 2002 and 2008 reported that NAFLD/NASH and diabetes are the most common risk factors (59% and 36%, respectively) (Sanyal et al., 2010). Multiple data sets in world have shown that about 27% of cases of NASH transform to HCC after the development of cirrhosis, although the overall occurrence of HCC in the setting of NAFLD remains a rare complication (Ratziu et al., 2002; Siegel and Zhu, 2009). Longitudinal outcome studies report the prevalence of HCC to be 0%–0.5% in NAFLD and 0%–2.8% in NASH over periods of up to 19.5 years (Adams et al., 2005; Ekstedt et al., 2006; Ong et al., 2008; Rafiq et al., 2009). The development of cirrhosis in NASH typically occurs at an older age than in other liver diseases, although once cirrhosis does develop in patients with NASH, their clinical course is comparable to patients with other causes of cirrhosis (Ratziu et al., 2002; Ong and Younossi, 2003).

Reports of HCC cases arising in the setting of NASH without underlying cirrhosis raises the interesting possibility that carcinogenesis can occur in NAFLD in the absence of advanced liver disease (Guzman et al., 2008).

Male Sex

The incidence of HCC is 2- to 3-fold higher in men than women (Davila et al. 2005). The reasons that men have higher rates of liver cancer are not completely understood but may be partly explained by the sex-specific prevalence of known risk factors. For example, men are more likely to be chronically infected with HCV and HBV, consume alcohol, smoke cigarettes, and have increased iron stores, which are risk factors for HCC (Kowdley, 2004; Yu and Yuan, 2004). Whether androgenic hormones or increased genetic susceptibility also predispose men to the development of liver cancer is not clear.

Summary of Risk Factors for HCC

The global risk of HCC has been largely driven by HBV infection for the past century. Contributions to risk have also been made by other factors, including HCV, aflatoxin, excessive alcohol consumption, diabetes, and obesity. The dominant effect of HBV on global HCC risk should decline in future generations as the population vaccinated against HBV advances in years. Infection with HCV should also decline as a major cause of HCC in future generations because this virus was removed from the blood supply of most countries in the early 1990s. Declining levels of alcohol consumption in many areas suggests that alcohol also may become less of a factor in HCC in coming years. However, high global prevalence of obesity and diabetes become even more important risk factors for HCC as the prevalence of other risk factors declines.

GENETICS OF HCC AND REVELANT MOUSE MODELS

Since the discovery of the first tumor suppressor gene 30 years ago, genetic altera-tions have been considered to be both the main features and the main causes of human carcinogenesis. The discovery of epigenetic control of tumor suppressor genes and oncogenes that may drive carcinogenesis revealed an additional level of complexity. Sequencing of the entire human genome and comparison of nor-mal and cancer genome sequence have provided the basis for comprehensive map-ping of cancer genome alterations and understanding the genetic events involved in carcinogenesis.

Liver carcinogenesis is a multistep process (Kitagawa et al., 1991). Genetic altera-tions, such as loss of heterozygosity and loss or gain of chromosome, have been described in a subset of dysplastic nodules. Global genomic analyses with microar-ray and microRNA studies have revealed that, in addition to the diverse risk fac-tors and underlying liver diseases, the etiologies and clinicopathological features of HCC are heterogeneous as well. Transgenic mouse models have been used to test the importance of oncogene or loss of tumor suppression in driving HCC mutations.

Wnt/Catenin Pathway

The Wnt/catenin pathway is involved in liver development, amino acid metabolism, regeneration, and oxidative stress (Monga et al., 2001; Cadoret et al., 2002; Monga et al., 2003; Micsenyi et al., 2004; Benhamouche et al., 2006; Thompson and Monga, 2007; Rebouissou et al., 2008). At baseline, β-catenin is associated with a nega-tive regulator complex in the cytoplasm that includes adenomatous polyposis coli (APC), AXIN1, and glycogen synthase kinase 3B (GSK3B). This complex phos-phorylates β-catenin at serine/threonine residues coded by exon 3. Phosphorylation of β-catenin leads to its cytoplasmic degradation by the proteasome machinery. When Wnt ligands bind to Frizzled receptors, they induce GSK3B inactivation via the activation of Disheveled. Unphosphorylated β-catenin is then stabilized in the cytoplasm and translocates into the nucleus to act as a transcription factor via its association with another transcription factor, the T-cell factor/lymphoid enhancing complex (TCF/LEF). This process leads to the transcription of a large number of genes involved in proliferation, metabolism, or hepatocyte function (Cadoret et al., 2002; Benhamouche et al., 2006; Thompson and Monga, 2007).

Activating mutations of β-catenin in HCC, which were first described by de la Coste et al., 1998) are found in 10%–40% of tumors, depending on the series (Legoix et al., 1999; Hsu et al., 2000; Laurent-Puig et al., 2001; Mao et al., 2001; Laurent-Puig and Zucman-Rossi, 2006; Audard et al., 2007; Imbeaud et al., 2010; Zucman-Rossi, 2010). The mutation targets exon 3 coding for the phosphorylation site by GSK3B, leading to the absence of β-catenin phosphorylation and its permanent acti-vation (de la Coste et al., 1998; Miyoshi et al., 1998). The role of β-catenin mutation in hepatocarcinogenesis has been studied in transgenic mouse model, which showed that a Wnt-activating β-catenin mutation alone causes hepatomegaly and that addi-tional mutations or epigenetic changes are required to induce hepatocarcinogenesis

(Harada et al., 2002). When mutations in both the β-catenin and H-ras genes were introduced by adenovirus-mediated Cre expression, early HCC was identified in all the mice killed 8 weeks after induction (Harada et al., 2004). High-grade HCC was established after approximately 26 weeks.

A study of the correlations between β-catenin mutation and features of HCC showed that HCC with β-catenin mutations was more frequently associated with to non-HBV infection and chromosomal stability (Laurent-Puig et al., 2001). Other teams have stressed a possible association with chronic hepatitis C (Hsu et al., 2000). Moreover, HCC with β-catenin activating mutations demonstrate a typical pathological phenotype of large, well-differentiated tumors associated with cholestasis frequently developed in noncirrhotic liver (Hsu et al., 2000; Audard et al., 2007; Cieply et al., 2009). AXIN1-inactivating mutations, which are the most second frequent genetic alteration in HCC, lead to the release of β-catenin inhibition by the APC/Axin1/GS3KB complex and induce permanent activation of the Wnt/catenin pathway. AXIN1 biallelic inactivating mutations have been found in 5%–15% of HCC cases (Satoh et al., 2000; Taniguchi et al., 2002; Ishizaki et al., 2004; Zucman-Rossi et al., 2007).

Moreover, overexpression of AXIN1 in HCC cell lines decreases proliferation via activation of apoptosis. In contrast with HCC with β-catenin-activating mutations, tumors demonstrating AXIN1 inactivation belong to a distinct subgroup by chromosomal instability and frequent chronic HBV infection (Boyault et al., 2007; Zucman-Rossi et al., 2007). Interestingly, AXIN1-inactivating mutations are not associated with transcriptomic overexpression of classical β-catenin target genes unlike HCC associated with β-catenin mutation (Zucman-Rossi et al., 2007). These findings suggest that hepatocarcinogenesis with different etiologies may cause mutations of different genes of the same pathway (Wnt/catenin pathway) and lead to different phenotypes.

CELL CYCLE REGULATORS

During carcinogenesis, the most common mutation is found in the tumor suppressor gene *TP53*, which leads to its inactivation. The corresponding protein, P53, is a classical cell cycle regulator at the G1/S regulation checkpoint that is also involved in the control of DNA repair and apoptosis. P53 is frequently inactivated in HCC (10%–61% of cases) via deletion, missense, or nonsense mutations and is often associated with loss of heterozygosity of the second allele (Puisieux et al., 1993). A mutation hotspot at codon 249 (R249S G:C to T:A transversion), which is specific to food contaminated with aflatoxin B1, was identified in more than 50% of African and Asian HCC patients (Bressac et al., 1991). Due to the rare exposure to aflatoxin B1 in Western countries, the rate of P53 mutations in HCC is lower (10%–20%) in Western countries than in Asian countries (40%–60%) and no specific mutation hotspot has been reported for Western countries (Karachristos et al., 1999; Laurent-Puig et al., 2001; Edamoto et al., 2003). The TP53 hotspot mutation at codon 249 illustrates how a tumor suppressor gene can be altered by an environmental carcinogen during hepatocarcinogenesis.

Among genes involved in the G1/S checkpoint are the classical tumor suppressor gene for retinoblastoma (Rb) and P16 (CDKN2A, a cyclin-dependent kinase inhibitor that encodes a G1 cell cycle inhibitor that modulates phosphorylation of the Rb gene product. Rb is rarely mutated in HCC (Zhang et al., 1994), whereas P16 is frequently inactivated in HCC. Promoter hypermethylation of P16 has been observed for 35%–60% of HCC cases. In addition, infrequent missense mutations or large in-frame deletions of P16 have been found in HCC (6%–17%) (Biden et al., 1997; Liew et al., 1999; Matsuda et al., 1999). In a study of HCC patients who had TP53-mutated tumors with inactivation of the Rb pathway via methylation of P16 (as determined with transcriptomic analysis results) genes involved in cell cycle control were markedly overexpressed and the prognosis was severe compared with patients with other HCC groups (Boyault et al., 2007).

IL-6/JAK/STAT PATHWAY

Chronic inflammation by viral infection and other risk factors is closely associated with HCC tumorigenesis. Activation of inflammatory signaling pathways is common among HCC patients with different etiologies (Tsai and Chung, 2010). The proinflammatory cytokine interleukin (IL) 6 (IL-6) can also greatly increase diethylnitrosamine (a chemical carcinogen)-induced HCC in male mice (Naugler et al., 2007). IL-6 binds to gp130, the co-receptor of IL-6, then recruits glycoprotein 80, which activates Janus kinases 1 and 2 (JAK1 and JAK2), respectively, which in turn phosphorylate signal transducer and activator of transcription 1 and 2 (STAT1 and STAT, respectively) (Grivennikov and Karin, 2008). STAT3 has been recognized as an oncogene for many years (Bromberg et al., 1999; Grivennikov et al., 2009; Grivennikov et al., 2010; Nault and Zucman-Rossi, 2010).

Activation of the IL-6/JAK/STAT pathway also induces the transcription of suppressor of cytokine signaling 1 and 3 (SOCS1 and SOCS3, respectively), two negative regulators of this pathway that constitute a negative feedback loop (Grivennikov and Karin, 2008). Silencing of SOCS1 due by methylation of its promoter has been described in 61% of HCC cases (Yoshikawa et al., 2001; Okochi et al., 2003). Similarly, 30%–38% of HCC cases exhibit epigenetic inactivation of SOCS3 due to promoter methylation (Niwa et al., 2005; Calvisi et al., 2006). However, it is unknown whether SOCS1 or SOCS3 inactivation alone serves as a driving mutation in HCC or whether an additional event, such as genetic alterations or autocrine/paracrine stimulation by cytokines, is required. Interestingly, glycoprotein 130 (gp130), and *Stat3* have been shown to be frequently mutated in inflammatory hepatocellular adenomas, a type of benign liver tumor (Rebouissou et al., 2009; Pilati et al., 2011). Although rare in HCC, the gp130-activating mutations are always accompanied by β-*catenin* gene mutations, suggesting that IL-6/STAT3 and WNT/β-*catenin* could promote the malignant conversion of hepatocytes in a cooperative manner (Rebouissou et al., 2009). The results also suggested that activation of the IL-6-JAK-STAT pathway alone could promote the development of benign liver tumors and that additional β-catenin activation can participate in malignant transformation.

The loss of β-II spectrin (SPTNB1, previously known as ELF, bIISP), an adapter protein to Smad3 in transforming growth factor (TGF) β signaling, is associated with increased IL-6/STAT3 signaling and HCC formation (Tang et al., 2008). Yet inhibition of IL-6/STAT3 markedly decreased the number of tumors observed in

ITIH4–Sptnb1 double heterozygotes (Tang et al., 2008). These findings suggest interaction of TGF-β signaling and IL-6/STAT3 in the development of HCC.

GROWTH FACTOR PATHWAYS

Growth factors and growth factor receptors (e.g., the ErbB family, insulin-like growth factors [IGF] and hepatocyte growth factor [HGF]/cMET) are pivotal growth signal regulators in solid tumors and hematologic malignancies. The growth signal transduced via the RAS/RAF/mitogen-activated protein (MAP) kinase pathway and the protein kinase B AKT/mammalian target of rapamycin (mTor) pathway downstream of the growth factors are frequently amplified or mutated in human cancer. The ErbB family, a tyrosine kinase receptor family involved in tumorigenesis, consist of four receptors: epidermal growth factor receptor (EGFR), ErbB2 (her2/neu), ErbB3, and ErbB4. EGFR- and ErbB2-activating mutations have been rarely described in HCC (1% and 2% of cases, respectively) (Su et al., 2005; Bekaii-Saab et al., 2006; Boyault et al., 2007; Wong et al., 2008), and amplification or overexpression of ErbB2, important mutation in the development of some breast or gastric cancer appears to be uncommon in HCC (0%–8% of cases) (Collier et al., 1992; Xian et al., 2005).

TGF-α and epidermal growth factor (EGF) are important hepatic mitogens that bind to EGFR. Half of the transgenic mice that overexpress human TGF-α under the inducible metallothionein 1 promoter develop liver tumors at 40–70 weeks (Jhappan et al., 1990). These tumors are genetically similar to human HCC associated with poor prognosis (Lee et al., 2004). Double transgenic mice carrying both c-myc (an albumin promoter) and TGF-α (a metallothionein promoter) have been shown to exhibit tremendous acceleration of tumor development compared with transgenic mice overexpressing only c-myc or TGF-α (Murakami et al., 1993; Ohgaki et al., 1996; Thorgeirsson and Santoni-Rugiu, 1996). After approximately 17 weeks, 20% of the double transgenic mice were diagnosed with HCC that consisted of multiple foci of carcinomas and adenomas, and at 40 weeks, 100% were diagnosed with the disease (Murakami, 1993). The faster occurrence of HCC in the double transgenic model, compared with the parental lines, suggests that the interaction of c-myc and TGF-α increases the likelihood of malignant transformation.

Overexpression of the secreted form of EGF following the albumin promoter in transgenic mice results in multiple highly malignant hepatic tumors at 24–36 weeks (Tonjes et al., 1995; Borlak et al., 2005). In double transgenic mice expressing both EGF and c-myc, tumor development is accelerated to as short as 17–18 weeks (Tonjes et al., 1995).

The IGF pathway is activated by the binding of IGF-1 and IGF-2, two small proteins secreted by the liver in an autocrine and paracrine manner, to IGF receptor 1 (IGFR1). This pathway promotes invasion, anchorage-independent cell growth, and inhibition of apoptosis (Nussbaum et al., 2008). Constitutive activation of the IGF pathway is observed in 20% of HCC cases predominantly via IGF-2 overexpression or IGFR1 overexpression (Tovar et al., 2010). IGF receptor 2 (IGFR2) inhibits cell growth by facilitating inactivation of IGF-2. The fact that as many as 20% of

HCC cases demonstrate inactivating mutations and deletions of IGFR2 that are associated with loss of heterozygosity highlights the tumor-suppressing role of IGFR2 (De Souza et al., 1995; Oka et al., 2002). Clinical trials are currently underway to assess the efficacy of an anti-IGF-1R monoclonal antibody against HCC (Abou-Alfa et al., 2014).

HGF is a cytokine involved in cell proliferation, cell migration, and angiogenesis in various types of human solid cancers. HGF binds to cMET, a membrane receptor, which phosphorylates the proteins GRB2 and GAB and recruits the protein son of sevenless (SOS). SOS therefore induces the RAS/RAF/MEK/ERK pathway. Induction of the cMET pathway has been noted in 20% to 40% of HCC cases (Ueki et al., 1997; Kaposi-Novak et al., 2006), and a cMET-regulated expression signature has been was associated with poor prognosis (Kaposi-Novak et al., 2006). In a randomized phase II study, the cMET tyrosine kinase inhibitor Tivantinib (ARQ, 197; ArQule, Inc.) has been shown to improve the survival of patients with increased cMET expression (Santoro et al., 2013).

The results are being confirmed in a phase III clinical trial (Rimassa et al., 2014). A monoclonal antibody directed against HGF is currently under investigation.

Members of the platelet-derived growth factor (PDGF) family are known to play an important role in cell proliferation and angiogenesis. Liver cirrhosis induced by overexpression of PDGF-A, PDGF-B, PDGF-C, or PDGF-D is associated with HSC activation possibly as a result of the induction of genes such as TGF-β1 (Campbell et al., 2005; Czochra et al., 2006; Borkham-Kamphorst et al., 2007; Thieringer et al., 2008). Long-term overexpression of the PDGF genes induces HCC after approximately 52 weeks (Campbell et al., 2005). Patients with increased level of PDGF have poor prognosis. PDGF inhibitors have been studied for the treatment of advanced HCC.

THE MAPKINASE PATHWAY

Ras proteins (Kras, Nras, Hras, and Braf) are responsible for signal transduction downstream of growth factor receptors. After binding and activation by GTP, these proteins recruit RAF, which activates MAP kinases (MEK1/2 and ERK1/2) by phosphorylation. MAP kinase pathway activation leads to cell proliferation and inhibition of apoptosis (Whittaker et al., 2010). A small subset of HCC exhibits Kras (0%–19%) or Nras (2%) activating mutations (Tsuda et al., 1989; Challen et al., 1992; Leon and Kew, 1995). HCC associated with vinyl chloride exposure appears to be more frequently associated with Kras mutations (33%–80%) (De Vivo et al., 1994; Weihrauch et al., 2001a, b). MEK inhibitor refametinib has been evaluated in HCC carrying KRAS mutation in a phase II study (Akinleye et al., 2013; Oh et al., 2005).

Most HCC cases (85%–90%) demonstrate promoter methylation of the Ras-association domain family 1A (RASSF1A), which codes for a protein involved in cell cycle regulation (Zhang et al., 2002; Yeo et al., 2005). Inactivation of RASSF1A could enhance cell proliferation and tumorigenesis as occurs in lung cancer (Li et al., 2003), but its relevance in hepatocarcinogenesis remains largely unclear.

PI3K/AKT/mTor Signaling Pathway

Phosphoinositide 3 kinase (PI3K)/AKT/mTor are downstream of the signaling pathways activated by growth factor receptors such as IGFR and EGFR (Whittaker et al., 2010). PIK3 is activated when growth factors bind to growth factor receptors and induce the production of phosphoinositotriphosphate (PIP3B), a second messenger PIP3B activates AKT, which then phosphorylates the mTor complex. The mTor complex controls cell proliferation, apoptosis, and angiogenesis.

Classically, the phosphatase and tensin homologue (PTEN) negatively regulates the PI3K/AKT/mTor pathway (Whittaker et al., 2010). The role of loss of PTEN in hepatocarcinogenesis has been studied with a transgenic mouse model. Liver-specific PTEN-deficient mice develop hepatic steatosis, inflammation, fibrosis, and tumors that are very similar to human NASH (Watanabe et al., 2007). Activation of the AKT/mTor pathway has been reported in 30%–40% of HCC cases (Villanueva et al., 2008). The use of everolimus to inhibit mTor in HCC cell lines was found to decrease cell proliferation, and this effect was enhanced by anti-EGFR antibody therapy (Villanueva et al., 2008). AKT/mTor pathway activation was associated with HCC patients who had PIK3CA and AXIN1 mutations, chromosomal instability, and HBV infection (as determined with transcriptomic analysis results) (Boyault et al., 2007).

A global phase III study showed that Afinitor® (everolimus) did not extend overall survival compared with placebo in patients with locally advanced or metastatic HCC after progression on or intolerance to sorafenib (http://clinicaltrials.gov/ct2/show/NCT01035229?term=EVOLVE-1&rank=1). The mechanism of AKT/mTor activation in HCC has not yet been elucidated. Understanding the activating mechanism may help in understanding how inhibition of AKT/mTor may not or may be effective in treating HCC. PTEN inactivating mutations, deletions, or insertions associated with loss of heterozygosity are found in 5%–8% of HCC samples and lead to AKT/mTor pathway activation by removal of PTEN, the inhibitor of the AKT/mTor pathway (Yao et al., 1999; Wang et al., 2007). Activating mutations of PIK3CA, an oncogene that codes for PIK3, have been described for a small subset of HCC cases (5%) (Lee et al., 2005; Tanaka et al., 2006; Boyault et al., 2007) and lead to permanent activation of the AKT/mTor pathway. Although small, this group of tumors is readily targetable using mTor inhibitors such as sirolimus. However, the majority of HCC with AKT/mTor activation do not present any genetic alterations. For these cases, activation could be explained by indirect activation of the PI3K/AKT/mTor pathway by growth factor receptors.

TGF-β Signaling

TGF-β is an important modulator of a broad spectrum of cellular processes, including cell growth, cell differentiation, wound repair, and apoptosis (Mishra et al., 2005; Massague, 2008). Functional genetics studies have demonstrate that the TGF-β signaling pathway suppresses the development of HCC as well as the promotion of liver fibrosis that precedes HCC formation, progression, and metastasis.

TGF-β binding activates type II and then type I receptors (TGFR-2 and TGFR-1, respectively) that in turn activate the eight SMAD homologues (Kimchi et al., 1988;

Chen et al., 1993; Feng and Derynck, 1997). Tissue-specific modulation of SMAD homologue function occurs through adaptors (including β-II spectrin [Sptbn1], filamin, or the zinc finger FYVE domain-containing protein 9 [ZFYVE9]), and E3 ligases (such as Smurfs, Nedd1, and Praja1) as well as by functional interactions within multiple signal transduction pathways (Heldin et al., 1997; Sporn, 1999; Wu et al., 2000; Derynck and Zhang, 2003; Mishra and Marshall, 2006). Adaptor proteins, such as β-II spectrin (Sptbn1) and ZFYVE9, have critical roles in mediating access to the receptors and SMAD homologue activation at the cell membrane, which controls the complex functions of TGF-β (Wu et al., 2000; Mishra and Marshall, 2006). The finding that 40% of Sptbn1$^{+/-}$ mice develop HCC supports the role of TGF-β signaling in the suppression of HCC development and serves as an excellent model in the studying the tumor suppressor function of TGF-β signaling (Tang et al., 2008). Activation of TGF-β/SMAD proteins results in transcriptional regulation and arrest of the cell cycle at G1/S phase through suppression of *MYC*, cyclin-dependent kinases, and induction *of CDKN1A* (also known as *p21*), *CDKN2B* (also known as *p15*), and *Serpine-1* (also known as *PAI-1*) (Kimchi et al., 1988; Chen et al., 1993; Feng and Derynck, 1997; Derynck and Zhang, 2003; Shi and Massague, 2003). TGF-β is an extracellular sensor of damage caused by injury from ultraviolet light and ionizing radiation (Barcellos-Hoff and Brooks, 2001; Barcellos-Hoff, 2005) and a potential guardian of genomic stability through modulation of the *Fanc* pathway at interstrand crosslinks (McMahon et al., 1999; Kumaresan et al., 2007; Bornstein et al., 2009). Extensive oxidative DNA damage in liver due to viral hepatitis, or NASH results in hepatocyte cell death, inflammation, and proliferation preceding HCC formation. TGF-β induces transcription factor nuclear respiratory factor 2–mediated synthesis of the gene encoding the antioxidant genes HO-1 and protect liver from oxidative damage (Churchman et al., 2009).

Meanwhile, TGF-β1 is also known to be important in the pathogenesis of fibrosis (Williams and Knapton, 1996). TGF-β1 enhances the production of several matrix components and decreases their degradation, thereby causing an accumulation of extracellular matrix, which is the basic underlying cause of fibrosis (Lechuga et al., 2004; Qi et al., 2006). In transgenic mice overexpressing TGF-β1, the most extensive liver fibrosis appears after approximately 10 weeks; nevertheless, fully developed cirrhosis is not seen, probably because of the high mortality rate in the transgenic strains (Sanderson et al., 1995). Repeated administration of anti-tuberculosis therapy (AAT) can induce cirrhosis after 18 weeks, which would lead to HCC if the experiment were to be continued for a prolonged period (Schnur et al., 2004). In addition, TGF-β promotes cancer progression and metastasis by inducing endothelial-to-mesenchymal transition (EMT). The level of TGF-β predicts the prognosis for patients with HCC.

Recent studies have shown that inhibition of TGF-β signaling results in multiple synergistic downstream effects, which will likely improve the clinical outcome in HCC (Giannelli et al., 2011). The TGF-β receptor inhibitor LY2157299 is currently being tested in patients with advanced HCC (http://www.clinicaltrials.gov/). In light of the complex role of TGF-β signaling in hepatocarcinogenesis, teasing out how complex pathways interplay with TGF-β signaling will be pivotal in designing therapeutic strategies targeting the TGF-β pathway to prevent and treat HCC.

Development of HCC in the Setting of NASH

High global prevalence rates of obesity and diabetes indicate that NASH will becomes an even more important risk factors for HCC as the prevalence of hepatitis B, hepatitis C, and alcoholic liver disease declines. The successful prevention and treatment of HCC due to NASH damage to the liver demands a better understanding of the mechanism by which HCC develop from NASH induced cirrhosis. The majority of basic and clinical evidence regarding the pathogenesis of HCC arises in the setting of chronic viral hepatitis. The exact mechanism behind the development of HCC in NASH remains unclear, although the pathophysiological mechanisms behind the development of NASH related to insulin resistance and the subsequent inflammatory cascade most likely contribute to the carcinogenic potential of NASH.

Insulin resistance associated with obesity, metabolic syndrome, and diabetes leads to increased release of free fatty acids from adipocytes, release of multiple proinflammatory cytokines including tumor necrosis factor α (TNF-α), IL-6, leptin, and resistin, and decreased amounts of adiponectin. These processes favor the development of hepatic steatosis and inflammation within the liver (Charlton et al., 2006; Milner et al., 2009). Adiponectin is an anti-inflammatory polypeptide specific to adipose tissue that is decreased in insulin-resistant states and has been shown to inhibit angiogenesis via modulation of apoptosis in the T241 fibrosarcoma—a syngeneic tumor in C57 BL/6J mice (Ukkola and Santaniemi, 2002; Brakenhielm et al., 2004). Hyperinsulinemia upregulates the production of IGF-1, which stimulates cellular proliferation and inhibition of apoptosis within the liver (Ish-Shalom et al., 1997; Calle and Kaaks, 2004; Page and Harrison, 2009). Insulin also activates insulin receptor substrate 1 (IRS-1), which is involved in cytokine signaling pathways and has been shown to be upregulated in HCC (Tanaka et al., 1997). Changes in cytokine, chemokine, and growth factor signaling related to an insulin-resistant state promote uninhibited cell growth and appear to play a significant role in the development of HCC in the setting of NASH.

The development of NASH is also associated with oxidative stress and the release of reactive oxygen species (ROS), which likely contributes to the development of HCC. An insulin-resistant obese mouse model was used to demonstrate that ROS production is increased in the mitochondria of hepatocytes with fatty infiltration, and that oxidative stress implicated in hepatic hyperplasia, which usually precedes cancer by many years (Yang et al., 2000; Milner et al., 2009). Furthermore, cancer-promoting mutations can be induced under oxidative stress trans-4-hydroxy-2-nonenal, a product of lipid peroxidation, has been shown to cause mutations of the tumor suppressor gene p53, which is associated with more than half of human cancers including HCC (Hu et al., 2002). Nuclear respiratory factor 1 (Nrf1) is a transcription factor essential in mediating oxidative stress. Hepatocytes lacking this transcription factor were shown to have increased susceptibility to oxidative stress in transgenic mouse model, which exhibited steatosis, apoptosis, necrosis, inflammation, and fibrosis, at finally the development of HCC (Xu et al., 2005).

Hepatocarcinogenesis in NASH may also be partially mediated by increased release of inflammatory and inhibitory cytokines such as TNF-α, IL-6, and nuclear factor (NF) κB (Ogata et al., 2006; Sakurai et al., 2006; Luedde et al., 2007).

Evidence suggests a complex interplay of the inflammatory cytokines and chemo-kines produced by hepatocytes and immune cells leads to hepatocyte death, com-pensatory proliferation, and ultimately carcinogenesis (Sakurai et al., 2006). NF-κB regulates immune and inflammatory responses and is activated in many tumors, inhibiting apoptosis (Luedde et al., 2007). Inhibition of this factor in mouse livers induced steatohepatitis and ultimately HCC by sensitizing the hepatocytes to spon-taneous apoptosis. This chronic cycle of injury, cell death, and regeneration through compensatory cellular proliferation likely contributes to the development of HCC (Luedde et al., 2007).

The c-Jun amino-terminal kinase 1 (JNK1) has also recently been linked to obe-sity, insulin resistance, NASH, and HCC development. Obesity is associated with abnormally elevated JNK activity (Hirosumi et al., 2002). Free fatty acids, TNF-α, and ROS released in the setting of hyperinsulinemia are all potent activators of JNK, which in turn phosphorylates IRS-1 leading to obesity-induced insulin resistance (Hirosumi et al., 2002). JNK activation is also known to increase hepatic inflamma-tion and apoptosis (Puri et al., 2008). JNK activation is specifically associated with the severity of NASH; a lower level of JNK activation is observed in NAFLD. Mouse models have also demonstrated that JNK1 promotes the development of steatohepa-titis (Schattenberg et al., 2006). Meanwhile, the absence of JNK1 prevented weight gain and the development of insulin resistance, protected against the development of hepatic steatosis, and reduced hepatic injury in mice compared with wild-type mice in response to a high-fat diet (Singh et al., 2009). JNK1 is overactivated in more than 50% of human HCC samples (Hui et al., 2008; Chang et al., 2009a, b; Chen et al., 2009; Chen and Castranova, 2009). The incidence of diethylnitrosamine/phenobar-bital-induced HCC was significantly reduced in $Jnk1^{-/-}$ (Hui et al., 2008). JNK1 as a therapeutic target for HCC warrant further investigation.

Accumulating evidence indicates that deregulation of the phosphatidylinositol 3 kinase (PI3K)/AKT pathway in hepatocytes is a common molecular event associated with metabolic dysfunctions including obesity, metabolic syndrome, and NAFLD. The liver of 40-week-old PTEN-deficient mice revealed macrovesicular steatosis, ballooning hepatocytes, lobular inflammatory cell infiltration, and perisinusoidal fibrosis that are characteristic of human NASH. By 80 weeks of age, 100% of PTEN-deficient livers from these mice had developed adenomas and 66% HCC (Watanabe et al., 2005). A tumor suppressor PTEN negatively regulates the PI3K/AKT path-ways through lipid phosphatase activity. PI3K/AKT may serve as a promising thera-peutic target for NASH and HCC.

Targeted Therapy for HCC

The development and approval of targeted therapy by the U.S. Food and Drug Administration in the treatment of cancer over the past 10 years highlights the con-siderable importance of understanding genetic and epigenetic alterations to adapt treatment to these diseases. Validation of sorafenib, a multikinase inhibitor targeting RAS, vascular endothelial growth factor receptor (VEGFR), and PDGF receptor, as the first systemic treatment for advanced-stage HCC has opened the way to other tar-geted therapies (Llovet et al., 2008; Cheng et al., 2009). Many targeted therapies are now being tested in phase II and III clinical trials; anti-VEGFR monoclonal antibody (bevacizumab), anti-EGFR monoclonal antibody (cetuximab), small molecule tyrosine kinase inhibitors (sunitib, gefitinib, brivanib, erlotinib), mTOR inhibitors (everolimus, sirolimus), or c-met inhibitor. Certainly, in the next few years, molecular character-ization of the tumor will directly impact the treatment of HCC. Molecular markers are able to predict treatment response or toxicity. As examples, HCCs that express high levels of c-met responds to the treatment with the c-met tyrosine kinase inhibi-tor tivantinib (ARQ, 197; ArQule, Inc.), and non–small-cell lung cancers with EGFR activating mutations show a good response to gefitinib or erlotinib, which are small molecule tyrosine kinase inhibitors that inhibit EGFR. However, only one targeted therapy, sorafenib is currently available for HCC and no molecular assays tests are used in clinical practice. With the rapid development of new biotherapies and the grow-ing numbers of clinical trials in HCC, the molecular features of these tumors will soon be used to determine appropriate treatment. The value and frequency of tumor biopsy to provide access to molecular features will need to be reevaluated in this setting.

CONCLUSION

This risk factors for HCC, the most common and deadly cancers worldwide, is slowly changing. With the increased prevalence of obesity and metabolic syndrome, fatty liver and NASH are emerging as an important risk factor for HCC. Understanding the molecular hepatocarcinogenesis is essential to the development of prevention and treatment strategies against HCC.

REFERENCES

Abou-Alfa, G. K., M. Capanu et al. (2014). A phase II study of cixutumumab (IMC-A12, NSC742460) in advanced hepatocellular carcinoma. *J Hepatol* 60: 319–324. doi: 10.1016/j.jhep.2013.09.008.

Adams, L. A., J. F. Lymp et al. (2005). The natural history of nonalcoholic fatty liver disease: A population-based cohort study. *Gastroenterology* 129: 113–121.

Akinleye, A., M. Furqan et al. (2013). MEK and the inhibitors: From bench to bedside. *J Hemol Oncol* 6: 1–11.

Altekruse, S. F., K. A. McGlynn et al. (2009). Hepatocellular carcinoma incidence, mortality, and survival trends in the United States from 1975 to 2005. *J Clin Oncol* 27: 1485–1491.

Audard, V., G. Grimber et al. (2007). Cholestasis is a marker for hepatocellular carcinomas displaying beta-catenin mutations. *J Pathol* 212: 345–352.

Barcellos-Hoff, M. H. (2005). Integrative radiation carcinogenesis: Interactions between cell and tissue responses to DNA damage. *Semin Cancer Biol* 15: 138–148.

Barcellos-Hoff, M. H. and A. L. Brooks (2001). Extracellular signaling through the microenvi-ronment: A hypothesis relating carcinogenesis, bystander effects, and genomic instabil-ity. *Radiat Res* 156: 618–627.

Bedogni, G., L. Miglioli et al. (2005). Prevalence of and risk factors for nonalcoholic fatty liver disease: The Dionysos nutrition and liver study. *Hepatology* 42: 44–52.

Bekaii-Saab, T., N. Williams et al. (2006). A novel mutation in the tyrosine kinase domain of ERBB2 in hepatocellular carcinoma. *BMC Cancer* 6: 278.

Benhamouche, S., T. Decaens et al. (2006). [Wnt/beta-catenin pathway and liver metabolic zonation: A new player for an old concept]. *Med Sci (Paris)* 22: 904–906.

Biden, K., J. Young et al. (1997). Frequency of mutation and deletion of the tumor suppressor gene CDKN2A (MTS1/p16) in hepatocellular carcinoma from an Australian population. *Hepatology* 25: 593–597.

Bordeaux, B., Bolen, S., and Brotman, D. J. (2006). Beyond cardiovascular risk: The impact of obesity on cancer death. *Cleveland Clin J Med* 73: 945–950.

Borkham-Kamphorst, E., C. R. van Roeyen et al. (2007). Pro-fibrogenic potential of PDGF-D in liver fibrosis. *J Hepatol* 46: 1064–1074.

Borlak, J., T. Meier et al. (2005). Epidermal growth factor-induced hepatocellular carcinoma: Gene expression profiles in precursor lesions, early stage and solitary tumours. *Oncogene* 24: 1809–1819.

Bornstein, S., R. White et al. (2009). Smad4 loss in mice causes spontaneous head and neck cancer with increased genomic instability and inflammation. *J Clin Invest* 119: 3408–3419.

Bosch, F. X., J. Ribes et al. (2004). Primary liver cancer: Worldwide incidence and trends. *Gastroenterology* 127: S5–S16.

Bostan, N. and T. Mahmood (2010). An overview about hepatitis C: A devastating virus. *Crit Rev Microbiol* 36: 91–133.

Boyault, S., D. S. Rickman et al. (2007). Transcriptome classification of HCC is related to gene alterations and to new therapeutic targets. *Hepatology* 45: 42–52.

Brakenhielm, E., N. Veitonmaki et al. (2004). Adiponectin-induced antiangiogenesis and anti-tumor activity involve caspase-mediated endothelial cell apoptosis. *Proc Natl Acad Sci USA* 101: 2476–2481.

Bressac, B., M. Kew et al. (1991). Selective G to T mutations of p53 gene in hepatocellular carcinoma from southern Africa. *Nature* 350: 429–431.

Bromberg, J. F., M. H. Wrzeszczynska et al. (1999). Stat3 as an oncogene. *Cell* 98: 295–303.

Bugianesi, E. (2007). Non-alcoholic steatohepatitis and cancer. *Clin Liver Dis* 11: 191–207, x–xi.

Bugianesi, E., N. Leone et al. (2002). Expanding the natural history of nonalcoholic steatohepatitis: From cryptogenic cirrhosis to hepatocellular carcinoma. *Gastroenterology* 123: 134–140.

Cadoret, A., C. Ovejero et al. (2002). New targets of beta-catenin signaling in the liver are involved in the glutamine metabolism. *Oncogene* 21: 8293–8301.

Caldwell, S. H., D. H. Oelsner et al. (1999). Cryptogenic cirrhosis: Clinical characterization and risk factors for underlying disease. *Hepatology* 29: 664–669.

Calle, E. E. and R. Kaaks (2004). Overweight, obesity and cancer: Epidemiological evidence and proposed mechanisms. *Nat Rev Cancer* 4: 579–591.

Calvisi, D. F., S. Ladu et al. (2006). Ubiquitous activation of Ras and Jak/Stat pathways in human HCC. *Gastroenterology* 130: 1117–1128.

Campbell, J. S., S. D. Hughes et al. (2005). Platelet-derived growth factor C induces liver fibrosis, steatosis, and hepatocellular carcinoma. *Proc Natl Acad Sci USA* 102: 3389–3394.

Challen, C., K. Guo et al. (1992). Infrequent point mutations in codons 12 and 61 of ras oncogenes in human hepatocellular carcinomas. *J Hepatol* 14: 342–346.

Chang, M. H., S. L. You et al. (2009a). Decreased incidence of hepatocellular carcinoma in hepatitis B vaccinees: A 20-year follow-up study. *J Natl Cancer Inst* 101: 1348–1355.

Chang, Q., Y. Zhang et al. (2009b). Sustained JNK1 activation is associated with altered histone H3 methylations in human liver cancer. *J Hepatol* 50: 323–333.

Charlton, M. R., P. J. Pockros et al. (2006). Impact of obesity on treatment of chronic hepatitis C. *Hepatology* 43: 1177–1186.

Chen, F., K. Beezhold et al. (2009). JNK1, a potential therapeutic target for hepatocellular carcinoma. *Biochim Biophys Acta* 1796: 242–251.

Chen, F. and V. Castranova (2009). Beyond apoptosis of JNK1 in liver cancer. *Cell Cycle* 8: 1145–1147.

Chen, R. H., R. Ebner et al. (1993). Inactivation of the type II receptor reveals two receptor pathways for the diverse TGF-beta activities. *Science* 260: 1335–1338.

Cheng, A. L., Y. K. Kang et al. (2009). Efficacy and safety of sorafenib in patients in the Asia-Pacific region with advanced hepatocellular carcinoma: A phase III randomised, double-blind, placebo-controlled trial. *Lancet Oncol* 10: 25–34.

Chitturi, S., S. Abeygunasekera et al. (2002). NASH and insulin resistance: Insulin hypersecretion and specific association with the insulin resistance syndrome. *Hepatology* 35: 373–379.

Chung, H., T. Ueda, M. Kudo. (2010). Changing trends in hepatitis C infection over the past 50 years in Japan. *Intervirology* 53: 39–43. doi:10.1159/000252782.

Churchman, A. T., A. A. Anwar et al. (2009). Transforming growth factor-beta1 elicits Nrf2-mediated antioxidant responses in aortic smooth muscle cells. *J Cell Mol Med* 13: 2282–2292.

Cieply, B., G. Zeng et al. (2009). Unique phenotype of hepatocellular cancers with exon-3 mutations in beta-catenin gene. *Hepatology* 49: 821–831.

Collier, J. D., K. Guo et al. (1992). c-erbB-2 oncogene expression in hepatocellular carcinoma and cholangiocarcinoma. *J Hepatol* 14: 377–380.

Colvin, H. M. and A. E. Mitchell (Eds.) (2010). Hepatitis and liver cancer: A national strategy for prevention and control of hepatitis B and C. Committee on the Prevention and Control of Viral Hepatitis Infections; Institute of Medicine, 252 pp.

Cortez-Pinto, H., M. E. Camilo et al. (1999). Non-alcoholic fatty liver: Another feature of the metabolic syndrome? *Clin Nutr* 18: 353–358.

Czochra, P., B. Klopcic et al. (2006). Liver fibrosis induced by hepatic overexpression of PDGF-B in transgenic mice. *J Hepatol* 45: 419–428.

Daniel, S., T. Ben-Menachem et al. (1999). Prospective evaluation of unexplained chronic liver transaminase abnormalities in asymptomatic and symptomatic patients. *Am J Gastroenterol* 94: 3010–3014.

Davila, J. A., R. O. Morgan et al. (2005). Diabetes increases the risk of hepatocellular carcinoma in the United States: A population based case control study. *Gut* 54: 533–539.

de la Coste, A., B. Romagnolo et al. (1998). Somatic mutations of the beta-catenin gene are frequent in mouse and human hepatocellular carcinomas. *Proc Natl Acad Sci USA* 95: 8847–8851.

De Souza, A. T., G. R. Hankins et al. (1995). M6P/IGF2R gene is mutated in human hepatocellular carcinomas with loss of heterozygosity. *Nat Genet* 11: 447–449.

De Vivo, I., M. J. Marion et al. (1994). Mutant c-Ki-ras p21 protein in chemical carcinogenesis in humans exposed to vinyl chloride. *Cancer Causes Control* 5: 273–278.

Derynck, R. and Y. E. Zhang (2003). Smad-dependent and Smad-independent pathways in TGF-beta family signalling. *Nature* 425: 577–584.

Donato, F., A. Tagger et al. (2002). Alcohol and hepatocellular carcinoma: The effect of lifetime intake and hepatitis virus infections in men and women. *Am J Epidemiol* 155: 323–331.

Edamoto, Y., A. Hara et al. (2003). Alterations of RB1, p53 and Wnt pathways in hepatocellular carcinomas associated with hepatitis C, hepatitis B and alcoholic liver cirrhosis. *Int J Cancer* 106: 334–341.

Ekstedt, M., L. E. Franzen et al. (2006). Long-term follow-up of patients with NAFLD and elevated liver enzymes. *Hepatology* 44: 865–873.

El-Serag, H. B. and A. C. Mason (1999). Rising incidence of hepatocellular carcinoma in the United States. *N Engl J Med* 340: 745–750.

El-Serag, H. B. and K. L. Rudolph (2007). Hepatocellular carcinoma: Epidemiology and molecular carcinogenesis. *Gastroenterology* 132: 2557–2576.

El-Serag, H., M. Johnson et al. (2009). Statins are associated with a reduced risk of hepatocellular carcinoma in a large cohort of patients with diabetes. *Gastroenterology* 136: 1601–1608.

Feng, X. H. and R. Derynck (1997). A kinase subdomain of transforming growth factor-beta (TGF-beta) type I receptor determines the TGF-beta intracellular signaling specificity. *EMBO J* 16: 3912–3923.

Giannelli, G., A. Mazzocca et al. (2011). Inhibiting TGF-b signaling in hepatcellular carcinoma. *Biochimica et Biophysica Acta (BBA)- Reviews on Cancer* 1815: 214–223.

Gomaa, A. I., S. A. Khan et al. (2008). Hepatocellular carcinoma: Epidemiology, risk factors and pathogenesis. *World J Gastroenterol* 14: 4300–4308.

Grivennikov, S., E. Karin et al. (2009). IL-6 and Stat3 are required for survival of intestinal epithelial cells and development of colitis-associated cancer. *Cancer Cell* 15: 103–113.

Grivennikov, S. and M. Karin (2008). Autocrine IL-6 signaling: A key event in tumorigenesis? *Cancer Cell* 13: 7–9.

Grivennikov, S. I., F. R. Greten et al. (2010). Immunity, inflammation, and cancer. *Cell* 140: 883–899.

Ground, K. E. (1982). Liver pathology in aircrew. *Aviat Space Environ Med* 53: 14–18.

Guzman, G., E. M. Brunt et al. (2008). Does nonalcoholic fatty liver disease predispose patients to hepatocellular carcinoma in the absence of cirrhosis? *Arch Pathol Lab Med* 132: 1761–1766.

Harada, N., H. Miyoshi et al. (2002). Lack of tumorigenesis in the mouse liver after adenovirus-mediated expression of a dominant stable mutant of beta-catenin. *Cancer Res* 62: 1971–1977.

Harada, N., H. Oshima et al. (2004). Hepatocarcinogenesis in mice with beta-catenin and Ha-ras gene mutations. *Cancer Res* 64: 48–54.

Heldin, C. H., K. Miyazono et al. (1997). TGF-beta signalling from cell membrane to nucleus through SMAD proteins. *Nature* 390: 465–471.

Hilden, M., P. Christoffersen et al. (1977). Liver histology in a 'normal' population—examinations of 503 consecutive fatal traffic casualties. *Scand J Gastroenterol* 12: 593–597.

Hirosumi, J., G. Tuncman et al. (2002). A central role for JNK in obesity and insulin resistance. *Nature* 420: 333–336.

Hsu, H. C., Y. M. Jeng et al. (2000). Beta-catenin mutations are associated with a subset of low-stage hepatocellular carcinoma negative for hepatitis B virus and with favorable prognosis. *Am J Pathol* 157: 763–770.

Hsu, I. C., R. A. Metcalf et al. (1991). Mutational hotspot in the p53 gene in human hepatocellular carcinomas. *Nature* 350: 427–428.

Hu, W., Z. Feng et al. (2002). The major lipid peroxidation product, *trans*-4-hydroxy-2-nonenal, preferentially forms DNA adducts at codon 249 of human p53 gene, a unique mutational hotspot in hepatocellular carcinoma. *Carcinogenesis* 23: 1781–1789.

Huang, Y. T., C. L. Jen et al. (2011). Lifetime risk and sex difference of hepatocellular carcinoma among patients with chronic hepatitis B and C. *J Clin Oncol* 29: 3643–3650.

Hui, L., K. Zatloukal et al. (2008). Proliferation of human HCC cells and chemically induced mouse liver cancers requires JNK1-dependent p21 downregulation. *J Clin Invest* 118: 3943–3953.

IARC, Ed. (1988). *Alcohol drinking*. IARC Working Group, Lyon, October 13–20, 1987. *IARC Monogr Eval Carcinog Risks Hum* 44: 1–378.

IARC, Ed. (2002). *Working Group on the Evaluation of Carcinogenic Risks to Humans, International Agency for Research on Cancer. Some traditional herbal medicines, some mycotoxins, naphthalene and styrene*. Lyon (France), IRACPress.

Iida, F., R. Iida et al. (1999). Chronic Japanese schistosomiasis and hepatocellular carcinoma: Ten years of follow-up in Yamanashi Prefecture, Japan. *Bull World Health Organ* 77: 573–581.

Imbeaud, S., Y. Ladeiro et al. (2010). Identification of novel oncogenes and tumor suppressors in hepatocellular carcinoma. *Semin Liver Dis* 30: 75–86.

Ish-Shalom, D., C. T. Christoffersen et al. (1997). Mitogenic properties of insulin and insulin analogues mediated by the insulin receptor. *Diabetologia* 40: S25–S31.

Ishizaki, Y., S. Ikeda et al. (2004). Immunohistochemical analysis and mutational analyses of beta-catenin, Axin family and APC genes in hepatocellular carcinomas. *Int J Oncol* 24: 1077–1083.

Jhappan, C., C. Stahle et al. (1990). TGF alpha overexpression in transgenic mice induces liver neoplasia and abnormal development of the mammary gland and pancreas. *Cell* 61: 1137–1146.

Kaposi-Novak, P., J. S. Lee et al. (2006). Met-regulated expression signature defines a subset of human hepatocellular carcinomas with poor prognosis and aggressive phenotype. *J Clin Invest* 116: 1582–1595.

Karachristos, A., T. Liloglou et al. (1999). Microsatellite instability and p53 mutations in hepatocellular carcinoma. *Mol Cell Biol Res Commun* 2: 155–161.

Kimchi, A., X. F. Wang et al. (1988). Absence of TGF-beta receptors and growth inhibitory responses in retinoblastoma cells. *Science* 240: 196–199.

Kitagawa, T., O. Hino et al. (1991). Multistep hepatocarcinogenesis in transgenic mice harboring SV40 T-antigen gene. *Princess Takamatsu Symp* 22: 349–360.

Kowdley K. V. (2004). Iron, hemochromatosis, and hepatocellular carcinoma. *Gastroenterology*. Nov; 127: S79–S86.

Kumaresan, K. R., D. M. Sridharan et al. (2007). Deficiency in incisions produced by XPF at the site of a DNA interstrand cross-link in Fanconi anemia cells. *Biochemistry* 46: 14359–14368.

Kuper, H., A. Tzonou et al. (2000). Tobacco smoking, alcohol consumption and their interaction in the causation of hepatocellular carcinoma. *Int J Cancer* 85: 498–502.

Lai, S. W., C. K. Tan et al. (2002). Epidemiology of fatty liver in a hospital-based study in Taiwan. *South Med J* 95: 1288–1292.

Laurent-Puig, P., P. Legoix et al. (2001). Genetic alterations associated with hepatocellular carcinomas define distinct pathways of hepatocarcinogenesis. *Gastroenterology* 120: 1763–1773.

Laurent-Puig, P. and J. Zucman-Rossi (2006). Genetics of hepatocellular tumors. *Oncogene* 25: 3778–3786.

Lawson, D. H., J. M. Gray et al. (1986). Diabetes mellitus and primary hepatocellular carcinoma. *Q J Med* 61: 945–955.

Lechuga, C. G., Z. H. Hernandez-Nazara et al. (2004). TGF-beta1 modulates matrix metalloproteinase-13 expression in hepatic stellate cells by complex mechanisms involving p38MAPK, PI3-kinase, AKT, and p70S6k. *Am J Physiol Gastrointest Liver Physiol* 287: G974–G987.

Lee, J. S., I. S. Chu et al. (2004). Application of comparative functional genomics to identify best-fit mouse models to study human cancer. *Nat Genet* 36: 1306–1311.

Lee, J. W., Y. H. Soung et al. (2005). PIK3CA gene is frequently mutated in breast carcinomas and hepatocellular carcinomas. *Oncogene* 24: 1477–1480.

Legoix, P., O. Bluteau et al. (1999). Beta-catenin mutations in hepatocellular carcinoma correlate with a low rate of loss of heterozygosity. *Oncogene* 18: 4044–4046.

Leon, M. and M. C. Kew (1995). Analysis of ras gene mutations in hepatocellular carcinoma in southern African blacks. *Anticancer Res* 15: 859–861.

Li, J., Z. Zhang et al. (2003). *RASSF1A* promoter methylation and *Kras2* mutations in non small cell lung cancer. *Neoplasia* July; 5: 362–366.

Liew, C. T., H. M. Li et al. (1999). High frequency of p16INK4A gene alterations in hepatocellular carcinoma. *Oncogene* 18: 789–795.

Llovet, J. M., S. Ricci et al. (2008). Sorafenib in advanced hepatocellular carcinoma. *N Engl J Med* 359: 378–390.

Ludwig, J., T. R. Viggiano et al. (1980). Nonalcoholic steatohepatitis: Mayo Clinic experiences with a hitherto unnamed disease. *Mayo Clin Proc* 55: 434–438.

Luedde, T., N. Beraza et al. (2007). Deletion of NEMO/IKKgamma in liver parenchymal cells causes steatohepatitis and hepatocellular carcinoma. *Cancer Cell* 11: 119–132.

Mao, T. L., J. S. Chu et al. (2001). Expression of mutant nuclear beta-catenin correlates with non-invasive hepatocellular carcinoma, absence of portal vein spread, and good prognosis. *J Pathol* 193: 95–101.

Marchesini, G., E. Bugianesi et al. (2003). Nonalcoholic fatty liver, steatohepatitis, and the metabolic syndrome. *Hepatology* 37: 917–923.

Massague, J. (2008). TGFbeta in Cancer. *Cell* 134: 215–230.

Matsuda, Y., T. Ichida et al. (1999). p16(INK4) is inactivated by extensive CpG methylation in human hepatocellular carcinoma. *Gastroenterology* 116: 394–400.

Mccullough, A. J., Ed. (2007). *The Epidemiology and Risk Factors of NASH, in Fatty Liver Disease: NASH and Related Disorders.ch3.* UK, Blackwell Publishing Ltd.

McKillop, I. H. and L. W. Schrum (2009). Role of alcohol in liver carcinogenesis. *Semin Liver Dis* 29: 222–232.

McMahon, L. W., C. E. Walsh et al. (1999). Human alpha spectrin II and the Fanconi anemia proteins FANCA and FANCC interact to form a nuclear complex. *J Biol Chem* 274: 32904–32908.

Micsenyi, A., X. Tan et al. (2004). Beta-catenin is temporally regulated during normal liver development. *Gastroenterology* 126: 1134–1146.

Milner, K. L., D. van der Poorten et al. (2009). Adipocyte fatty acid binding protein levels relate to inflammation and fibrosis in nonalcoholic fatty liver disease. *Hepatology* 49: 1926–1934.

Mishra, L., R. Derynck et al. (2005). Transforming growth factor-beta signaling in stem cells and cancer. *Science* 310: 68–71.

Mishra, L. and B. Marshall (2006). Adaptor proteins and ubiquinators in TGF-beta signaling. *Cytokine Growth Factor Rev* 17: 75–87.

Miyoshi, Y., K. Iwao et al. (1998). Activation of the beta-catenin gene in primary hepatocellular carcinomas by somatic alterations involving exon 3. *Cancer Res* 58: 2524–2527.

Monga, S. P., H. K. Monga et al. (2003). Beta-catenin antisense studies in embryonic liver cultures: Role in proliferation, apoptosis, and lineage specification. *Gastroenterology* 124: 202–216.

Monga, S. P., P. Pediaditakis et al. (2001). Changes in WNT/beta-catenin pathway during regulated growth in rat liver regeneration. *Hepatology* 33: 1098–1109.

Murakami, H., N. D. Sanderson et al. (1993). Transgenic mouse model for synergistic effects of nuclear oncogenes and growth factors in tumorigenesis: Interaction of c-myc and transforming growth factor alpha in hepatic oncogenesis. *Cancer Res* 53: 1719–1723.

Naugler, W. E., T. Sakurai et al. (2007). Gender disparity in liver cancer due to sex differences in MyD88-dependent IL-6 production. *Science* 317: 121–124.

Nault, J. C. and J. Zucman-Rossi (2010). Building a bridge between obesity, inflammation and liver carcinogenesis. *J Hepatol* 53: 777–779.

Niwa, Y., H. Kanda et al. (2005). Methylation silencing of SOCS-3 promotes cell growth and migration by enhancing JAK/STAT and FAK signalings in human hepatocellular carcinoma. *Oncogene* 24: 6406–6417.

Nomura, H., S. Kashiwagi et al. (1988). Prevalence of fatty liver in a general population of Okinawa, Japan. *Jpn J Med* 27: 142–149.

Nonomura, A., Y. Mizukami et al. (1992). Clinicopathologic study of alcohol-like liver disease in non-alcoholics; non-alcoholic steatohepatitis and fibrosis. *Gastroenterol Jpn* 27: 521–528.

Nussbaum, T., J. Samarin et al. (2008). Autocrine insulin-like growth factor-II stimulation of tumor cell migration is a progression step in human hepatocarcinogenesis. *Hepatology* 48: 146–156.

Ogata, H., T. Kobayashi et al. (2006). Deletion of the SOCS3 gene in liver parenchymal cells promotes hepatitis-induced hepatocarcinogenesis. *Gastroenterology* 131: 179–193.

Oh, S. W., Y. S. Yoon, and S.-A. Shin (2005). Effects of excess weight on cancer incidences depending on cancer sites and histologic findings among men: Korea National Health Insurance Corporation Study. *J Clinical Oncol* 23: 4742–4754.

Ohgaki, H., N. D. Sanderson et al. (1996). Molecular analyses of liver tumors in c-myc transgenic mice and c-myc and TGF-alpha double transgenic mice. *Cancer Lett* 106: 43–49.

Oka, Y., R. A. Waterland et al. (2002). M6P/IGF2R tumor suppressor gene mutated in hepatocellular carcinomas in Japan. *Hepatology* 35: 1153–1163.

Okochi, O., K. Hibi et al. (2003). Methylation-mediated silencing of SOCS-1 gene in hepatocellular carcinoma derived from cirrhosis. *Clin Cancer Res* 9: 5295–5298.

Omagari, K., Y. Kadokawa et al. (2002). Fatty liver in non-alcoholic non-overweight Japanese adults: Incidence and clinical characteristics. *J Gastroenterol Hepatol* 17: 1098–1105.

Ong, J. P., A. Pitts et al. (2008). Increased overall mortality and liver-related mortality in non-alcoholic fatty liver disease. *J Hepatol* 49: 608–612.

Ong, J. P. and Z. M. Younossi (2003). Nonalcoholic fatty liver disease (NAFLD)—two decades later: Are we smarter about its natural history? *Am J Gastroenterol* 98: 1915–1917.

Ong, J. P. and Z. M. Younossi (2007). Epidemiology and natural history of NAFLD and NASH. *Clin Liver Dis* 11: 1–16, vii.

Ozturk, M. (1991). p53 mutation in hepatocellular carcinoma after aflatoxin exposure. *Lancet* 338: 1356–1359.

Pagano, G., G. Pacini et al. (2002). Nonalcoholic steatohepatitis, insulin resistance, and metabolic syndrome: Further evidence for an etiologic association. *Hepatology* 35: 367–372.

Page, J. M. and S. A. Harrison (2009). NASH and HCC. *Clin Liver Dis* 13: 631–647.

Parkin, D. M. (2001). Global cancer statistics in the year 2000. *Lancet Oncol* 2: 533–543.

Pilati, C., M. Amessou et al. (2011). Somatic mutations activating STAT3 in human inflammatory hepatocellular adenomas. *J Exp Med* 208: 1359–1366.

Plymoth, A., S. Viviani et al. (2009). Control of hepatocellular carcinoma through hepatitis B vaccination in areas of high endemicity: Perspectives for global liver cancer prevention. *Cancer Lett* 286: 15–21.

Poonawala, A., S. P. Nair et al. (2000). Prevalence of obesity and diabetes in patients with cryptogenic cirrhosis: A case–control study. *Hepatology* 32: 689–692.

Powell, E. E., W. G. Cooksley et al. (1990). The natural history of nonalcoholic steatohepatitis: A follow-up study of forty-two patients for up to 21 years. *Hepatology* 11: 74–80.

Puisieux, A., F. Ponchel et al. (1993). p53 as a growth suppressor gene in HBV-related hepatocellular carcinoma cells. *Oncogene* 8: 487–490.

Puri, P., F. Mirshahi et al. (2008). Activation and dysregulation of the unfolded protein response in nonalcoholic fatty liver disease. *Gastroenterology* 134: 568–576.

Qi, W., X. Chen et al. (2006). Tranilast attenuates connective tissue growth factor-induced extracellular matrix accumulation in renal cells. *Kidney Int* 69: 989–995.

Qian, G. S., R. K. Ross et al. (1994). A follow-up study of urinary markers of aflatoxin exposure and liver cancer risk in Shanghai, People's Republic of China. *Cancer Epidemiol Biomarkers Prev* 3: 3–10.

Rafiq, N., C. Bai et al. (2009). Long-term follow-up of patients with nonalcoholic fatty liver. *Clin Gastroenterol Hepatol* 7: 234–238.

Ratziu, V., L. Bonyhay et al. (2002). Survival, liver failure, and hepatocellular carcinoma in obesity-related cryptogenic cirrhosis. *Hepatology* 35: 1485–1493.

Rebouissou, S., M. Amessou et al. (2009). Frequent in-frame somatic deletions activate gp130 in inflammatory hepatocellular tumours. *Nature* 457: 200–204.

Rebouissou, S., G. Couchy et al. (2008). The beta-catenin pathway is activated in focal nodular hyperplasia but not in cirrhotic FNH-like nodules. *J Hepatol* 49: 61–71.

Rimassa, L., C. Porta et al. (2014). Tivantinib in MET-high hepatocellular carcinoma patients and the ongoing Phase III clinical trial. *Hepatic Oncol* 1: 181–188. doi:10.2217/HEP.14.3.

Ross, R. K., J. M. Yuan et al. (1992). Urinary aflatoxin biomarkers and risk of hepatocellular carcinoma. *Lancet* 339: 943–946.

Sakurai, T., S. Maeda et al. (2006). Loss of hepatic NF-kappa B activity enhances chemical hepatocarcinogenesis through sustained c-Jun N-terminal kinase 1 activation. *Proc Natl Acad Sci USA* 103: 10544–10551.

Sanderson, N., V. Factor et al. (1995). Hepatic expression of mature transforming growth factor beta 1 in transgenic mice results in multiple tissue lesions. *Proc Natl Acad Sci USA* 92: 2572–2576.

Santoro, A., L. Rimassa et al. (2013). Tivanitib for second-line treatment of advanced hepatocellular carcinoma: A randomized, placebo-controlled phase 2 study. *The Lancet Oncology* 14: 55–63.

Sanyal, A., A. Poklepovic et al. (2010). Population-based risk factors and resource utilization for HCC: US perspective. *Curr Med Res Opin* 26: 2183–2191.

Satoh, S., Y. Daigo et al. (2000). AXIN1 mutations in hepatocellular carcinomas, and growth suppression in cancer cells by virus-mediated transfer of AXIN1. *Nat Genet* 24: 245–250.

Schattenberg, J. M., R. Singh et al. (2006). JNK1 but not JNK2 promotes the development of steatohepatitis in mice. *Hepatology* 43: 163–172.

Schnur, J., J. Olah et al. (2004). Thioacetamide-induced hepatic fibrosis in transforming growth factor beta-1 transgenic mice. *Eur J Gastroenterol Hepatol* 16: 127–133.

Seeff, L. B., R. N. Miller et al. (2000). 45-year follow-up of hepatitis C virus infection in healthy young adults. *Ann Intern Med* 132: 105–111.

Seitz, H. K., G. Poschl et al. (1998). Alcohol and cancer. *Recent Dev Alcohol* 14: 67–95.

Shen, L., J. G. Fan et al. (2003). Prevalence of nonalcoholic fatty liver among administrative officers in Shanghai: An epidemiological survey. *World J Gastroenterol* 9: 1106–1110.

Shi, Y. and J. Massague (2003). Mechanisms of TGF-beta signaling from cell membrane to the nucleus. *Cell* 113: 685–700.

Siegel, A. B. and A. X. Zhu (2009). Metabolic syndrome and hepatocellular carcinoma: Two growing epidemics with a potential link. *Cancer* 115: 5651–5661.

Singh, R., Y. Wang et al. (2009). Differential effects of JNK1 and JNK2 inhibition on murine steatohepatitis and insulin resistance. *Hepatology* 49: 87–96.

Skelly, M. M., P. D. James et al. (2001). Findings on liver biopsy to investigate abnormal liver function tests in the absence of diagnostic serology. *J Hepatol* 35: 195–199.

Sporn, M. B. (1999). TGF-beta: 20 years and counting. *Microbes Infect* 1: 1251–1253.

Su, M. C., H. C. Lien et al. (2005). Absence of epidermal growth factor receptor exon 18–21 mutation in hepatocellular carcinoma. *Cancer Lett* 224: 117–121.

Tanaka, S., L. Mohr et al. (1997). Biological effects of human insulin receptor substrate-1 overexpression in hepatocytes. *Hepatology* 26: 598–604.

Tanaka, Y., F. Kanai et al. (2006). Absence of PIK3CA hotspot mutations in hepatocellular carcinoma in Japanese patients. *Oncogene* 25: 2950–2952.

Tang, Y., K. Kitisin et al. (2008). Progenitor/stem cells give rise to liver cancer due to aberrant TGF-beta and IL-6 signaling. *Proc Natl Acad Sci USA* 105: 2445–2450.

Taniguchi, K., L. R. Roberts et al. (2002). Mutational spectrum of beta-catenin, AXIN1, and AXIN2 in hepatocellular carcinomas and hepatoblastomas. *Oncogene* 21: 4863–4871.

Thieringer, F., T. Maass et al. (2008). Spontaneous hepatic fibrosis in transgenic mice overexpressing PDGF-A. *Gene* 423: 23–28.

Thompson, M. D. and S. P. Monga (2007). WNT/beta-catenin signaling in liver health and disease. *Hepatology* 45: 1298–1305.

Thorgeirsson, S. S. and E. Santoni-Rugiu (1996). Transgenic mouse models in carcinogenesis: Interaction of c-myc with transforming growth factor alpha and hepatocyte growth factor in hepatocarcinogenesis. *Br J Clin Pharmacol* 42: 43–52.

Tonjes, R. R., J. Lohler et al. (1995). Autocrine mitogen IgEGF cooperates with c-myc or with the Hcs locus during hepatocarcinogenesis in transgenic mice. *Oncogene* 10: 765–768.

Torres, D. M. and S. A. Harrison (2008). Diagnosis and therapy of nonalcoholic steatohepatitis. *Gastroenterology* 134: 1682–1698.

Tovar, V., C. Alsinet et al. (2010). IGF activation in a molecular subclass of hepatocellular carcinoma and pre-clinical efficacy of IGF-1R blockage. *J Hepatol* 52: 550–559.

Tsai, W. L. and R. T. Chung (2010). Viral hepatocarcinogenesis. *Oncogene* 29: 2309–2324.

Tsuda, H., S. Hirohashi et al. (1989). Low incidence of point mutation of c-Ki-ras and N-ras oncogenes in human hepatocellular carcinoma. *Jpn J Cancer Res* 80: 196–199.

Ueki, T., J. Fujimoto et al. (1997). Expression of hepatocyte growth factor and its receptor c-met proto-oncogene in hepatocellular carcinoma. *Hepatology* 25: 862–866.

Ukkola, O. and M. Santaniemi (2002). Adiponectin: A link between excess adiposity and associated comorbidities? *J Mol Med (Berl)* 80: 696–702.

Villanueva, A., D. Y. Chiang et al. (2008). Pivotal role of mTOR signaling in hepatocellular carcinoma. *Gastroenterology* 135: 1972–1983, 1983 e1971–1911.

Wang, L., W. L. Wang et al. (2007). Epigenetic and genetic alterations of PTEN in hepatocellular carcinoma. *Hepatol Res* 37: 389–396.

Watanabe, S., Y. Horie et al. (2007). Non-alcoholic steatohepatitis and hepatocellular carcinoma: Lessons from hepatocyte-specific phosphatase and tensin homolog (PTEN)-deficient mice. *J Gastroenterol Hepatol* 22: S96–S100.

Watanabe, S., Y. Horie et al. (2005). Hepatocyte-specific Pten-deficient mice as a novel model for nonalcoholic steatohepatitis and hepatocellular carcinoma. *Hepatol Res* 33: 161–166.

Weihrauch, M., M. Benick et al. (2001a). High prevalence of K-ras-2 mutations in hepatocellular carcinomas in workers exposed to vinyl chloride. *Int Arch Occup Environ Health* 74: 405–410.

Weihrauch, M., M. Benicke et al. (2001b). Frequent k- ras –2 mutations and p16(INK4A)methylation in hepatocellular carcinomas in workers exposed to vinyl chloride. *Br J Cancer* 84: 982–989.

Whittaker, S., R. Marais et al. (2010). The role of signaling pathways in the development and treatment of hepatocellular carcinoma. *Oncogene* 29: 4989–5005.

Wild, C. P. and A. J. Hall (2000). Primary prevention of hepatocellular carcinoma in developing countries. *Mutat Res* 462: 381–393.

Williams, A. O. and A. D. Knapton (1996). Hepatic silicosis, cirrhosis, and liver tumors in mice and hamsters: Studies of transforming growth factor beta expression. *Hepatology* 23: 1268–1275.

Wong, C. I., H. L. Yap et al. (2008). Lack of somatic ErbB2 tyrosine kinase domain mutations in hepatocellular carcinoma. *Hepatol Res* 38: 838–841.

World Cancer Research Fund, AICR, Ed. (2007). *Food, Nutrition, Physical Activity, and the Prevention of Cancer: A Global Perspective.* Washington, DC: AICR.

World Health Organization (2010a). Mortality database. Available at: http://www.who.int/whosis/en. Accessed July 30, 2013.

World Health Organization (2010b). Hepatitis B. Available at: http://www.who.int/immunization/topics/hepatits_b/en/index.html. Accessed November 20, 2010.

World Health Organization (2013). Available at: http://www.cdc.gov/cancer/dcpc/data/. Accessed July 20, 2013.

Wu, G., Y. G. Chen et al. (2000). Structural basis of Smad2 recognition by the Smad anchor for receptor activation. *Science* 287: 92–97.

Xian, Z. H., S. H. Zhang et al. (2005). Overexpression/amplification of HER-2/neu is uncommon in hepatocellular carcinoma. *J Clin Pathol* 58: 500–503.

Xu, Z., L. Chen et al. (2005). Liver-specific inactivation of the Nrf1 gene in adult mouse leads to nonalcoholic steatohepatitis and hepatic neoplasia. *Proc Natl Acad Sci USA* 102: 4120–4125.

Yang, S., H. Zhu et al. (2000). Mitochondrial adaptations to obesity-related oxidant stress. *Arch Biochem Biophys* 378: 259–268.

Yao, Y. J., X. L. Ping et al. (1999). PTEN/MMAC1 mutations in hepatocellular carcinomas. *Oncogene* 18: 3181–3185.

Yeo, W., N. Wong et al. (2005). High frequency of promoter hypermethylation of RASSF1A in tumor and plasma of patients with hepatocellular carcinoma. *Liver Int* 25: 266–272.

Yoshikawa, H., K. Matsubara et al. (2001). SOCS-1, a negative regulator of the JAK/STAT pathway, is silenced by methylation in human hepatocellular carcinoma and shows growth-suppression activity. *Nat Genet* 28: 29–35.

Yu, M. C., J. M. Yuan (2004). Environmental factors and risk for hepatocellular carcinoma. *Gastroenterology* 127: S72–S78.

Yuan, J. M., S. Govindarajan et al. (2004). Synergism of alcohol, diabetes, and viral hepatitis on the risk of hepatocellular carcinoma in blacks and whites in the U.S. *Cancer* 101: 1009–1017.

Zhang, X., H. J. Xu et al. (1994). Deletions of chromosome 13q, mutations in Retinoblastoma 1, and retinoblastoma protein state in human hepatocellular carcinoma. *Cancer Res* 54: 4177–4182.

Zhang, Y. J., H. Ahsan et al. (2002). High frequency of promoter hypermethylation of RASSF1A and p16 and its relationship to aflatoxin B1-DNA adduct levels in human hepatocellular carcinoma. *Mol Carcinog* 35: 85–92.

Zucman-Rossi, J. (2010). Molecular classification of hepatocellular carcinoma. *Dig Liver Dis* 42: S235–S241.

Zucman-Rossi, J., S. Benhamouche et al. (2007). Differential effects of inactivated Axin1 and activated beta-catenin mutations in human hepatocellular carcinomas. *Oncogene* 26: 774–780.

4 Cellular Stress Responses in the Regulation of Drug-Induced Liver Steatosis

Dotan Uzi, Duah Alkam, and Boaz Tirosh

CONTENTS

INTRODUCTION TO DRUG-INDUCED LIVER INJURY

Drug-induced liver injury (DILI) is a general term for a liver injury caused by exposure to xenobiotics and drugs. These exposures constitute the majority of DILI incidents. In most cases, it is not the parent drug that causes DILI but rather the products of its metabolism, making it difficult to study DILI in animal models. Drugs that cause DILI in high percentage of individuals and in a dose-dependent manner, with few exceptions, are excluded in clinical trials. Hence, most hepatotoxic drugs are termed idiosyncratic, meaning the response to said drugs depends on the individual's specific constitution, often apparent at very low frequency in the population. Whether DILI is a result of a complex genetic makeup and/or acquired factors, such as nutrition and psychological parameters, has not yet been established, and to date, no genetic, metabolic, or other characteristic has been found to reliably predict severe DILI. As such, clinical trials often fail to predict idiosyncratic DILI, and in many instances, DILI is reported in retrospective studies only after the drug has been approved for clinical use. In the last 50 years, DILI has been the most frequent single cause of safety-related drug marketing withdrawals. Hepatotoxicity discovered following approval for marketing has limited the use of many drugs (Holt and Ju, 2006). DILI is a major cause of acute liver failure and is estimated to be the leading cause of liver transplantation in the United States and other Western countries (Davern, 2012).

Although the mechanisms of DILI vary among different drugs and develop in an unpredictable manner, cellular stress signaling pathways have been recently recognized to be shared by many DILI etiologies. In this chapter, we will address the major cellular stress pathways that contribute to DILI with special consideration to drug induced hepatic steatosis.

Fat accumulation (or steatosis) is a leading cause for liver injury. The leading causes of liver steatosis are obesity and glucose tolerance, infection with hepatitis viruses, and alcohol consumption. However, some drugs are also implicated in liver steatosis, such as aspirin, tetracycline, amiodarone, valproic acid, and several antiviral nucleoside analogues (Fromenty and Pessayre, 1997).

MECHANISM AND CELLULAR PATHWAYS IN DILI

MITOCHONDRIAL DYSFUNCTION AND LIVER STEATOSIS

Mitochondria are responsible for ATP production by the oxidative phosphorylation system, a process that constitutively generates reactive oxygen species (ROS). Mitochondria integrity is crucial for cell survival. Thus, disruption of mitochondrial outer membrane initiates a series of events that result in apoptosis.

Impairment of mitochondrial respiratory functions may lead to lipid accumulation. The mechanisms involve increase in ROS formation, changes in the $NADH/NAD^+$ ratios, and attenuation of β-oxidation of fatty acids. This causes the accumulation of fatty acids in the form of triglycerides in cytoplasmic fat deposits (Watmough et al., 1990). Drugs that inhibit mitochondrial respiration, increase ROS, or impair β-oxidation of fatty acids may confer hepatic steatosis.

Prominent examples for drugs that affect mitochondrial respiration are antidiabetic drugs from the PPAR-γ agonists family (ciglitazone, troglitazone, and darglitazone) and a few of the statin family, which are used to treat hypercholesterinemia (Nadanaciva et al., 2007). Amiodarone, a widely used anti-arrhythmic drug, has a lipophilic moiety and amine function, which may by positively charged. Therefore, it might easily cross cellular membrane and interfere with the mitochondrial function by uncoupling protons (Kodavanti and Mehendale, 1990). Overdose of amoidarone partially hampers electron transfer along the respiratory chain causing electrons to be passed to oxygen to form many ROS types (Fromenty et al., 1990a, b). Moreover, the mitochondrial ROS accumulation may lead to lipid peroxidation (Berson et al., 1998). Isolated hepatocytes exposed to amiodarone show liver damage manifested by Mallory-Denk bodies, typical for chronic damage of alcoholics (Robin et al., 2008).

Aspirin (or salicylic acid) is also known to uncouple mitochondrial respiration and favor mitochondrial permeability transition and cellular death (Oh et al., 2003). Although, in rare cases, aspirin leads to spotty liver, there are no indications for development of NAFLD, suggesting that the relationship between mitochondrial respiration and liver steatosis is not straightforward (Zimmerman, 1981).

Another prominent mitochondrial respiration attenuator is efavirenz, a reverse transcriptase inhibitor, used as part of drug cocktail therapy in patients carrying the human immunodeficiency virus (HIV). Efavirenz is a potent mitochondrial complex I inhibitor and therefore causes ATP depletion in hepatocyes, which carry activated AMPK and increased fatty acid uptake contributing to hepatic steatosis (Blas-Garcia et al., 2010). In addition, efavirenz increases mitochondrial superoxide formation and triggers MMP and hepatocellular apoptosis (Apostolova et al., 2010).

Efavirenz is not the only anti-HIV drug that confers steatosis. Reverse transcriptase dideoxynucleoside analogues, such as zalcitabine, didanosine, and stavudine, carry 5′-hydroxyl group of deoxyribose but lack the normal 3′-hydroxyl group (Walker et al., 2004). These nucleic acid analogues can form triphosphate derivatives, which can be incorporated to growing mtDNA (Mitsuya and Broder, 1986). Incorporation of these analogues to the mtDNA is carried out by DNA polymerase γ, which acts at the mitochondria. This depletion of mtDNA carries transcriptional attenuation of mitochondrial proteins and damages respiratory complexes that depend upon mtDNA transcription (Brivet et al., 2000). Dideoxynucleoside analogues not only prevent mtDNA replication but can trigger mtDNA damage using other targets as well. The best studied example is zidovudine (AZT), which can compete on phosphorylation with thymidine, limit TMP and TTP flow and slow DNA replication (Lynx and McKee, 2006). Moreover, dideoxynucleoside analogues induce ROS-mediated mitochondrial damage. These analogues impair ADP entry into the mitochondrial matrix and therefore prevent protons from entering through ATP synthase, causing high mitochondrial potential (Esposito et al., 1999). The latter leads to electron flow blockage in the respiratory chain further increasing respiratory chain complex production, which causes additional ROS formation and further exacerbates mtDNA deletion (Esposito et al., 1999).

The reversible cholinesterase inhibitor tacrine is a drug given to slow the development of Alzheimer's disease. Tacrine selectively injures liver tissue mitochondria by multiple mechanisms. At the mitochondria, tacrine metabolites accumulate and damage mtDNA (Berson et al., 1996) by intercalating between mtDNA bases, attenuating topoisomerase, and decreasing mtDNA synthesis (Mansouri et al., 2003). These cooperate to progressively deplete mtDNA, and subsequently cause of hepatocellular death. The fact that tacrine is able to form reactive metabolites adds cumulative cause to liver injury (Woolf et al., 1993).

Tamoxifen, an anti-estrogenic drug, is given to estrogen receptor–positive breast cancer patients. The cationic nature of the molecule allows it to accumulate at the mitochondria owing to its strong negative charge. Tamoxifen intercalates between DNA bases, inhibits topoisomerase, and decreases mtDNA synthesis, leading to severe hepatic mtDNA depletion in the liver (Larosche et al., 2007).

THE JNK PATHWAY

c-Jun-N-terminal kinase (JNK) is a member of the mitogen-activated protein kinase (MAPK) family. In mammalian livers, two different JNK isoforms are expressed (JNK1, JNK2). JNK is activated by its phosphorylation by three types of enzymes: MAP3Ks (such as MLK3, MEKK1, and TAK1) are known as JNKs activators, MAP2Ks (MKK4 and MKK7) phosphorylates JNKs at threonine and tyrosine residues, and autophosphorylation by MAP kinase themselves. JNK activation and induction occurs in response to many types of stimulations, both intracellular and extracellular such as ROS accumulation, toxins, drugs, endoplasmic reticulum (ER) stress, and metabolic changes.

JNK is directly linked to the development of liver steatosis in the forms of NAFLD and NASH. Strong activation of JNK has been observed in the liver, fat, and muscle tissues in mice placed on a high-fat diet (HFD). Moreover, HFD causes obesity in wild-type, but not in $Jnk1^{-/-}$ mice (Hirosumi et al., 2002; Solinas et al., 2006; Singh et al., 2009). However, $Jnk2^{-/-}$ mice placed on the HFD displayed a similar degree of hepatic steatosis as wild type mice, but have increased hepatocyte injury, obesity, and insulin resistance (Singh et al., 2009). This may be explained by the fact that livers from $Jnk2^{-/-}$ mice have greater JNK activity, indicating that JNK1 overcompensation damages the liver. The roles of JNK in NASH have been studied using mice placed on methionine–choline-deficient (MCD) diets. Again, JNK1 deficiency protected mice from the effects of the MCD diet, but JNK2 deficiency had no effect (Schattenberg et al., 2006). These data implicate JNK1 as a target in the treatment of NAFLD and NASH.

Because JNK activation is sensitive to oxidative stress and ER stress and is potently induced by TNF signaling, it is not surprising that drugs can modulate JNK activity by diverse mechanisms. Acetaminophen (APAP) accounts for almost half of DILI cases in the United States. Upon exposure to APAP overdose (due to cytochrome P450-mediated conversion to the electrophilic metabolite NAPQI) GSH is depleted by covalent binding to NAPQI. When depletion exceeds 90%, mitochondrial ROS is vastly induced. Under these conditions, JNK translocates to the mitochondria where it undergoes activation in a GSK3β- and MEKK1-dependent mechanism (Hanawa et al., 2008). The outcome of APAP intoxication is severe centrilobular necrosis that can develop into acute liver failure. Provision of JNK inhibitors can prevent APAP hepatotoxicity, implicating JNK as a main regulator of hepatocyte survival following acute oxidative stress. Although APAP is an extreme example of JNK activation leading to cell death rather than to development of fatty liver, when JNK is activated more mildly and in a chronic fashion, it promotes NAFLD. The best example for this hypothesis is elevated serum fatty acid (SFA) levels. Although the connection between SFA and JNK has been clearly demonstrated in humans and rodents, the precise cellular and molecular mechanisms resulting in JNK activation have not been fully revealed. One of the mechanisms is ER stress, which will be addressed separately below. However, ER stress-independent mechanisms also operate, including (apoptosis signal-regulating kinase 1) ASK1 (Tobiume et al., 2001), mixed lineage kinases (MLK) (Jaeschke and Davis, 2007), (GSK) 3α and β (Coso et al., 1995). Recently, the double-stranded RNA-dependent protein kinase (PKR) has also shown to be a required component of JNK activation in response to SFA (Nakamura et al., 2010). Thus, multiple pathways converge in JNK activation in the etiology of NAFLD.

CYTOCHROME P450 METABOLISM

The cytochrome P450 system (CYP) is comprised of many isoenzymes with over-lapping chemical specificity and overlapping functions (Williams et al., 2004). For many drugs, CYP metabolism occurs first, and metabolites are then exposed to fur-ther metabolism. The CYP450 family is divided into three major groups: CYP1, CYP2, and CYP3. Each group is further divided to subgroups based on sequence similarity. Although most of the known CYP450 family members are expressed in the liver, their expression is diverse among the population and undergoes further changes during NAFLD. We will describe the primary CYP isoforms in drug metab-olism and address their involvement in NAFLD and NASH.

CYP3A4

CYP3A subfamily members are considered to be the most abundant proteins among CYP450 family. CYP3A4, for example, participates in the metabolism of about 50% of all drugs, and is able to metabolize drugs from almost all classes (Hewitt et al., 2007). CYP3A4 is subjected to induction, activation, and inhibition by drugs and other xenobiotics. A number of important drugs have been identified as substrates, inducers, and/or inhibitors of CYP3A4. CYP3A4 inducers include drugs such as rifampin, phenytoin, and ritonavir (Zhou, 2008). As inducers, these drugs target the orphan nuclear receptor, pregnane X receptor (PXR), which was found to play a critical role in CYP3A4 induction. The inhibition or induction of CYP3A4, how-ever, is carried out by various drugs, often caused by unfavorable and long-lasting drug–drug interactions. Clinically important drugs that act as CYP3A4 inhibitors include macrolide antibiotics (clarithromycin and erythromycin), anti-HIV agents (ritonavir and delavirdine), antidepressants (fluoxetine and fluvoxamine), calcium channel blockers (verapamil and diltiazem), and steroids and their modulators (ges-todene and mifepristone). CYP3A4 involves the formation of reactive metabolites; therefore, inactivation or inhibition leads to cellular metabolism alteration. However, induction of CYP3A4 results in ROS accumulation and extensive cellular damage.

CYP2C Family

CYP2C enzymes are responsible for metabolizing approximately 20% of clinical drugs (Nebert and Russell, 2002). Hepatocytes express several CYP2C isoforms including 2C8, 2C9, and 2C, 19 (Hewitt et al., 2007), which metabolize various sets of drug substrates such as anticonvulsant drugs, anticoagulants, antidiabetic drugs, proton pump inhibitors, anticancer drugs, and nonsteroidal anti-inflammatory drugs. CYP2C enzymes are also subjected to transcriptional alteration and modifications (Chen and Goldstein, 2009). Some drugs bind nuclear receptors at their *cis*-elements within CYP2C promoters, and regulate the transcription of CYP2C genes. In this regard, HNF4α plays a key role in CYP2C gene regulation. However, the cross-talk between HNF4α sites and PXR/CAR sites is necessary for induction in response to drugs such as rifampicin, artemisinin, and hyperforin (Chen and Goldstein, 2009). The glucocorticoid dexamethasone activates the CYP2C promoters via the glucocorticoid receptor. Other regulatory factors such as coactivators, corepressors, and signal pathways indirectly modulate the expression of human CYP2C genes.

CYP1A2

CYP1A2 is one of the major CYPs in human liver (approximately 13%) and metabolizes a variety of clinically important drugs, carcinogens, and important endogenous compounds including steroids, retinols, melatonin, uroporphyrinogen, and arachidonic acid (Zhou et al., 2009). Clozapine, lidocaine, theophylline, tacrine, and leflunomide are some of the most well-known drugs metabolized by CYP1A2. Although CYP1A2 is critical for the metabolism of many subtrates, the mechanism of its activation and attenuation is very limited. To date, the regulation of CYP1A2 is mostly related to the aromatic hydrocarbon receptor, similar to other CYPs such as CYP1A1 and 1B1 (Zhou et al., 2009).

CYP2B6

CYP2B6 has been recently proven important in drug metabolism. This cytochrome is polymorphic, carrying more than 28 allelic variants and subvariants (1B through 29), and as a result, is expressed differently in different ethnic groups (Mo et al., 2009). Human CYP2B6 activation depends upon either the constitutive and rostane receptor (CAR/NR1I3) or the pregnane X receptor and glucocorticoid receptor upon ligand binding. CYP2B6 is known to metabolize approximately 8% of drugs, such as cyclophosphamide, ifosfamide, tamoxifen, ketamine, artemisinin, nevirapine, efavirenz, bupropion, sibutramine, and propofol. In addition, CYP2B6 has the ability to bioactivate few procarcinogens and toxicants; therefore, its upregulation is consistent with DILI (Mo et al., 2009).

CYP2E1

CYP2E1 has a relatively small part in hepatic–drug metabolism. However, CYP2E1 is the most conserved drug-related CYP and is known for its ability to metabolize several clinically important drugs, chemical toxins, and carcinogens. Although drugs metabolized by CYP2E1 are limited, their hepatotoxicity is constantly studied such as anesthetics (sulfadiazine), pain killers (acetaminophen), antiepileptics (phenobarbital), antidepressants (fluoxetine), bronchodilator (theophylline), and muscle relaxant (chlorzoxazone) (Tanaka et al., 2000). Activation of CYP2E1 depends upon its stabilization via substrate–protein interaction and does not involve transcriptional upregulation of CYP2E1 (Gonzalez, 2007).

The metabolism of chlorzoxazone, a skeletal muscle relaxant, is also used as an indicator of exposure to organic solvents (Jayyosi et al., 1995; Nedelcheva, 1996; Ernstgard et al., 1999) and to monitor liver function before and after transplantation and as an indicator severity of liver disease. Chlorzoxazone is metabolized by CYP2E1 and cause 6-hydroxychlorzoxazone accumulation in liver microsomes (Vesell et al., 1995; Bachmann and Sarver, 1996). However, CYP2E1 plays an almost identical role to CYP1A2, in 6-hydroxychlorzoxazone formation at physiological chlorzoxazone concentrations (Ono et al., 1995). Trimethadione, an antiepileptic drug, is another suitable candidate for estimating DILI. In human liver, CYP2C9, 2E1, and 3A4 metabolize trimethadione to dimethadione, which allows monitoring hepatic microsomal function through blood samples (Tanaka and Funae, 1996; Kurata et al., 1998).

The connection between CYP activity and NASH is poorly understood. Immuno-histological analyses indicated an increased expression of CYP2E1 in livers from patients with NASH, irrespective of the etiologic association. As in the rat model, hepatic distribution of CYP2E1 corresponded to that of steatosis. In contrast to CYP2E1, CYP3A immunostaining was decreased in patients with NASH (Weltman et al., 1998). However, analysis of ducks fed with HFD yielded the reverse pheno-types, i.e., decrease in CYP expression and activity (Leclercq et al., 1998), whereas a similar approach in rats was associated with an increase in CYP2E1 (Bahcecioglu et al., 2010). These data highlight the complexities involved in drug metabolism-related predisposition to liver steatosis and the fact that when liver disease develops, drug metabolism is affected.

ENDOPLASMIC RETICULUM STRESS

The ER is the major cellular site of protein folding and modification. ER stress occurs when the amount of protein entering the ER exceeds its folding capacity. This imbalance induces a cytoprotective reaction collectively termed the unfolded protein response (UPR) (Ron and Walter, 2007). The mammalian UPR is trans-duced by three major sensors (IRE1, PERK, and ATF6) that reside in the ER and undergo activation under ER stress conditions. IRE1 and PERK are activated by autophosphorylation, whereas ATF6 is activated by intramembrane cleavage, which releases its N-terminal fragment for transcription transactivation. Activated IRE1 splices the mRNA of XBP1 in a noncanonical fashion, yielding the potent transcription factor XBP1s (Yoshida et al., 2001; Calfon et al., 2002). Activated PERK phosphorylates eIF2α, inducing selective translation of ATF4 and transcription of ATF3 and CCAAT-enhancer-binding protein homologous protein (CHOP) in a sequential manner (Jiang et al., 2004). Targets of ATF6 have been recently characterized using the ATF6α knockout mouse and include elements of the ER associated degradation pathway.

Activation of the UPR leads initially to attenuation of protein synthesis and protein translocation into the ER, thus preventing further accumulation of misfolded proteins. This initial step is followed by an increase in the capacity of the ER to handle unfolded proteins. If the stress is not relieved in a timely fashion, cell death is triggered in an intricate mechanism that involves caspase activation, calcium leakage from the ER and mitochondrial damage (Kim et al., 2008). Interestingly, UPR itself plays an important role in the life or death decision. For example, CHOP promotes cell death by utilizing various mechanisms (McCullough et al., 2001; Chen et al., 1996; Sylvester et al., 1994). Moreover, deletion of CHOP protects mice from various liver-specific challenges, such as diet-induced steatohepatitis, bile duct ligation, and alcohol intoxication (Ji et al., 2005; Rahman et al., 2007; Tamaki et al., 2008). A second pro-apoptotic arm of the UPR is the activation of JNK by the kinase activity of IRE1α (Urano et al., 2000). Recently, the nuclease activity of IRE1α

was implicated in ER stress-mediated apoptosis primarily through the cleavage of miRNA directed against pro-apoptotic molecules and, thus, reversing their inhibition of the apoptotic machinery (Upton et al., 2012).

The discovery that homocyteine elicits ER stress suggested a mechanistic explanation to the hepatic steatosis that develops in patients having severe hyperhomocysteinemia. Indeed, the first indication that ER stress plays a role in liver steatosis came from in vitro and in vivo studies with homocysteine. Homocysteine-fed mice developed biochemical signature of ER stress accumulation of cholesterol and triglycerides in livers, but not plasmas (Werstuck et al., 2001). Further support for this hypothesis came from the analysis of various mouse models deficient in the UPR. Disruption of either of the ER stress-sensing pathways included the development of hepatic microvesicular steatosis upon challenge with the ER stress-causing drug tunicamycin (Rutkowski et al., 2008; Zhang et al., 2011; Yamamoto et al., 2010). The mechanisms that connect ER stress to liver steatosis are not entirely clear and major ones include increased lipoprotein delivery to the liver (Jo et al., 2013), decreased VLDL release, and dysregulation of the SREBP transcription factors (Lee et al., 2008).

The role of ER stress in drug-induced steatosis is gaining interest particularly in the context of anti-HIV therapy. In addition to its effect on mitochondrial function, zidovudine (AZT) also causes oxidative stress and ER stress in mice treated with the drug (Banerjee et al., 2013). Mice treated with the HIV protease inhibitors lopinavir or ritonavir, which, in the clinic, causes lipodystrophy and dyslipidemia at a high percentage of HIV-positive patients, exhibit activation of ER stress and inhibition of autophagy (Zha et al., 2013). Interestingly, ER stress is not restricted to hepatocytes and occurs in gut epithelium and in adipocytes, suggesting that the concerted consequences of ER stress in various cell types is responsible for liver steatosis.

NUCLEAR FACTOR ERYTHROID 2–RELATED FACTOR 2 (NRF2)–KELCH ECH ASSOCIATING PROTEIN 1 (KEAP1) PATHWAY

The Keap1–Nrf2 pathway is the major regulator of cytoprotective transcription responses to endogenous and exogenous stresses caused by ROS and electrophiles. Keap1 is a very cysteine-rich protein, with mouse Keap1 having a total of 25 and human 27 cysteine residues. Three of these residues have been shown to play a functional role by altering the conformation of Keap1, leading to nuclear translocation of Nrf2 and subsequent target gene expression. Examination of Nrf2 KO mice for diet-induced NASH showed a substantial increase in macrovesicular and microvesicularsteatosis and a massive increase in the number of neutrophil polymorphs, compared with livers from wild-type mice treated similarly. As expected, livers of Nrf2$^{-/-}$ mice on the MCD diet had more oxidative stress and heightened inflammation relative to their wild-type counterparts (Chowdhry et al., 2010). In support of these data, overactivation of Nrf2 (by limiting the amount of keap1) protected the mice from diet-induced NASH (Zhang et al., 2010).

It is now clear that Nrf2 controls an important program that accompanies mitochondrial dysfunction and ROS accumulation aiming at protection against liver steatosis and primarily the development of NAFLD into NASH. Nrf2-dependent program limits triglyceride accumulation in the liver, helping to restore mitochondrial respiration, limit ROS production, and prevent lipid peroxidation (Yang et al., 2013). However, the exact components of this program await clarification.

REFERENCES

Apostolova, N., L. J. Gomez-Sucerquia, A. Moran, A. Alvarez, A. Blas-Garcia, and J. V. Esplugues. 2010. Enhanced oxidative stress and increased mitochondrial mass during efavirenz-induced apoptosis in human hepatic cells. *Br J Pharmacol* 160:2069–84.

Bachmann, K., and J. G. Sarver. 1996. Chlorzoxazone as a single sample probe of hepatic CYP2E1 activity in humans. *Pharmacology* 52:169–77.

Bahcecioglu, I. H., N. Kuzu, K. Metin et al. 2010. Lycopene prevents development of steatohepatitis in experimental nonalcoholic steatohepatitis model induced by high-fat diet. *Vet Med Int* 2010:8. doi: 10.4061/2010/262179.

Banerjee, A., M. A. Abdelmegeed, S. Jang, and B. J. Song. 2013. Zidovudine (AZT) and hepatic lipid accumulation: Implication of inflammation, oxidative and endoplasmic reticulum stress mediators. *PLoS One* 8:e76850.

Berson, A., V. De Beco, P. Letteron et al. 1998. Steatohepatitis-inducing drugs cause mitochondrial dysfunction and lipid peroxidation in rat hepatocytes. *Gastroenterology* 114:764–74.

Berson, A., S. Renault, P. Letteron et al. 1996. Uncoupling of rat and human mitochondria: A possible explanation for tacrine-induced liver dysfunction. *Gastroenterology* 110:1878–90.

Blas-Garcia, A., N. Apostolova, D. Ballesteros et al. 2010. Inhibition of mitochondrial function by efavirenz increases lipid content in hepatic cells. *Hepatology* 52:115–25.

Brivet, F. G., I. Nion, B. Megarbane et al. 2000. Fatal lactic acidosis and liver steatosis associated with didanosine and stavudine treatment: A respiratory chain dysfunction? *J Hepatol* 32:364–5.

Calfon, M., H. Zeng, F. Urano et al. 2002. IRE1 couples endoplasmic reticulum load to secretory capacity by processing the XBP-1 mRNA. *Nature* 415:92–6.

Chen, B. P., C. D. Wolfgang, and T. Hai. 1996. Analysis of ATF3, a transcription factor induced by physiological stresses and modulated by gadd153/Chop10. *Mol Cell Biol* 16:1157–68.

Chen, Y., and J. A. Goldstein. 2009. The transcriptional regulation of the human CYP2C genes. *Curr Drug Metab* 10:567–78.

Chowdhry, S., M. H. Nazmy, P. J. Meakin et al. 2010. Loss of Nrf2 markedly exacerbates nonalcoholic steatohepatitis. *Free Radic Biol Med* 48:357–71.

Coso, O. A., M. Chiariello, J. C. Yu et al. 1995. The small GTP-binding proteins Rac1 and Cdc42 regulate the activity of the JNK/SAPK signaling pathway. *Cell* 81:1137–46.

Davern, T. J. 2012. Drug-induced liver disease. *Clin Liver Dis* 16:231–45.

Ernstgard, L., E. Gullstrand, G. Johanson, and A. Lof. 1999. Toxicokinetic interactions between orally ingested chlorzoxazone and inhaled acetone or toluene in male volunteers. *Toxicol Sci* 48:189–96.

Esposito, L. A., S. Melov, A. Panov, B. A. Cottrell, and D. C. Wallace. 1999. Mitochondrial disease in mouse results in increased oxidative stress. *Proc Natl Acad Sci USA* 96:4820–5.

Fromenty, B., C. Fisch, A. Berson, P. Letteron, D. Larrey, and D. Pessayre. 1990a. Dual effect of amiodarone on mitochondrial respiration. Initial protonophoric uncoupling effect followed by inhibition of the respiratory chain at the levels of complex I and complex II. *J Pharmacol Exp Ther* 255:1377–84.

Fromenty, B., C. Fisch, G. Labbe et al. 1990b. Amiodarone inhibits the mitochondrial beta-oxidation of fatty acids and produces microvesicular steatosis of the liver in mice. *J Pharmacol Exp Ther* 255:1371–6.

Fromenty, B., and D. Pessayre. 1997. Impaired mitochondrial function in microvesicular steatosis. Effects of drugs, ethanol, hormones and cytokines. *J Hepatol* 26:43–53.

Gonzalez, F. J. 2007. The 2006 Bernard B. Brodie Award Lecture. Cyp2e1. *Drug Metab Dispos* 35:1–8.

Hanawa, N., M. Shinohara, B. Saberi, W. A. Gaarde, D. Han, and N. Kaplowitz. 2008. Role of JNK translocation to mitochondria leading to inhibition of mitochondria bioenergetics in acetaminophen-induced liver injury. *J Biol Chem* 283:13565–77.

Hewitt, N. J., M. J. Lechon, J. B. Houston et al. 2007. Primary hepatocytes: Current understanding of the regulation of metabolic enzymes and transporter proteins, and pharmaceutical practice for the use of hepatocytes in metabolism, enzyme induction, transporter, clearance, and hepatotoxicity studies. *Drug Metab Rev* 39:159–234.

Hirosumi, J., G. Tuncman, L. Chang et al. 2002. A central role for JNK in obesity and insulin resistance. *Nature* 420:333–6.

Holt, M. P., and C. Ju. 2006. Mechanisms of drug-induced liver injury. *AAPS J* 8:E48–54.

Jaeschke, A., and R. J. Davis. 2007. Metabolic stress signaling mediated by mixed-lineage kinases. *Mol Cell* 27:498–508.

Jayyosi, Z., D. Knoble, M. Muc, J. Erick, P. E. Thomas, and M. Kelley. 1995. Cytochrome P-450 2E1 is not the sole catalyst of chlorzoxazone hydroxylation in rat liver microsomes. off. *J Pharmacol Exp Ther* 273:1156–61.

Ji, C., R. Mehrian-Shai, C. Chan, Y. H. Hsu, and N. Kaplowitz. 2005. Role of CHOP in hepatic apoptosis in the murine model of intragastric ethanol feeding. *Alcohol Clin Exp Res* 29:1496–503.

Jiang, H. Y., S. A. Wek, B. C. McGrath et al. 2004. Activating transcription factor 3 is integral to the eukaryotic initiation factor 2 kinase stress response. *Mol Cell Biol* 24:1365–77.

Jo, H., S. S. Choe, K. C. Shin et al. 2013. Endoplasmic reticulum stress induces hepatic steatosis via increased expression of the hepatic very low-density lipoprotein receptor. *Hepatology* 57:1366–77.

Kim, I., W. Xu, and J. C. Reed. 2008. Cell death and endoplasmic reticulum stress: Disease relevance and therapeutic opportunities. *Nat Rev Drug Discov* 7:1013–30.

Kodavanti, U. P., and H. M. Mehendale. 1990. Cationic amphiphilic drugs and phospholipid storage disorder. *Pharmacol Rev* 42:327–54.

Kurata, N., Y. Nishimura, M. Iwase et al. 1998. Trimethadione metabolism by human liver cytochrome P450: Evidence for the involvement of CYP2E1. *Xenobiotica* 28:1041–7.

Larosche, I., P. Letteron, B. Fromenty et al. 2007. Tamoxifen inhibits topoisomerases, depletes mitochondrial DNA, and triggers steatosis in mouse liver. *J Pharmacol Exp Ther* 321:526–35.

Leclercq, I., Y. Horsmans, J. P. Desager, N. Delzenne, and A. P. Geubel. 1998. Reduction in hepatic cytochrome P-450 is correlated to the degree of liver fat content in animal models of steatosis in the absence of inflammation. *J Hepatol* 28:410–6.

Lee, A. H., E. F. Scapa, D. E. Cohen, and L. H. Glimcher. 2008. Regulation of hepatic lipogenesis by the transcription factor XBP1. *Science* 320:1492–6.

Lynx, M. D., and E. E. McKee. 2006. 3′-Azido-3′-deoxythymidine (AZT) is a competitive inhibitor of thymidine phosphorylation in isolated rat heart and liver mitochondria. *Biochem Pharmacol* 72:239–43.

Mansouri, A., D. Haouzi, V. Descatoire et al. 2003. Tacrine inhibits topoisomerases and DNA synthesis to cause mitochondrial DNA depletion and apoptosis in mouse liver. *Hepatology* 38:715–25.

McCullough, K. D., J. L. Martindale, L. O. Klotz, T. Y. Aw, and N. J. Holbrook. 2001. Gadd153 sensitizes cells to endoplasmic reticulum stress by down-regulating Bcl2 and perturbing the cellular redox state. *Mol Cell Biol* 21:1249–59.

Mitsuya, H., and S. Broder. 1986. Inhibition of the in vitro infectivity and cytopathic effect of human T-lymphotrophic virus type III/lymphadenopathy-associated virus (HTLV-III/ LAV) by 2′,3′-dideoxynucleosides. *Proc Natl Acad Sci USA* 83:1911–5.

Mo, S. L., Y. H. Liu, W. Duan, M. Q. Wei, J. R. Kanwar, and S. F. Zhou. 2009. Substrate specificity, regulation, and polymorphism of human cytochrome P450 2B6. *Curr Drug Metab* 10:730–53.

Nadanaciva, S., A. Bernal, R. Aggeler, R. Capaldi, and Y. Will. 2007. Target identification of drug induced mitochondrial toxicity using immunocapture based OXPHOS activity assays. *Toxicol In Vitro* 21:902–11.

Nakamura, T., M. Furuhashi, P. Li et al. 2010. Double-stranded RNA-dependent protein kinase links pathogen sensing with stress and metabolic homeostasis. *Cell* 140:338–48.

Nebert, D. W., and D. W. Russell. 2002. Clinical importance of the cytochromes P450. *Lancet* 360:1155–62.

Nedelcheva, V. 1996. Effects of acetone on the capacity of o-xylene and toluene to induce several forms of cytochrome P450 in rat liver. *Cent Eur J Public Health* 4:119–22.

Oh, K. W., T. Qian, D. A. Brenner, and J. J. Lemasters. 2003. Salicylate enhances necrosis and apoptosis mediated by the mitochondrial permeability transition. *Toxicol Sci* 73:44–52.

Ono, S., T. Hatanaka, H. Hotta, M. Tsutsui, T. Satoh, and F. J. Gonzalez. 1995. Chlorzoxazone is metabolized by human CYP1A2 as well as by human CYP2E1. *Pharmacogenetics* 5:143–50.

Rahman, S. M., J. M. Schroeder-Gloeckler, R. C. Janssen et al. 2007. CCAAT/enhancing binding protein beta deletion in mice attenuates inflammation, endoplasmic reticulum stress, and lipid accumulation in diet-induced nonalcoholic steatohepatitis. *Hepatology* 45:1108–17.

Robin, M. A., V. Descatoire, D. Pessayre, and A. Berson. 2008. Steatohepatitis-inducing drugs trigger cytokeratin cross-links in hepatocytes. Possible contribution to Mallory-Denk body formation. *Toxicol In Vitro* 22:1511–9.

Ron, D., and P. Walter. 2007. Signal integration in the endoplasmic reticulum unfolded protein response. *Nat Rev Mol Cell Biol* 8:519–29.

Rutkowski, D. T., J. Wu, S. H. Back et al. 2008. UPR pathways combine to prevent hepatic steatosis caused by ER stress-mediated suppression of transcriptional master regulators. *Dev Cell* 15:829–40.

Schattenberg, J. M., R. Singh, Y. Wang et al. 2006. JNK1 but not JNK2 promotes the development of steatohepatitis in mice. *Hepatology* 43:163–72.

Singh, R., Y. Wang, Y. Xiang, K. E. Tanaka, W. A. Gaarde, and M. J. Czaja. 2009. Differential effects of JNK1 and JNK2 inhibition on murine steatohepatitis and insulin resistance. *Hepatology* 49:87–96.

Solinas, G., W. Naugler, F. Galimi, M. S. Lee, and M. Karin. 2006. Saturated fatty acids inhibit induction of insulin gene transcription by JNK-mediated phosphorylation of insulin-receptor substrates. *Proc Natl Acad Sci USA* 103:16454–9.

Sylvester, S. L., C. M. ap Rhys, J. D. Luethy-Martindale, and N. J. Holbrook. 1994. Induction of GADD153, a CCAAT/enhancer-binding protein (C/EBP)-related gene, during the acute phase response in rats. Evidence for the involvement of C/EBPs in regulating its expression. *J Biol Chem* 269:20119–25.

Tamaki, N., E. Hatano, K. Taura et al. 2008. CHOP deficiency attenuates cholestasis-induced liver fibrosis by reduction of hepatocyte injury. *Am J Physiol Gastrointest Liver Physiol* 294:G498–505.

Tanaka, E., and Y. Funae. 1996. Trimethadione: Metabolism and assessment of hepatic drug-oxidizing capacity. *Methods Enzymol* 272:163–9.

Tanaka, E., M. Terada, and S. Misawa. 2000. Cytochrome P450 2E1: Its clinical and toxico-logical role. *J Clin Pharm Ther* 25:165–75.

Tobiume, K., A. Matsuzawa, T. Takahashi et al. 2001. ASK1 is required for sustained activa-tions of JNK/p38 MAP kinases and apoptosis. *EMBO Rep* 2:222–8.

Upton, J. P., L. Wang, D. Han et al. 2012. IRE1alpha cleaves select microRNAs during ER stress to derepress translation of proapoptotic caspase-2. *Science* 338:818–22.

Urano, F., X. Wang, A. Bertolotti et al. 2000. Coupling of stress in the ER to activation of JNK protein kinases by transmembrane protein kinase IRE1. *Science* 287:664–6.

Vesell, E. S., T. D. Seaton, and A. Rahim YI. 1995. Studies on interindividual variations of CYP2E1 using chlorzoxazone as an in vivo probe. *Pharmacogenetics* 5:53–7.

Walker, U. A., J. Bauerle, M. Laguno et al. 2004. Depletion of mitochondrial DNA in liver under antiretroviral therapy with didanosine, stavudine, or zalcitabine. *Hepatology* 39: 311–7.

Watmough, N. J., L. A. Bindoff, M. A. Birch-Machin et al. 1990. Impaired mitochondrial beta-oxidation in a patient with an abnormality of the respiratory chain. Studies in skeletal muscle mitochondria. *J Clin Invest* 85:177–84.

Weltman, M. D., G. C. Farrell, P. Hall, M. Ingelman-Sundberg, and C. Liddle. 1998. Hepatic cytochrome P450 2E1 is increased in patients with nonalcoholic steatohepatitis. *Hepatology* 27:128–33.

Werstuck, G. H., S. R. Lentz, S. Dayal et al. 2001. Homocysteine-induced endoplasmic reticu-lum stress causes dysregulation of the cholesterol and triglyceride biosynthetic path-ways. *J Clin Invest* 107:1263–73.

Williams, J. A., R. Hyland, B. C. Jones et al. 2004. Drug-drug interactions for UDP-glucuronosyltransferase substrates: A pharmacokinetic explanation for typically observed low exposure (AUCi/AUC) ratios. *Drug Metab Dispos* 32:1201–8.

Woolf, T. F., W. F. Pool, S. M. Bjorge et al. 1993. Bioactivation and irreversible binding of the cognition activator tacrine using human and rat liver microsomal preparations. Species difference. *Drug Metab Dispos* 21:874–82.

Yamamoto, K., K. Takahara, S. Oyadomari et al. 2010. Induction of liver steatosis and lipid droplet formation in ATF6alpha-knockout mice burdened with pharmacological endo-plasmic reticulum stress. *Mol Biol Cell* 21:2975–86.

Yang, J. J., H. Tao, C. Huang, and J. Li. 2013. Nuclear erythroid 2-related factor 2: A novel potential therapeutic target for liver fibrosis. *Food Chem Toxicol* 59:421–7.

Yoshida, H., T. Matsui, A. Yamamoto, T. Okada, and K. Mori. 2001. XBP1 mRNA is induced by ATF6 and spliced by IRE1 in response to ER stress to produce a highly active tran-scription factor. *Cell* 107:881–91.

Zha, B. S., X. Wan, X. Zhang et al. 2013. HIV protease inhibitors disrupt lipid metabolism by activating endoplasmic reticulum stress and inhibiting autophagy activity in adipocytes. *PLoS One* 8:e59514.

Zhang, K., S. Wang, J. Malhotra et al. 2011. The unfolded protein response transducer IRE1alpha prevents ER stress-induced hepatic steatosis. *EMBO J* 30:1357–75.

Zhang, Y. K., R. L. Yeager, Y. Tanaka, and C. D. Klaassen. 2010. Enhanced expression of Nrf2 in mice attenuates the fatty liver produced by a methionine- and choline-deficient diet. *Toxicol Appl Pharmacol* 245:326–34.

Zhou, S. F. 2008. Drugs behave as substrates, inhibitors and inducers of human cytochrome P450 3A4. *Curr Drug Metab* 9:310–22.

Zhou, S. F., E. Chan, Z. W. Zhou, C. C. Xue, X. Lai, and W. Duan. 2009. Insights into the structure, function, and regulation of human cytochrome P450 1A2. *Curr Drug Metab* 10:713–29.

Zimmerman, H. J. 1981. Effects of aspirin and acetaminophen on the liver. *Arch Intern Med* 141:333–42.

5 The Role of the Keap1/Nrf2 Pathway in the Development and Progression of Nonalcoholic Fatty Liver Disease

Dionysios V. Chartoumpekis
and Thomas W. Kensler

CONTENTS

Keap1–Nrf2 PATHWAY

Nrf2 (Nf-e2-related factor 2–like 2) is a transcription factor that is a central mediator of the adaptive response to endogenous and exogenous oxidative or electrophilic stresses (Kensler et al., 2007). It belongs to the family of the cap n' collar transcription factors with a basic leucine zipper along with its invertebrate homologues SKN-1 (*Caenorhabditis elegans*) and CncC (*Drosophila melanogaster*). They are all of essential importance in cytoprotective responses against stressors (Sykiotis and Bohmann, 2010; Kobayashi and Yamamoto, 2006). Nrf2 structurally consists of six conserved Nrf2–ECH homology domains (Neh 1–6). Small avian musculoaponeurotic fibrosarcoma AS42 oncogene homologue (Maf) proteins mainly form heterodimers with Nrf2 through interaction with its Neh1 domain that also contains the basic leucine zipper that binds to the antioxidant response element (ARE) sequences (5′-NTGAG/CNNNGC-3′) in the regulatory domains of the Nrf2 target genes and leads to their expression. Nrf2 target genes regulate conjugation/detoxication reactions (e.g., glutathione S-transferases [Gsts]), antioxidative responses, such as NADPH quinine oxidoreductase (Nqo1), and proteasome function (proteasome subunits), among many gene functions (Kwak et al., 2003).

The major negative regulator of Nrf2 is the Kelch-like ECH-associated protein 1 (Keap1) (Itoh et al., 1999), which is a cysteine-rich zinc metalloprotein that binds to the Neh2 Nrf2 domain in the cytoplasm through its double glycine repeat domain (DGR). When Nrf2 is bound to Keap1, it is marked for proteasomal degradation after a Keap1-facilitated ubiquitin conjugation. Other elements of the complex that facilitate Nrf2 ubiquitination include the ring-box 1 E3 ubiquitin protein ligase (Rbx1) and cullin 3 (Cul3), which binds to the BTB domain (Drosophila broad-complex C, Tramtrack, and Bric-a-brac) of Keap1 (Kobayashi et al., 2004). Upon oxidative or electrophilic stress, reactive cysteines of Keap1 are modified and Keap1 undergoes conformational changes that lead to disruption or dissociation of the Keap1-Nrf2 complex and thus to rescue of Nrf2 from Keap1-mediated proteasomal degradation (Wakabayashi et al., 2004). The "hinge and latch" model for the Keap1–Nrf2 complex structure suggests that one Nrf2 molecule interacts with 2 Keap1 molecules; the "hinge" represents a high-affinity interaction of Nrf2 with the one Keap1 molecule, whereas the "latch" represents a low-affinity interaction of Nrf2 with the other Keap1 molecule (Tong et al., 2006). The latter is the one that is disrupted by the modification of the Keap1-reactive cysteines, and consequently, Nrf2 is not properly presented for ubiquitination/proteasomal degradation. Hence, in response to stress signals, Nrf2 accumulates and can translocate to the nucleus and induce the expression of its target genes.

Acetylation and/or phosphorylation of Nrf2 have been described to affect the nuclear levels of Nrf2 after its release from Keap1. Specifically, CREB-binding protein induces Nrf2 acetylation and enhances its binding to the ARE sequences in the regulatory regions of its target genes. On the contrary, sirtuin 1 decreases Nrf2 acetylation and facilitates its nuclear export (Kawai et al., 2011). Nrf2 phosphorylation by PKR-like endoplasmic reticulum kinase (PERK) (Cullinan et al., 2003) or by phosphoinositide 3 kinase (PI3K) (Lee et al., 2001) has been described to enhance Nrf2-driven transcription, but its phosphorylation by Fyn enhances nuclear export of Nrf2 (Niture et al., 2011). Figure 5.1 summarizes the dynamic elements of the Keap1/Nrf2 pathway.

The regulation of cytoprotective enzymes by Nrf2 and its seemingly ubiquitous expression in mammalian cells has intrigued researchers to study the role of Nrf2 in a variety of pathologies. The main model used so far has been the Nrf2$^{-/-}$ mouse (Chan et al., 1996; Itoh et al., 1997). Nrf2$^{-/-}$ mice are viable, but they have been shown to have increased sensitivity to acetaminophen-induced hepatoxicity (Enomoto et al., 2001; Chan et al., 2001), cigarette smoke–induced emphysema (Rangasamy et al., 2004), chemical-induced gastric carcinogenesis (Ramos-Gomez et al., 2001), and neurodegenerative inflammatory diseases (Johnson et al., 2008). Systemic

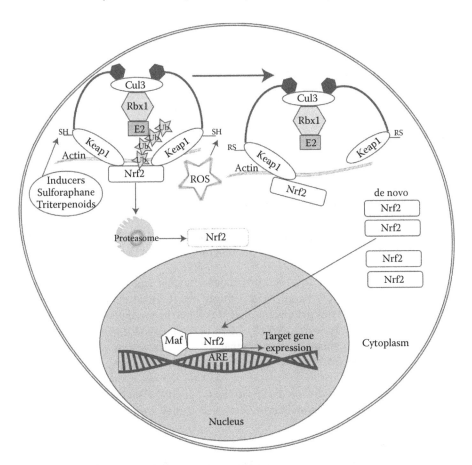

FIGURE 5.1   A brief schematic representation of the Keap1/Nrf2 pathway. Under basal conditions, one Nrf2 molecule is bound to two Keap1 molecules with different affinities according to the hinge and latch model; "hinge" represents a high-affinity interaction and "latch" represents a low-affinity interaction. Nrf2 is marked for proteasomal degradation after a Keap1-facilitated ubiquitination. Upon exposure to inducers (sulforaphane, triterpenoids) or to ROS, which reacts with specific Keap1 cysteines, the low-affinity Keap1–Nrf2 interaction is disrupted, rendering the Keap1–Nrf2 complex inactive and sparing Nrf2 from proteasomal degradation. Thus, de novo–synthesized Nrf2 escapes the Keap1-mediated proteasomal degradation and can enter the nucleus and induce the expression of its target genes.

Keap1$^{-/-}$ mice were established to verify in vivo the negative regulation of Keap1 on Nrf2, but resulted in mice that, although viable, die within 2 weeks postnatally due to malnutrition because of esophageal hyperkeratosis (Wakabayashi et al., 2003). Interestingly, this phenotype is rescued in double knockout mice (Keap1$^{-/-}$:Nrf2$^{-/-}$).

Given the postnatal lethality of the Keap1$^{-/-}$ mice and the need for a genetic model of Nrf2 activation, Keap1$^{flox/flox}$ mice were generated to conditionally delete Keap1 in tissues of interest (Okawa et al., 2006). However, the resultant Keap1^{flox} allele is hypomorphic, and this mouse can be used as a gain of Nrf2 function model (Taguchi et al., 2010). This genetic activation of the Keap1/Nrf2 pathway resulted in protective effects against toxic insults such as acetaminophen (Okawa et al., 2006).

This protective effect increased the interest in the evaluation of small-molecule inducers of the Keap1/Nrf2 pathway as they could be potentially used in clinical trials in disease prevention settings. Triterpenoids, dithiolethiones, and isothiocyanates are chemical inducers of Nrf2 that mainly modify reactive cysteines in Keap1 (Wakabayashi et al., 2004). The triterpenoid CDDO-Me (Pergola et al., 2011) and the isothiocyanate sulforaphane (in the form of broccoli sprouts extracts) (Egner et al., 2011; Kensler et al., 2013) have been used in clinical trials and have proved the feasibility of pharmacological activation of the Keap1/Nrf2 pathway in humans. However, the early termination of a phase III clinical study (NCT01351675) using CDDO-Me in patients with stage 4 chronic kidney disease and type 2 diabetes for the assessment of the prevention of the progression to end-stage renal disease revealed the need for further investigation in the safety/efficacy of triterpenoids in a variety of clinical settings. Whether the adverse events were "on" or "off" target effects has not been revealed as yet.

The use of the genetically modified mouse models and the pharmacological interventions affecting the Keap1/Nrf2 pathway has revealed the potential of Nrf2 involvement in a variety of pathologies that are related to susceptibility to oxidative/electrophilic stresses. However, Nrf2 has also been shown to cross-talk with other transcription factor–regulated molecular pathways (Wakabayashi et al., 2010) that influence cellular metabolism and especially lipogenesis and obesity (Chartoumpekis and Kensler, 2013). Therefore, the role of Nrf2 on the development and progression of NAFLD, which will be discussed next, cannot be limited only to its well described cytoprotective/antioxidant effects, but it may include direct or indirect metabolic effects.

ROLE OF Nrf2 IN MURINE MODELS OF FATTY LIVER DISEASE

COMMON MODELS OF DIET-INDUCED STEATOSIS

The majority of the studies on the role of the Keap1/Nrf2 pathway in the development and progression of fatty liver disease have been performed using mouse models. Initial focus will be on the most common diets that are used to induce fatty liver in mice, as different diets cause accumulation of fat in the liver through different mechanisms. Therefore, it is important to evaluate the data emanating from the various studies on diet-induced fatty liver taking into account the diet type and the underlying molecular mechanisms of fat accumulation in the liver.

The methionine–choline-deficient diet (MCD) is the most common diet used in mouse experiments, as it can cause a fatty liver phenotype within a short feeding period (within 3–4 weeks). The MCD diet can also lead to inflammation (steatohepatitis) and ultimately fibrosis if the feeding period is extended to about 6 weeks or more. This liver injury caused by MCD in mice recapitulates histologically the features of human nonalcoholic steatohepatitis (NASH), namely steatosis, intralobular inflammation, and hepatocellular ballooning (Takahashi et al., 2012). It appears that one of the major mechanisms of triglyceride accumulation after MCD feeding in mice involves the impaired secretion of very-low-density lipoproteins (VLDL) because of the lack of phosphatidyl-choline synthesis that is the main phospholipid that coats the VLDL particles (Rinella et al., 2008). However, mice fed an MCD diet lose weight (50% weight loss after 10 weeks on the regimen compared with the mice fed a control diet), have low plasma triglycerides, and reduced liver to body weight ratios (Anstee and Goldin, 2006). Therefore, even though the histological liver characteristics of MCD-fed mice resemble human NAFLD and NASH, the phenotype is unrelated to the obese, insulin-resistant, dyslipidemic, and diabetic phenotype in humans with NAFLD.

The high-fat diet (HFD) is also another commonly used regimen that induces obesity and insulin resistance in the C57BL6J mice along with liver steatosis (Surwit et al., 1988). However, the time required to induce liver steatosis in mice fed a HFD is considerably longer (months) than the mice fed an MCD diet (weeks), but it has the advantage that the resulting obese, glucose intolerant phenotype is similar to the majority of humans with NAFLD. The HFDs are usually characterized by the percentage of calories that comes from the fat content of the diet with 40 and 60 kcal% fat diets being the most frequently used. A disadvantage of using the HFD as a model of dietary liver steatosis lies in the fact that the degree of steatosis, inflammation, and fibrosis is highly variable and is dependent on the percentage of calories from fat, the source, and type of fat (animal, plant, or combined, saturated or polyunsaturated) and of course the duration of feeding (Takahashi et al., 2012). Moreover, the degree of steatosis produced by a HFD is usually milder when compared with the MCD diet (Anstee and Goldin, 2006). Hence, it is of high importance to state the exact ingredients of the diet used in each experiment as some discrepancies that exist among different studies may be due to differences in the composition of the diet.

EFFECT OF MANIPULATION OF THE KEAP1/NRF2 PATHWAY ON NAFLD DEVELOPMENT AND PROGRESSION

MCD-Induced Steatosis

It has been described that mice with deletion of *Nrf2* develop more severe steatosis and steatohepatitis when fed an MCD diet than wild-type mice. Specifically, when male Nrf2$^{-/-}$ mice were fed an MCD diet for 2 weeks, they accumulated about twice as many lipids in their livers and had increased inflammation (NASH) as evidenced by increased accumulation of neutrophils and Councilman's bodies (Chowdhry et al., 2010). A longer-term MCD feeding (3 and 6 weeks) resulted in a comparable but more pronounced phenotype of liver lipid accumulation, inflammation and fibrosis (Sugimoto et al., 2010). When the Keap1$^{flox/flox}$ mice, whose Keap1^{flox} allele is hypomorphic and, thus, a model of intermediate gain of Nrf2 function, were fed an MCD diet for 5 days, they accumulated significantly less fat in their livers compared with their wild-type counterparts (Zhang et al., 2010). Therefore, it can be concluded that Nrf2 can have a protective effect against the development of MCD-induced hepatic steatosis and steatohepatitis in mice. The exact mechanisms underlying this protective effect of Nrf2 remain to be elucidated.

However, based on the already available data, it is possible to describe the role of Nrf2 in the accumulation of triglycerides in the liver (simple steatosis) and in the progression to steatohepatitis. Nrf2 is a well described central orchestrator of antioxidant and cytoprotective gene expression, and the progression from simple steatosis to NASH is associated with the toxic effects of lipid peroxidation products and the production of reactive oxygen species (ROS) (Seki et al., 2002). Thus, it has been hypothesized that Nrf2 can delay the progression from simple steatosis to NASH by inducing cytoprotective enzymes and minimizing the deleterious effects of oxidative stress. Indeed, the Nrf2$^{-/-}$ mice had lower reduced glutathione levels (GSH) and increased oxidized glutathione levels (GSSG) than the wild type after MCD feeding (Chowdhry et al., 2010; Sugimoto et al., 2010). The lower GSH levels in the Nrf2$^{-/-}$ after MCD may be caused by the lower levels of γ-glutamyl cysteine synthetase (γ-GCS) and of glutamate cysteine ligase catalytic subunit (GCLC) in these mice. Moreover, the reduced expression of catalase and superoxide dismutase (SOD), two enzymes that can eliminate ROS, in the Nrf2$^{-/-}$ livers after MCD contributes to the increased sensitivity of tissues in the Nrf2$^{-/-}$ mice to oxidative damage. Thus, loss of Nrf2 makes the hepatocytes more vulnerable to their exposure to oxidative stress after MCD. This increased hepatocyte damage in the Nrf2$^{-/-}$ mice after MCD treatment is reflected by the higher alanine transaminase (ALT) and aspartate aminotransferase (AST) levels in serum of these mice (Sugimoto et al., 2010).

Besides the apparent cytoprotective effect of Nrf2 in the hepatocytes after MCD feeding that can at least partially protect from the development of steatohepatitis, Nrf2 can also play a role in the initial step of lipid accumulation in the liver that leads to simple steatosis. Studies using mRNA microarray analysis in liver from mice with an activated Nrf2 pathway (Yates et al., 2009) or proteomic analysis in livers of Nrf2$^{-/-}$ mice (Kitteringham et al., 2010) have shown that Nrf2 may repress the expression of genes involved in lipid metabolism. Specifically, such a gene is the one encoding the adipose differentiation-related protein (ADRP), which is known to increase in fatty liver disease in humans and mice and plays a role in lipid accumulation and lipid droplet formation (Okumura, 2011). Expression of ADRP was found elevated in the livers of Nrf2$^{-/-}$ mice under MCD (Chowdhry et al., 2010) and decreased in mice with activated Nrf2 signaling in their livers fed a standard diet (Yates et al., 2009). Although the exact molecular mechanism through which Nrf2 may repress the expression of these genes is not clear yet, the existing data support an interesting role of Nrf2 during the development of simple liver steatosis beyond the well-described cytoprotective one.

HFD-Induced Steatosis

As described earlier, HFD feeding of C57BL6J mice leads to a phenotype relevant to humans with NAFLD (obesity, insulin resistance). However, the degree of HFD-induced steatosis in mice is much lower compared with the MCD model and requires longer feeding periods. The use of high-fat diets of different compositions by various research groups has made it even more complicated to draw conclusions by comparing the different studies. Although the number of studies on Nrf2 and obesity is significant, they have focused more in describing the resulting phenotype and less on the

liver steatosis itself. Briefly, it has been shown that Nrf2 deletion may partially protect from obesity and insulin resistance (Chartoumpekis et al., 2011; Pi et al., 2010;
Meher et al., 2012) through reduced expression of peroxisome proliferator–activated
receptor γ (PPAR-γ) in adipose tissue (Pi et al., 2010) or increased levels of fibroblast growth factor 21 (FGF21) in serum, adipose tissue, and liver (Chartoumpekis
et al., 2011). Interestingly, the genetic gain of Nrf2 function (Uruno et al., 2013) or
the pharmacological activation of Keap1/Nrf2 pathway with CDDO-Im (Shin et al.,
2009) also partially prevent HFD-induced obesity through increased energy expenditure via mechanisms that require further investigation.

As far as the degree of liver steatosis is concerned in the HFD-induced obesity
mouse models, treatment with CDDO-Im (30 μmol/kg body weight) 3 times a week
resulted in about 50% less hepatic lipid accumulation, as judged by oil-red-O staining, compared with the vehicle-treated mice when fed a 60 kcal% fat HFD for 3
months (Shin et al., 2009). Similarly, mice that have been rendered obese after being
fed a 40 kcal% fat HFD for 3 months and then treated with CDDO-Me for 2 weeks,
had lower total lipids levels in their livers than the vehicle-treated animals (Saha et
al., 2010).

Meanwhile, when Nrf2$^{-/-}$ mice were challenged with an atherogenic plus high-
fat diet, which is a modified high-fat diet (Matsuzawa et al., 2007), they developed
significantly more hepatic steatosis after 24 weeks on this diet than the wild-type
under the same regimen as evidenced by increased hepatic triglycerides levels
(Okada et al., 2013). Moreover, the Nrf2$^{-/-}$ mice developed more severe steatohepatitis and more fibrosis as shown by the elevated inflammatory cell counts and
a larger fibrotic area.

The underlying molecular mechanisms through which Nrf2 may mediate this
effect on hepatic steatosis after HFD are not clarified yet. Nevertheless, there are
some proposed pathways described in these studies involving Nrf2 cross-talk.
Specifically, deletion of Nrf2 leads to increased hepatic levels of sterol regulatory
element-binding protein 1c (SREBP-1c), fatty acid synthase (FAS), and acetyl-CoA
carboxylase 1 (ACC1) after an atherogenic plus HFD (Okada et al., 2013), whereas
pharmacological activation of the Keap1/Nrf2 pathway with CDDO-Me in already
HFD-induced obese mice led to the opposite results with reference to the expression
of the above genes (Saha et al., 2010). These three genes that seem to be repressed
by Nrf2 activity encode proteins that catalyze pivotal steps in fatty acid synthesis
or regulate transcription of genes implicated in this process. SREBP-1c enhances
transcription of genes required for fatty acid synthesis such as ATP citrate lyase
(acetyl-CoA production) and acetyl-CoA carboxylase and FAS (Horton et al., 2002).
ACC1 catalyzes the carboxylation of acetyl-CoA to malonyl-CoA, which is the rate-
limiting step in fatty acid biosynthesis. FAS mainly catalyzes the synthesis of palmitate from acetyl-CoA and malonyl-CoA, in the presence of NADPH, into long-chain
saturated fatty acids. Moreover, another interesting finding that may contribute to
the reduction in liver steatosis after treatment with CDDO-Me is that treatment with
this triterpenoid can increase the phosphorylation of AMP-activated protein kinase
(AMPK) (Saha et al., 2010). AMPK is a heterotrimeric protein complex that consists
of an α catalytic subunit and two (β and γ) regulatory subunits and acts as a cellular
energy sensor that is activated by an increased AMP/ATP ratio (Hardie, 2004). The

primary phosphorylation of the α catalytic subunit occurs at Thr172. The activated AMPK can phosphorylate ACC1 at Ser79 (Brownsey et al., 2006) and SREBP-1c at Ser 372 (Li et al., 2011). Both these phosphorylations have an inhibitory effect and lead to reduced lipogenesis in the liver.

Keap1/Nrf2 PATHWAY ACTIVATION IN HUMANS WITH NAFLD

Studies on the role of Nrf2 in the development and progression of NAFLD in humans are limited and retrospective and rely on liver samples from tissue banks. Characterization of the expression of Nrf2 and its target genes in different stages of NAFLD, ranging from normal livers to steatotic, NASH (fatty) and NASH (non-fatty), gave an insight on the potential role of Nrf2 during the progression of this disease (Hardwick et al., 2010). First, Nrf2-positive hepatocyte nuclei were 10 times more frequent in the various stages of NAFLD compared with the normal livers. The expression and activity of NQO1, a prototypical target gene of Nrf2, were also significantly increased, mainly in the NASH stages of NAFLD. Second, the ratio of GSH/GSSG in the liver tended to decrease and levels of malondialdehyde (a product of lipid peroxidation and thus an indirect indicator of oxidative stress) tended to increase through the progressive NAFLD stages. This evidence would lead to the conclusion that as oxidative stress is increased during NAFLD progression, the Keap1/Nrf2 pathway is activated, but GSH is depleted due to the increasing oxidative stress. GSH synthesis itself did not seem to be dysregulated during NAFLD. In another study, NASH livers were compared with normal ones and increased oxidative stress levels (as estimated indirectly by 8-hydroxydeoxyguanosine,an oxidized DNA nucleoside) were found as well (Takahashi et al., 2014). Increased nuclear Nrf2 protein levels along with enhanced expression of some potential Nrf2 target genes such as γ-GCS and glutathione peroxidase 2 showed that the Keap1/Nrf2 pathway is also activated in these NASH liver samples presumably due to the increased oxidative stress.

CONCLUSIONS

All the studies in the mouse models of NAFLD and in the human samples converge to the fact that oxidative stress is increased during the progression of NAFLD, and this stress, in turn, can cause activation of the Keap1/Nrf2 pathway. However, this adaptive response of pathway activation is not sufficient enough to counteract the deleterious effects of oxidative stress and NAFLD gradually progresses. The importance of Nrf2 as a brake in the progression of NAFLD is highlighted by observations that Nrf2$^{-/-}$ mice undergo a rapid transition to NASH compared with the wild type. Another role of Nrf2, beyond its cytoprotective one, as a putative repressor of lipogenic gene expression is highlighted in the mouse models in the initial stages of NAFLD that lead to simple steatosis. The potential roles of Nrf2 during the progression of NAFLD are shown in Figure 5.2. Therefore, Nrf2 appears to be an attractive target for preventing the progression of NAFLD. Pharmacological intervention with triterpenoids or isothiocyanates may be considered a therapeutic/preventive option for NAFLD in the future.

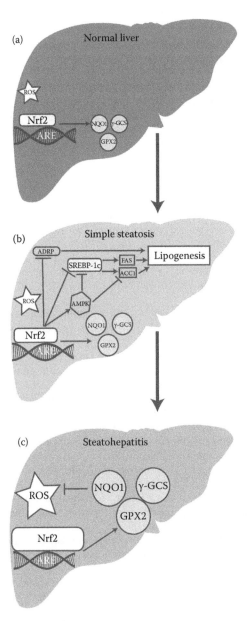

FIGURE 5.2   Main roles of Nrf2 during the progression of NAFLD. (a) Under basal conditions, Nrf2 regulates the constitutive expression of its target genes (mainly antioxidant/cytoprotective genes). (b) As NAFLD progresses to simple steatosis, Nrf2 may also cross-talk with pathways that lead to the repression of genes that favor lipogenesis. (c) When NAFLD has progressed to the steatohepatitis stage, which is characterized by increased oxidative stress and activation of inflammatory pathways, the role of Nrf2 as an orchestrator of antioxidant/cytoprotective gene expression is accentuated. Induction, →; repression, ⊥. The different sizes of the drawings are representative of the differential level of expression of the depicted genes during the progression of NAFLD.

REFERENCES

Anstee, Q. M., and R. D. Goldin. 2006. Mouse models in non-alcoholic fatty liver disease and steatohepatitis research. *Int J Exp Pathol* 87:1–16.

Brownsey, R. W., A. N. Boone, J. E. Elliott, J. E. Kulpa, and W. M. Lee. 2006. Regulation of acetyl-CoA carboxylase. *Biochem Soc Trans* 34:223–7.

Chan, K., X. D. Han, and Y. W. Kan. 2001. An important function of Nrf2 in combating oxidative stress: Detoxification of acetaminophen. *Proc Natl Acad Sci USA* 98:4611–6.

Chan, K., R. Lu, J. C. Chang, and Y. W. Kan. 1996. NRF2, a member of the NFE2 family of transcription factors, is not essential for murine erythropoiesis, growth, and development. *Proc Natl Acad Sci USA* 93:13943–8.

Chartoumpekis, D. V., and T. W. Kensler. 2013. New player on an old field; the keap1/Nrf2 pathway as a target for treatment of type 2 diabetes and metabolic syndrome. *Curr Diabetes Rev* 9:137–45.

Chartoumpekis, D. V., P. G. Ziros, A. I. Psyrogiannis et al. 2011. Nrf2 represses FGF21 during long-term high-fat diet-induced obesity in mice. *Diabetes* 60:2465–73.

Chowdhry, S., M. H. Nazmy, P. J. Meakin et al. 2010. Loss of Nrf2 markedly exacerbates nonalcoholic steatohepatitis. *Free Radic Biol Med* 48:357–71.

Cullinan, S. B., D. Zhang, M. Hannink, E. Arvisais, R. J. Kaufman, and J. A. Diehl. 2003. Nrf2 is a direct PERK substrate and effector of PERK-dependent cell survival. *Mol Cell Biol* 23:7198–209.

Egner, P. A., J. G. Chen, J. B. Wang et al. 2011. Bioavailability of Sulforaphane from two broccoli sprout beverages: Results of a short-term, cross-over clinical trial in Qidong, China. *Cancer Prev Res (Phila)* 4:384–95.

Enomoto, A., K. Itoh, E. Nagayoshi et al. 2001. High sensitivity of Nrf2 knockout mice to acetaminophen hepatotoxicity associated with decreased expression of ARE-regulated drug metabolizing enzymes and antioxidant genes. *Toxicol Sci* 59:169–77.

Hardie, D. G. 2004. The AMP-activated protein kinase pathway—New players upstream and downstream. *J Cell Sci* 117:5479–87.

Hardwick, R. N., C. D. Fisher, M. J. Canet, A. D. Lake, and N. J. Cherrington. 2010. Diversity in antioxidant response enzymes in progressive stages of human nonalcoholic fatty liver disease. *Drug Metab Dispos* 38:2293–301.

Horton, J. D., J. L. Goldstein, and M. S. Brown. 2002. SREBPs: Activators of the complete program of cholesterol and fatty acid synthesis in the liver. *J Clin Invest* 109:1125–31.

Itoh, K., T. Chiba, S. Takahashi et al. 1997. An Nrf2/small Maf heterodimer mediates the induction of phase II detoxifying enzyme genes through antioxidant response elements. *Biochem Biophys Res Commun* 236:313–22.

Itoh, K., N. Wakabayashi, Y. Katoh et al. 1999. Keap1 represses nuclear activation of antioxidant responsive elements by Nrf2 through binding to the amino-terminal Neh2 domain. *Genes Dev* 13:76–86.

Johnson, J. A., D. A. Johnson, A. D. Kraft et al. 2008. The Nrf2-ARE pathway: An indicator and modulator of oxidative stress in neurodegeneration. *Ann N Y Acad Sci* 1147:61–9.

Kawai, Y., L. Garduno, M. Theodore, J. Yang, and I. J. Arinze. 2011. Acetylation-deacetylation of the transcription factor Nrf2 (nuclear factor erythroid 2-related factor 2) regulates its transcriptional activity and nucleocytoplasmic localization. *J Biol Chem* 286:7629–40.

Kensler, T. W., P. A. Egner, A. S. Agyeman et al. 2013. Keap1-nrf2 signaling: A target for cancer prevention by sulforaphane. *Top Curr Chem* 329:163–77.

Kensler, T. W., N. Wakabayashi, and S. Biswal. 2007. Cell survival responses to environmental stresses via the Keap1-Nrf2-ARE pathway. *Annu Rev Pharmacol Toxicol* 47:89–116.

Kitteringham, N. R., A. Abdullah, J. Walsh et al. 2010. Proteomic analysis of Nrf2 deficient transgenic mice reveals cellular defence and lipid metabolism as primary Nrf2-dependent pathways in the liver. *J Proteomics* 73:1612–31.

Kobayashi, A., M. I. Kang, H. Okawa et al. 2004. Oxidative stress sensor Keap1 functions as an adaptor for Cul3-based E3 ligase to regulate proteasomal degradation of Nrf2. *Mol Cell Biol* 24:7130–9.

Kobayashi, M., and M. Yamamoto. 2006. Nrf2-Keap1 regulation of cellular defense mechanisms against electrophiles and reactive oxygen species. *Adv Enzyme Regul* 46:113–40.

Kwak, M. K., N. Wakabayashi, K. Itoh, H. Motohashi, M. Yamamoto, and T. W. Kensler. 2003. Modulation of gene expression by cancer chemopreventive dithiolethiones through the Keap1-Nrf2 pathway. Identification of novel gene clusters for cell survival. *J Biol Chem* 278:8135–45.

Lee, J. M., J. M. Hanson, W. A. Chu, and J. A. Johnson. 2001. Phosphatidylinositol 3-kinase, not extracellular signal-regulated kinase, regulates activation of the antioxidant-responsive element in IMR-32 human neuroblastoma cells. *J Biol Chem* 276:20011–6.

Li, Y., S. Xu, M. M. Mihaylova et al. 2011. AMPK phosphorylates and inhibits SREBP activity to attenuate hepatic steatosis and atherosclerosis in diet-induced insulin-resistant mice. *Cell Metab* 13:376–88.

Matsuzawa, N., T. Takamura, S. Kurita et al. 2007. Lipid-induced oxidative stress causes steatohepatitis in mice fed an atherogenic diet. *Hepatology* 46:1392–403.

Meher, A. K., P. R. Sharma, V. A. Lira et al. 2012. Nrf2 deficiency in myeloid cells is not sufficient to protect mice from high-fat diet-induced adipose tissue inflammation and insulin resistance. *Free Radic Biol Med* 52:1708–15.

Niture, S. K., A. K. Jain, P. M. Shelton, and A. K. Jaiswal. 2011. Src subfamily kinases regulate nuclear export and degradation of transcription factor Nrf2 to switch off Nrf2-mediated antioxidant activation of cytoprotective gene expression. *J Biol Chem* 286:28821–32.

Okada, K., E. Warabi, H. Sugimoto et al. 2013. Deletion of Nrf2 leads to rapid progression of steatohepatitis in mice fed atherogenic plus high-fat diet. *J Gastroenterol* 48:620–32.

Okawa, H., H. Motohashi, A. Kobayashi, H. Aburatani, T. W. Kensler, and M. Yamamoto. 2006. Hepatocyte-specific deletion of the keap1 gene activates Nrf2 and confers potent resistance against acute drug toxicity. *Biochem Biophys Res Commun* 339:79–88.

Okumura, T. 2011. Role of lipid droplet proteins in liver steatosis. *J Physiol Biochem* 67:629–36.

Pergola, P. E., P. Raskin, R. D. Toto et al. 2011. Bardoxolone methyl and kidney function in CKD with type 2 diabetes. *N Engl J Med* 365:327–36.

Pi, J., L. Leung, P. Xue et al. 2010. Deficiency in the nuclear factor E2-related factor-2 transcription factor results in impaired adipogenesis and protects against diet-induced obesity. *J Biol Chem* 285:9292–300.

Ramos-Gomez, M., M. K. Kwak, P. M. Dolan et al. 2001. Sensitivity to carcinogenesis is increased and chemoprotective efficacy of enzyme inducers is lost in nrf2 transcription factor-deficient mice. *Proc Natl Acad Sci USA* 98:3410–5.

Rangasamy, T., C. Y. Cho, R. K. Thimmulappa et al. 2004. Genetic ablation of Nrf2 enhances susceptibility to cigarette smoke-induced emphysema in mice. *J Clin Invest* 114:1248–59.

Rinella, M. E., M. S. Elias, R. R. Smolak, T. Fu, J. Borensztajn, and R. M. Green. 2008. Mechanisms of hepatic steatosis in mice fed a lipogenic methionine choline-deficient diet. *J Lipid Res* 49:1068–76.

Saha, P. K., V. T. Reddy, M. Konopleva, M. Andreeff, and L. Chan. 2010. The triterpenoid 2-cyano-3,12-dioxooleana-1,9-dien-28-oic-acid methyl ester has potent anti-diabetic effects in diet-induced diabetic mice and Lepr(*db/db*) mice. *J Biol Chem* 285:40581–92.

Seki, S., T. Kitada, T. Yamada, H. Sakaguchi, K. Nakatani, and K. Wakasa. 2002. In situ detection of lipid peroxidation and oxidative DNA damage in non-alcoholic fatty liver diseases. *J Hepatol* 37:56–62.

Shin, S., J. Wakabayashi, M. S. Yates et al. 2009. Role of Nrf2 in prevention of high-fat diet-induced obesity by synthetic triterpenoid CDDO-imidazolide. *Eur J Pharmacol* 620:138–44.

Sugimoto, H., K. Okada, J. Shoda et al. 2010. Deletion of nuclear factor-E2-related factor-2 leads to rapid onset and progression of nutritional steatohepatitis in mice. *Am J Physiol Gastrointest Liver Physiol* 298:G283–94.

Surwit, R. S., C. M. Kuhn, C. Cochrane, J. A. McCubbin, and M. N. Feinglos. 1988. Diet-induced type II diabetes in C57BL/6J mice. *Diabetes* 37:1163–7.

Sykiotis, G. P., and D. Bohmann. 2010. Stress-activated cap'n'collar transcription factors in aging and human disease. *Sci Signal* 3:doi:10.1126/scisignal.3112re3.

Taguchi, K., J. M. Maher, T. Suzuki, Y. Kawatani, H. Motohashi, and M. Yamamoto. 2010. Genetic analysis of cytoprotective functions supported by graded expression of Keap1. *Mol Cell Biol* 30:3016–26.

Takahashi, Y., Y. Kobayashi, K. Kawata et al. 2014. Does hepatic oxidative stress enhance activation of nuclear factor-E2-related factor in patients with non-alcoholic steatohepatitis? *Antioxid Redox Signal* 20:538–43.

Takahashi, Y., Y. Soejima, and T. Fukusato. 2012. Animal models of nonalcoholic fatty liver disease/nonalcoholic steatohepatitis. *World J Gastroenterol* 18:2300–8.

Tong, K. I., A. Kobayashi, F. Katsuoka, and M. Yamamoto. 2006. Two-site substrate recognition model for the Keap1-Nrf2 system: A hinge and latch mechanism. *Biol Chem* 387:1311–20.

Uruno, A., Y. Furusawa, Y. Yagishita et al. 2013. The Keap1-Nrf2 system prevents onset of diabetes mellitus. *Mol Cell Biol* 33:2996–3010.

Wakabayashi, N., A. T. Dinkova-Kostova, W. D. Holtzclaw et al. 2004. Protection against electrophile and oxidant stress by induction of the phase 2 response: Fate of cysteines of the Keap1 sensor modified by inducers. *Proc Natl Acad Sci USA* 101:2040–5.

Wakabayashi, N., K. Itoh, J. Wakabayashi et al. 2003. Keap1-null mutation leads to postnatal lethality due to constitutive Nrf2 activation. *Nat Genet* 35:238–45.

Wakabayashi, N., S. L. Slocum, J. J. Skoko, S. Shin, and T. W. Kensler. 2010. When NRF2 talks, who's listening? *Antioxid Redox Signal* 13:1649–63.

Yates, M. S., Q. T. Tran, P. M. Dolan et al. 2009. Genetic versus chemoprotective activation of Nrf2 signaling: Overlapping yet distinct gene expression profiles between Keap1 knock-out and triterpenoid-treated mice. *Carcinogenesis* 30:1024–31.

Zhang, Y. K., R. L. Yeager, Y. Tanaka, and C. D. Klaassen. 2010. Enhanced expression of Nrf2 in mice attenuates the fatty liver produced by a methionine- and choline-deficient diet. *Toxicol Appl Pharmacol* 245:326–34.

6 Methionine Adenosyltransferase Genes in Liver Health and Disease

Komal Ramani and Shelly C. Lu

CONTENTS

INTRODUCTION

Methionine is an essential amino acid whose metabolism in the liver is mediated by its conversion to S-adenosylmethionine (AdoMet), the methyl donor in mammalian cells. This reaction is catalyzed by methionine adenosyltransferases (MAT) (Lu and Mato, 2012). Three types of MAT proteins, MATα1, MATα2, and MATβ are encoded by *MAT1A*, *MAT2A*, and *MAT2B* genes, respectively (Mato et al., 2002). Variations in the expression of MAT isoenzymes have a long-standing relationship with liver diseases such as nonalcoholic steatohepatitis (NASH) (Martínez-Chantar et al., 2002a), liver cirrhosis (Martin-Duce et al., 1988), and hepatocellular carcinoma (HCC) (Cai et al., 1998). Mutations in the human *MAT1A* gene have been linked to hepatic MAT deficiency (OMIM number 250850), an inborn error of methionine metabolism in which patients have presented with isolated persistent hypermethioninemia (Gaull et al., 1981). In this chapter, we will describe the current knowledge on regulation and function of MAT genes in normal and diseased liver.

THE METHIONINE METABOLIC PATHWAY

The first step of the methionine metabolic pathway is the ATP-dependent conversion of dietary methionine to AdoMet that is catalyzed by MAT enzymes (EC 2.5.1.6) (Lu and Mato, 2012). AdoMet contains a high-energy sulfonium ion, which activates each of the attached carbons toward nucleophilic attack and confers on AdoMet the ability to participate in three major types of reactions: transmethylation, transsulfuration, and aminopropylation (Lu and Mato, 2012). In transmethylation reactions, AdoMet serves as the universal methyl donor to acceptors such as nucleic acids, proteins, phospholipids, and biologic amines (Mato et al., 1997). Although different enzymes catalyze these reactions, the common product of all methylation reactions is S-adenosylhomocysteine (AdoHcy). AdoMet-dependent methylation reactions are strongly inhibited by high AdoHcy and low AdoMet concentrations (Mato et al., 1997). Hence, AdoHcy needs to be rapidly removed after synthesis. AdoHcy is hydrolyzed to homocysteine and adenosine by AdoHcy hydrolase. This reaction is reversible and favors AdoHcy formation. It progresses toward hydrolysis only if the products, adenosine and homocysteine, are removed rapidly (Finkelstein, 1990). In transsulfuration reactions, cystathionine β-synthase catalyzes the vitamin-B6-dependent conversion of homocysteine and serine to form cystathionine. Cystathionine is further hydrolyzed by γ-cystathionase to form cysteine and α-ketobutyrate. Cysteine reacts with glutamate and glycine to form glutathione (GSH), an essential antioxidant (Lu, 2013). Homocysteine can also be used in remethylation pathways where it acquires a methyl group from N-5-methyltetrahydrofolate or from betaine to regenerate methionine (Lu and Mato, 2012). Aminopropylation for the synthesis of polyamines (spermine and spermidine) is another important function of AdoMet (Lu and Mato, 2012). AdoMet is decarboxylated by AdoMet decarboxylase and its aminopropyl group is transferred, first to putrescine to form spermidine and methylthioadenosine (MTA) and then to spermidine to form spermine and a second molecule of MTA (Mato et al., 2002). MTA produced during the synthesis of polyamines, is an inhibitor of methylation (Clarke, 2006). Under normal conditions, this pathway accounts for <5% of the available AdoMet, but this percentage is markedly enhanced under conditions of increased polyamine synthesis, such as liver regeneration (Lieber and Packer, 2002).

METHIONINE ADENOSYLTRANSFERASES

MAT Structure and Properties

Mammalian systems express three forms of MAT genes, namely *MAT1A*, *MAT2A*, and *MAT2B* (Kotb et al., 1997). The *MAT1A* gene encodes the 396 amino acid MATα1 catalytic subunit, which organizes into homodimers (MATIII) or homotetramers (MATI) (Kotb et al., 1997). The gene *MAT2A* encodes for a 395–amino acid MATα2 catalytic subunit that combines with a noncatalytic 334 amino acid regulatory β subunit encoded by *MAT2B* to form the MATII isoform of the enzyme. Data from isothermal titration calorimetry shows that MATα2 and β subunits form heterotrimers in which α2 dimers associate with a single β subunit (González et al., 2012). MATβ regulates the activity of MATII by lowering the inhibition constant (K_i) for AdoMet and the Michaelis constant (K_m) for methionine (Halim et al., 1999). In humans, four variants of the *MAT2B* gene have been described (Yang et al., 2008). Out of these, two main splicing forms, V1 and V2, are different in their transcription initiation sites located at positions −203 and −2372 upstream of the ATG codon, respectively. Thus, V2 uses a different exon 1, and the resulting proteins diverge in the initial 20 amino acids at their N-terminal (Yang et al., 2008). Isoforms of MAT differ in kinetic and regulatory properties and sensitivities to inhibitors (Mato et al., 2002). MAT II has the lowest K_m (~4–10 µM), MAT I has intermediate K_m (23 µM–1 µM), and MAT III has the highest K_m (215 µM–7 µM) for methionine (Sullivan and Hoffman, 1983). Although MAT isoenzymes catalyze the same reaction, they are differentially regulated by their product, AdoMet. AdoMet strongly inhibits MATII (50% inhibitory concentration [IC_{50}] = 60 µM), which is close to the normal intracellular AdoMet concentration (Finkelstein, 1990), whereas it minimally inhibits MATI (IC_{50} = 400 µM) and stimulates MATIII (up to 8-fold at 500 µM AdoMet) (Sullivan and Hoffman, 1983). Thus, the type of MAT isoform expressed in cells controls the steady state AdoMet level. Under normal physiological conditions, MATII activity is thought to contribute little to hepatic methionine metabolism in healthy, adult liver as opposed to MATI/III that maintains high levels of AdoMet synthesis (approximately 6–8 g/day) (Mato et al., 2002). Consistently, hepatic cell lines overexpressing *MAT1A* have increased accumulation of AdoMet as compared with cells expressing *MAT2A* (Cai et al., 1998; Li et al., 2010). Increased expression of *MAT2B* can further lower steady state AdoMet level due to influence of MATβ on the K_i of MATII for AdoMet (Martínez-Chantar et al., 2003).

MAT Expression and Subcellular Localization

MAT1A is expressed mostly in liver (Gil et al., 1996) and pancreas with high level of expression seen in pancreatic acinar cells (Lu et al., 2003). *MAT2A* is widely expressed in extrahepatic tissues and is also expressed in fetal liver, but is replaced by *MAT1A* during development (Horikawa and Tsukada, 1992). Hence, *MAT1A* can be considered as a marker of adult, differentiated liver. Within the liver, there is differential expression of MAT proteins in various cell types. Hepatocytes express the MATα1 isoenzyme only, whereas Kupffer cells and endothelial cells express both MATα1 and MATα2 proteins (Shimizu-Saito et al., 1997). Hepatic stellate cells (HSCs) express the MATα2 isoenzyme, but not MATα1 (Shimizu-Saito et al., 1997). HSCs also express the MATβ regulatory subunit (Ramani et al. 2010).

Reytor et al. (2009) have shown that the MATI/III enzyme exhibits two partially overlapping areas in its carboxy terminal that regulate cytoplasmic and nuclear localization of this protein. The group also identified tetrameric and monomeric forms of MATα1 subunit in the nucleus. These findings support the role of MATα1 in providing a source of nuclear AdoMet. Accumulation of active MATα1 protein in the nucleus correlates with higher levels of histone H3K27 trimethylation, an epigenetic modification associated with gene repression and DNA methylation (Reytor et al., 2009). The MATII isoenzyme is localized both in the cytoplasm and the nucleus. A functional effect of MATII nuclear localization has recently been described. Nuclear MATα2 in conjunction with MATβ acts as a corepressor of the small maf oncoprotein, mafK, by its interaction with chromatin regulators and by supplying AdoMet for histone methylation (Katoh et al., 2011).

Variants of MATβ are localized both in the cytoplasm and the nucleus of human HCC cell lines. They also interact with the mRNA stabilizing protein, human RNA binding (HuR) (Xia et al., 2010). HuR is essentially a nuclear protein (Fan and Steitz, 1998). Forced expression of MATβ in liver cancer cells increases the cytoplasmic content of HuR and enhances the expression of HuR target genes (Xia et al., 2010). Interactions between MATβ and sirtuin 1 (a protein known to contribute to HCC tumorigenicity and chemotherapy resistance) have been shown in the nucleus as well as the cytoplasm of human HCC cell lines (Yang et al., 2013a). Interestingly, cross-talk among MATβ, sirtuin 1, and HuR impacts the pro-apoptotic and growth suppressive effects of a small molecule, resveratrol, in HCC (Yang et al., 2013a). Overall, these findings show that subcellular localization of MAT proteins has distinct functional impact on liver cancer cells.

MAT PROTEIN MODIFICATIONS

Covalent modifications of rat and human MATα1 on cysteine at position 121 have been described (Perez-Mato et al., 1999). This residue is present in a flexible loop over the active site cleft of rat MATα1. Nitrosylation or oxidation of cysteine 121 of MATα1 inactivates this enzyme (Avila et al., 1997; Perez-Mato et al., 1999). GSH and other thiol-reducing agents are known to reverse this inactivation (Corrales et al., 1990). GSH maintains the normal redox potential and scavenges peroxides and free radicals in the liver (Kaplowitz, 1981). Under normal conditions, oxidation of the sulfhydryl groups of MATI/III might be protected by the cellular levels of glutathione (Corrales et al., 1990). Glutathione and cysteine levels are diminished in patients with liver diseases such as cirrhosis (Chawla et al., 1984). Although glutathione does not affect the enzyme directly, a reduction in liver glutathione might leave the sulfhydryl groups of MATI/III susceptible to oxidation and might cause the marked decrease in MATI/III activity observed in liver disease.

Pajares et al. (1994) have described the phosphorylation of MATI/III by protein kinase C (PKC) at threonine 342. This phosphorylation event does not alter the kinetic parameters of MATI/III. However, dephosphorylation of this site by alkaline phosphatase lowers the activity of both MATI and MATIII forms. Unpublished work from Ramani et al. (2013) suggests that MATα2 and β subunits are also phosphorylated. The implications of these findings are discussed later in this chapter.

MAT DYSREGULATION IN HCC DEVELOPMENT

Mechanisms of *MAT1A* Silencing during HCC

The human and rat *MAT1A* promoters contain several consensus binding sites for hepatocyte nuclear factor (HNF), glucocorticoid response elements (GRE), one or more binding sites for interleukin 6 (IL-6), and activator protein 1 (AP-1) (Zeng et al., 2000). The human *MAT1A* promoter also contains consensus binding sites for CCAAT enhancer binding protein (C/EBP) and one or more sites for cyclic AMP response element-binding protein (CRE-BP), E2F, signal transducers and activators of transcription (STAT), c-Myc, and v-Myb. HNF and C/EBP are transcriptional factors important in liver-specific gene expression (Zeng et al., 2000). However, functional analysis by transient transfection has shown that the rat *MAT1A* promoter is active not only in hepatocytes and liver-type cells such as the human hepatoblastoma cell line HepG2, but also in a nonhepatic cells such as the CHO cell line (Mato et al., 2002). These data suggest that the liver-specific expression of this gene is not mediated by tissue-specific factors.

Experimental evidence suggests that epigenetic changes in *MAT1A* genomic profile as well as post-transcriptional effects on its mRNA control this gene in HCC. In normal rat liver, hyperacetylation of a 750-bp region above the transcription initiation site along with hypomethylation of cytosines located at positions −13 and −755 of the rat *MAT1A* promoter favor increased expression of this gene (Torres et al., 2000). Treatment of HepG2 cells with 5-aza-2′-deoxycytidine, a demethylating agent or with a histone deacetylase inhibitor induced *MAT1A* expression (Torres et al., 2000). Promoter hypermethylation of *MAT1A* has also been reported in livers of F344 rats genetically predisposed to hepatocarcinogenesis versus slow-progressing HCC of resistant BN strain rats (Frau et al., 2012). Moreover, reduced MATI/III activity was a significant prognostic factor in human HCC patient samples compared with surrounding normal liver (Frau et al., 2012). Apart from promoters, coding region methylation at sites +10 and +88 relative to the transcription start site has also been reported to downregulate *MAT1A* transcription in human HCC cell lines (Tomasi et al., 2012a).

MAT1A is also known to be post-transcriptionally controlled by AU-rich RNA-binding factor 1 (AUF1) protein, a known destabilizer of target mRNAs (Antic and Keene, 1997). AUF1 was shown to be associated with the *MAT1A* 3′-untranslated region (UTR) and decrease *MAT1A* mRNA stability and steady-state abundance. Silencing AUF1 enhanced *MAT1A* mRNA levels in rat hepatocytes (Vázquez-Chantada et al., 2010).

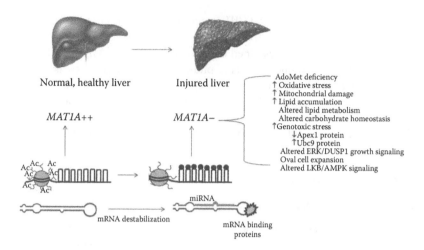

FIGURE 6.1 Mechanisms and outcome of *MAT1A* silencing in liver disease. Liver injury leads to silencing of *MAT1A* by histone deacetylation, DNA hypermethylation, and mRNA destabilization. The outcomes of *MAT1A* downregulation are summarized. Ac, acetylated histone; 🔴, methylated DNA; miRNA, microRNA.

Recently, mechanisms of *MAT1A* regulation via microRNAs have been described in HCC. MicroRNAs are a class of small noncoding RNAs that regulate gene expression in eukaryotic organisms by targeting the 3′-UTR of mRNAs leading to decreased protein translation and/or increased mRNA degradation (Bartel, 2004). In early pre-neoplastic livers in rats induced by 2-acetylaminofluorene, an induction of miR-22 and miR-29b has been observed (Koturbash et al., 2013). Induction of these micro-RNAs substantially downregulated *MAT1A* mRNA expression (Koturbash et al., 2013). MicroRNAs miR-485-3p, miR-495, and miR-664 have recently been shown to be induced in HCC (Yang et al., 2013b). These microRNAs were also shown to downregulate *MAT1A* expression in the human hepatoblastoma cell line, HepG2, and in the HCC cell line, Hep3B. Moreover, silencing these microRNAs induced *MAT1A* expression along with reduced growth and enhanced apoptosis (Yang et al., 2013b). The various mechanisms regulating *MAT1A* are summarized in Figure 6.1.

CONSEQUENCES OF HEPATIC *MAT1A* DOWNREGULATION IN LIVER

Hepatic AdoMet deficiency is a major risk factor in the development of HCC and an important contributing factor is the fall in *MAT1A* expression and MATI/III activity in pre-neoplastic and neoplastic liver (Martínez-Chantar et al., 2002a). The *MAT1A*-KO mouse model (*MAT1A*-KO) was developed to address how AdoMet deficiency and altered methionine metabolism can contribute to HCC development (Lu et al., 2001). Three-month-old *MAT1A*-KO mice have hepatic hyperplasia and are more prone to develop steatosis in response to a choline-deficient diet. By 8 months, they spontaneously develop NASH on a normal diet, and by 18 months many of the mice develop HCC (Lu et al., 2001). The outcomes of *MAT1A* deficiency are described below and listed in Figure 6.1.

Oxidative Stress

Oxidative stress is an important contributor of liver carcinogenesis. Recurrence-free survival of patients with high-serum-reactive oxygen metabolites is low after curative treatment for HCC is done (Suzuki et al., 2013). The *MAT1A*-KO mouse exhibits enhanced oxidative stress. The reasons for increased oxidative stress include lowering of GSH levels, increased cytochrome P450 2E1 (*CYP2E1*) and mitochondrial dysfunction (Martínez-Chantar et al., 2002a). Low hepatic content of AdoMet in *MAT1A*-KO favors methionine conservation, and there is less conversion of homocysteine through the transsulfuration pathway that leads to GSH synthesis. Hence AdoMet reduction depletes hepatic GSH content (Corrales et al., 1992; Martínez-Chantar et al., 2002a). CYP2E1 is known to metabolize and activate many important toxicological substrates including ethanol, carbon tetrachloride, acetaminophen, and *N*-nitrosodimethylamine to more toxic products, including reactive oxygen species (Cederbaum, 2010). *MAT1A*-KO mice have enhanced expression and activity of CYP2E1 and exhibit severe liver injury in response to carbon tetrachloride compared with normal mice (Martínez-Chantar et al., 2002a).

MAT1A-KO mice show a decrease in prohibitin 1 (PHB1), a well-known mitochondrial chaperone protein, from time of birth to NASH development at 8 months (Santamaría et al., 2003). Mitochondrial dysfunction in *MAT1A*-KO mice has been attributed to the decrease in PHB1 protein. Recently, it has been shown that *PHB1* KO mice have severe liver injury, abnormal mitochondria and increased oxidative stress (Ko et al., 2010).

Altered Lipid Homeostasis

MAT1A-KO mice have elevated levels of hepatic triglyceride and hyperglycemia (Martínez-Chantar et al., 2002a). Recently, it was deciphered that *MAT1A* was required for normal very-low-density lipoprotein (VLDL) assembly and plasma lipid homeostasis in mice (Cano et al., 2011). Impaired VLDL synthesis, mainly due to AdoMet depletion, contributes to nonalcoholic fatty liver disease (NAFLD) in *MAT1A*-KO mice (Cano et al., 2011). It is known that methylation is critical for synthesis of phosphatidylcholine (PC), a major membrane component (Hagen et al., 2010). Walker et al. (2011) recently showed that blocking PC production through siRNA-mediated depletion of *MAT1A* (causing AdoMet depletion/limiting methylation) in human hepatoblastoma cell line, HepG2, resulted in accumulation of large lipid droplets along with increased nuclear concentration of activated sterol regulatory element-binding protein 1a (SREBP-1a), a transcription factor that regulates transcription of many genes involved in fatty acid biosynthesis. Thus, conditions that limit AdoMet production such as *MAT1A* deficiency activate SREBP-1, contributing to lipid accumulation in fatty liver disease.

Genotoxic Stress

The genome is exposed to genotoxic events that can damage DNA. Endogenous factors include errors in DNA replication/repair and alterations in cellular metabolism. Exogenous factors are exposure to exogenous genotoxic agents such as ultraviolet light, oxidative stress, and chemical mutagens, leading to a variety of nucleotide modifications and DNA strand breaks. DNA hypomethylation may generate genomic instability (GI) during carcinogenesis (Eden et al., 2003). Changes in AdoMet metabolism and global DNA methylation may have a prognostic value for hepatocarcinogenesis in the majority of individuals and the mechanisms could be via GI (Calvisi et al., 2007). The apurinic/apyrimidinic endonuclease 1 (APEX1) protein is a cellular defense mechanism against GI. It is a multifunctional protein possessing both DNA repair and redox regulatory activities (Mol et al., 2000) and is upregulated by oxidative stress (Ramana et al., 1998). The expression of APEX1 is downregulated in *MAT1A*-KO mice along with increased GI (Tomasi et al., 2009). The decrease in APEX1 has been attributed to AdoMet deficiency in these mice. Exogenous treatment of primary hepatocytes with pharmacological doses of AdoMet prevents AdoMet depletion and stabilizes APEX1 protein (Tomasi et al., 2009). Therefore, AdoMet depletion can lead to decreased APEX1 protein stability and increased GI, contributing to malignant degeneration.

Another cellular mechanism known to respond to genotoxic stress is sumoylation (Romanenko et al., 2006). Sumoylation is an ubiquitin-like modification of proteins mediated by the class of enzymes called SUMO, that influences protein stability, enzymatic activity, nucleocytoplasmic trafficking, and protein–protein interactions (Moschos and Mo, 2006). Ubiquitin conjugating enzyme 9 (Ubc9), the only SUMO E2 enzyme catalyzing the conjugation of SUMO to target proteins, is overexpressed in several cancers such as lung adenocarcinoma, melanoma, and ovarian carcinoma (Moschos and Mo, 2006). Recently, Ubc9 phosphorylation and total level were shown to be induced in human HCC tissues compared with their normal controls (Tomasi et al., 2012b). *MAT1A*-KO tumors also exhibited increased Ubc9 protein expression and phosphorylation (Tomasi et al., 2012b). Enhanced interaction between Ubc9 and cell division cycle 2 (Cdc2) protein has been observed in *MAT1A*-KO liver specimens, and based on the above results, it has been suggested that Cdc2 interaction with Ubc9 induces Ubc9 phosphorylation and enhances its stability. Replenishing AdoMet in *MAT1A*-KO mice lowered the interaction between Cdc2 and Ubc9 to wild-type levels and also decreased phosphorylated and total Ubc9 levels (Tomasi et al., 2012b).

Deregulated Growth Signaling

Several aspects of deregulated growth signaling are associated with *MAT1A* deficiency. Some of these are described below.

Extracellular Signal Regulated Kinase (ERK) Activation

ERK is a survival protein deregulated in several different cancers (Roberts and Der, 2007). A mechanism by which ERK activity is controlled in normal cells is by the influence of a dual-specificity MAPK phosphatase 1 (DUSP1). DUSP1 can dephosphorylate both serine/threonine and tyrosine residues (Tonks and Neel, 1996). ERK and DUSP1 regulate each other. Prolonged ERK activation phosphorylates DUSP1 at serine 296 and makes it susceptible to proteasomal degradation (Lin et al., 2003). However, transient ERK activation increases the catalytic activity of DUSP1, and in this state, DUSP1 causes ERK inactivation (Lin et al., 2003). In human HCC, DUSP1 expression is negatively correlated to cell proliferation and positively correlated to apoptotic index (Calvisi et al., 2008). Liver DUSP1 expression was low in *MAT1A*-KO mice both at the mRNA and protein level, with the protein lower than its mRNA level (Tomasi et al., 2010). Exogenous administration of AdoMet to *MAT1A*-KO mice normalized DUSP1 mRNA and protein levels (Tomasi et al., 2010). At the transcriptional level, AdoMet depletion was shown to reduce binding of p53 to the DUSP1 promoter in *MAT1A*-KO animals and AdoMet replenishment partly corrected this interaction.

Enhanced proteasomal activity and increased expression of an E3 ubiquitin ligase, SKP2 in *MAT1A*-KO animals are two mechanisms for degradation of DUSP1 protein. Consistently, AdoMet replenishment in *MAT1A*-KO mice normalized proteasomal activity, increased DUSP1 protein level, and reduced ERK activity back to baseline (Tomasi et al., 2010). Thus, *MAT1A*/AdoMet deficiency predisposes to HCC by allowing for uncontrolled ERK activity due to decreased DUSP1 expression.

Oval Cell Expansion

Oval cells are hepatic stem cells found in the nonparenchymal fraction of the liver. They are few in number, but proliferate extensively during prolonged liver injury and in models of hepatocarcinogenesis (Jelnes et al., 2007). *MAT1A*-KO mice have expansion of a population of oval cells that behave like liver cancer stem cells as they age (Rountree et al., 2008). These cells are CD49f+ and exhibit high level of oncogenic gene expression such as that of K-ras and survivin. A subpopulation of the CD49f+ cells that is also CD133+ is tumorigenic to nude mice. Also, liver cancer stem cells from *MAT1A*-KO mice possess increased level and activity of ERK (Ding et al., 2009). This is consistent with previous reports that show alterations in the ERK pathway in *MAT1A*-KO mice (Mato et al., 2002). As compared with the CD133− cell populations, constitutive ERK activation in CD133+ CD49f+ cells allows them to evade the apoptotic effect of transforming growth factor β (TGF-β), a well-known growth inhibitor in hepatocytes (Ding et al., 2009).

LKB1/AMPK Signaling

The LKB1/AMPK signaling protein kinase pathway consists of serine/threonine 11 (LKB1) and its downstream player, AMP-activated protein kinase (AMPK). Although AMPK is primarily known for maintenance of energy homeostasis and LKB1 is a known tumor suppressor, in hepatocytes, the mitogenic growth factor hepatocyte growth factor (HGF) exerts its mitogenic effect by activating LKB1 and AMPK (Vázquez-Chantada et al., 2009). AMPK activation in hepatocytes leads to nuclear to cytoplasmic translocation of HuR protein that can stabilize several cyclin mRNAs to result in growth (Vázquez-Chantada et al., 2009). AMPK is also known to activate endothelial nitric oxide synthase (eNOS), leading to increased nitric oxide (NO) formation. NO is an inhibitor of MATI/III and its action results in lowering of AdoMet level, which may release the inhibitory tone exerted on mitogens such as HGF (Vázquez-Chantada et al., 2009). AdoMet can facilitate the interaction between protein phosphatase 2A (PP2A) and AMPK, thereby causing dephosphorylation and inactivation of AMPK (Martínez-Chantar et al., 2006). Consistently, AdoMet deficiency in *MAT1A*-KO mice results in enhanced basal LKB1 and AMPK activity, cytoplasmic HuR level, increased cyclin D1 expression, and basal proliferation (Vázquez-Chantada et al., 2009). It has also been demonstrated that the increase in LKB1 activity in HCC cells isolated from

MAT1A-KO livers is required for cell survival. LKB1 activity is also enhanced in human HCC tissues (Martínez-López et al., 2010). These findings support the role of LKB1 in facilitating proliferation and promoting carcinogenesis in *MAT1A*-KO cells.

RESTORATION OF *MAT1A* EXPRESSION IN HCC

Because *MAT1A* deficiency facilitates tumor growth, we and others have examined the effect of restoring *MAT1A* expression on growth parameters in HCC. Forced expression of *MAT1A* in vitro is associated with induction of tumor suppressor genes and apoptosis and downregulation of angiogenesis genes and cell growth (Li et al., 2010). *MAT1A*-overexpressing tumors in nude mice exhibited reduced tumor growth rate, low microvessel density, and higher apoptotic rates (Li et al., 2010). Using proteomics, Schröder et al. (2012) reported HCC cell line Huh-7-overexpressing *MAT1A* had lower level of the human Dead-box protein 3 (DDX3X) (Schröder et al., 2012). DDX3X is a RNA helicase that regulates RNA splicing, export, transcription, and translation, and it has been shown to be upregulated in HCC tissues (Huang et al., 2004; Schröder, 2010). It has been speculated that reduced AdoMet levels in HCC cause DDX3X upregulation and contribute to HCC pathogenesis. Replenishing AdoMet via *MAT1A* re-expression might prove to have beneficial effects, at least in part by reducing DDX3X levels (Schröder et al., 2012).

Increased *MAT1A* expression can also be achieved in vitro and in vivo in liver tumors by blocking the expression of microRNAs, specifically miR-485-3p, miR-495, and miR-664, which are upregulated in HCC and negatively regulate *MAT1A* at the mRNA level (Yang et al., 2013b). Forced expression of *MAT1A* in these tumors along with silencing of the above microRNAs reduced tumor growth, invasion, and metastasis (Yang et al., 2013b). Interestingly, higher *MAT1A* expression resulted in higher MATα1 protein in the nuclear compartment in the cancer cell, leading to epigenetic changes and silencing of *LIN28B*, a known oncogene implicated in HCC invasion and metastasis (Yang et al., 2013b).

MECHANISMS OF *MAT2A/MAT2B* DEREGULATION DURING HCC

MAT2A is a marker for rapid liver growth and de-differentiation and is induced in human HCC (Cai et al., 1996). Several transcriptional and post-transcriptional regulatory elements control the *MAT2A* gene in HCC. The *MAT2A* promoter contains *cis*-acting elements that respond to the *trans*-activating factors, specificity protein 1 (Sp1), c-Myb, nuclear factor κB (NF-κB), AP-1, and E2F. These factors contribute to transcriptional upregulation of *MAT2A* during HCC (Yang et al., 2001b). During liver regeneration in rats, *MAT2A* was found to be upregulated during G_0–G_1 transition and during G_1–S transition. Cooperative binding of E2F and Sp1 to two adjacent sites on the *MAT2A* promoter positively regulated its expression during the G_1–S phase (Rodríguez et al., 2007). Tumor necrosis factor α (TNF-α), a pleiotropic cytokine involved in preserving liver homeostasis (Wullaert et al., 2007), upregulated *MAT2A* via NF-κB and AP-1 elements in HCC (Yang et al., 2003).

MAT2A expression is also regulated by promoter methylation and histone acetylation. The promoter is hypomethylated in HCC, but hypermethylated in normal liver and hyperacetylation of histones favors higher *MAT2A* expression (Yang et al., 2001a). Hypoxia-inducible factor 1α (HIF-1α), an important prognostic factor in HCC (Dai et al., 2009), has been shown to induce *MAT2A* promoter activity in HCC by positively regulating a putative HIF-1α element on the promoter (Liu et al., 2011).

Post-transcriptionally, *MAT2A* mRNA is regulated at its 3′-UTR by the binding of HuR protein and its methylated counterpart, methyl-HuR (Vázquez-Chantada et al., 2010). In HCC and in hepatocyte de-differentiation, an induction in HuR levels was associated with a decrease in its methylated form, methyl-HuR. While HuR stabilizes target mRNAs, methyl-HuR destabilizes them (Vázquez-Chantada et al., 2010). A switch from methyl-HuR to HuR binding on the *MAT2A* 3′-UTR enhanced *MAT2A* expression in HCC and in de-differentiated hepatocytes.

Recently, a cross-talk between *MAT2A* and polyamines has been reported to enhance liver cancer cell growth (Tomasi et al., 2013). Increased *MAT2A* expression in liver cancer cells was shown to promote polyamine biosynthesis and increased polyamine levels *trans*-activated the *MAT2A* promoter via binding of the c-jun proto-oncogene to a putative AP-1 *cis*-acting element (Tomasi et al., 2013).

Like *MAT2A, MAT2B* is expressed at very low levels in normal liver but is induced in HCC (Yang et al., 2008; Martínez-Chantar et al., 2003). In human HepG2 cells, TNF-α transcriptionally upregulated *MAT2B-V1* mRNA, but not *MAT2B-V2* mRNA via an AP-1 and NF-κB-dependent mechanism (Yang et al., 2008). In normal hepatocytes, TNF-α has no cytotoxic effect because NF-κB is also induced to protect from TNF-α–mediated apoptosis by inducing the expression of protective genes against apoptotic cell death (Schwabe and Brenner, 2006). One of these protective genes in liver cancer cells is *MAT2B-V1*. Indeed, silencing *MAT2B-V1* but not *V2* sensitized HepG2 cells to TNF-α–induced apoptosis (Yang et al., 2008). Hence, *MAT2B-V1* acts as a NF-κB–dependent survival factor in liver cancer cells.

Studies on the effect of growth factors on *MAT2A* and *MAT2B* expression emphasize the role played by these genes in proliferating liver. It is known that *MAT2A* expression is induced in the liver after partial hepatectomy. Latasa et al. (2001) have shown that HGF strongly induces *MAT2A* transcription in rat hepatocytes via histone H4 promoter acetylation. In addition, liver HGF levels are induced after partial hepatectomy that is responsible for *MAT2A* induction. Moreover, *MAT2A* induction is required for HGF to mediate its proliferative action in human hepatoma cells (Paneda et al., 2002).

Another growth factor associated with *MAT2A* and *MAT2B* induction is leptin (Ramani et al., 2008). It is known to induce growth and invasive potential of liver cancer cells (Ramani et al., 2008; Saxena et al., 2007). We have previously demonstrated that leptin induced *MAT2A* and *MAT2B* transcription in HepG2 cells and silencing of either *MAT2A* or *MAT2B* blocked the mitogenic potential of leptin (Ramani et al., 2008). MATα2 promoted leptin-mediated growth by increasing the intracellular AdoMet levels to promote polyamine biosynthesis. MATβ, meanwhile, played a novel role in promoting leptin signaling. Gene silencing studies demonstrated that MATβ was required for leptin-mediated growth signaling involving ERK and phosphatidyl inositol 3 kinase (PI3-K) activation. In addition, MATβ stimulated STAT3 activation, an upstream event in leptin signaling (Saxena et al., 2007). These findings suggest that apart from its role as a regulatory subunit of MATII, MATβ is involved in multiple growth-associated functions in the cell. The mechanism of

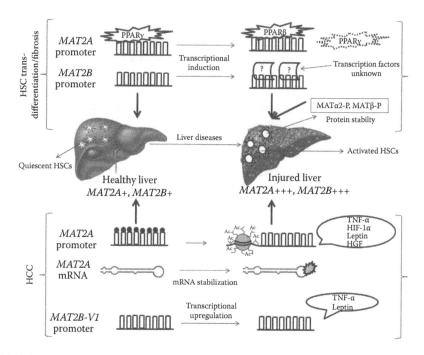

FIGURE 6.2 Mechanisms of *MAT2A/MAT2B* upregulation in liver disease. Normal hepatocytes express only the MATα1 enzyme, whereas other liver cell types such as HSCs express *MAT2A* and *MAT2B* only. Liver injury leads to upregulation of both *MAT2A* and *MAT2B* in the liver. In HCC, mechanisms of *MAT2A* induction include histone acetylation of promoter regions, DNA hypomethylation, and transcriptional upregulation mediated by TNF-α, HIF-1α, leptin, and HGF. *MAT2A* mRNA is stabilized by mRNA-binding proteins in HCC. *MAT2B-V1* promoter is transcriptionally induced by TNF-α and leptin. In quiescent HSCs from normal liver, *MAT2A* promoter is negatively controlled by PPAR-γ. Loss of PPAR-γ and induction by PPARβ promotes *MAT2A* in *trans*-differentiated HSCs from injured liver. *MAT2B* is also transcriptionally upregulated in activated HSCs from injured liver. However, mechanisms of transcriptional control are not yet known. In activated HSCs, both MATα2 and MATβ are post-translationally stabilized by phosphorylation. MATα2-P, MATα2-phosphorylated; MATβ-P, MATβ-phosphorylated.

how MATβ regulates these pathways is under investigation. Recently, it was found that the MATβ forms a scaffold with G-protein–coupled receptor kinase-interacting protein 1 (GIT1), and this complex recruits and activates mitogen-activated protein kinase/ERK kinase (MEK) and ERK to promote growth and tumorigenesis (Peng et al., 2013). The findings provide mechanistic insight into how MATβ influences survival-signaling pathways. The mechanisms of *MAT2A/MAT2B* upregulation in HCC are summarized in Figure 6.2.

MAT DEREGULATION IN LIVER FIBROSIS/CIRRHOSIS

Progression of NASH to fibrosis, cirrhosis, and end-stage liver disease is associated with alterations in methionine metabolism (Lu and Mato, 2012). Liver injury leads to lowering of *MAT1A* and overexpression of *MAT2A* and *MAT2B*. In the following section, we will review the current information on how these genes are influenced during liver fibrosis/cirrhosis. The mechanisms of regulation of *MAT2A/MAT2B* in liver fibrosis/cirrhosis and HSC activation are summarized in Figure 6.2.

MAT1A Silencing during Liver Cirrhosis

Liver cirrhosis is associated with an abnormal metabolism of methionine, a state that was discovered more than half a century ago (Kinsell et al., 1948). In cirrhotic patients, independent of the etiology (alcohol, hepatitis B, hepatitis C), the rate of clearance of methionine from the blood is markedly impaired compared with normal subjects (Martín-Duce et al., 1988; Avila et al., 2000). The failure to metabolize methionine in cirrhosis has been attributed to the low expression of *MAT1A* and diminished activity of MATI/III (Martínez-Chantar et al., 2002b; Avila et al., 2000). Two mechanisms for this drop have been identified. The *MAT1A* promoter is hypermethylated in cirrhotic livers that silences this gene (Avila et al., 2000). Also, there is a high level of reactive oxygen metabolites and NO in cirrhotic livers that are capable of inactivating the MATI/III enzyme (Ruiz et al., 1998; Avila et al., 1997; Perez-Mato et al., 1999). Inactivation of MATI/III via enhanced production of free radicals has also been observed in experimental models of liver injury such as alcohol intoxication in baboons (Lieber et al., 1990), carbon tetrachloride in rats (Corrales et al., 1992), paracetamol in rats (Stramentinoli et al., 1979), buthionine, and sulfoximine intoxication in rats (Corrales et al., 1991).

MAT2A and *MAT2B* Deregulation in Liver Fibrosis/Cirrhosis

The regulation of *MAT2A* and *MAT2B* during liver fibrosis is an emerging area of study. Previous work has shown that in experimental models of liver fibrosis (carbon tetrachloride), an induction of *MAT2A* mRNA is observed (Fang et al., 2007). This is consistent with a decrease in *MAT1A* expression in these animals. MATβ subunit expression is induced in human cirrhotic tissues versus normal controls, indicating that this protein is associated with human liver dysfunction (Martínez-Chantar et al., 2003).

Recent work from our laboratory sheds light on the expression and regulation of *MAT2A* and *MAT2B* during HSC activation. HSCs are fibrogenic cells that are normally storage sites for vitamin A in the adult liver. Following chronic liver injury, HSCs undergo activation with increased proliferation, loss of vitamin A and production of excessive matrix proteins and enhanced expression of α-smooth muscle actin (α-SMA) and collagen (Maher and McGuire, 1990). Development of liver fibrosis entails major alterations in the quantity and quality of hepatic extracellular matrix (ECM), and there is overwhelming evidence that activated HSCs are the major producers of the fibrotic neomatrix (Burt, 1993). Among the large number of factors identified as inducers of matrix production and HSC activation are transforming growth β (TGF-β), connective tissue growth factor (CTGF), leptin, and platelet-derived growth factor (PDGF) (Burt, 1993). Normal, quiescent HSCs of the liver express *MAT2A* and *MAT2B* mRNA and their corresponding proteins (Shimizu-Saito et al., 1997;

Ramani et al., 2010); however, these cells lack the expression of *MATα1*, encoded by *MAT1A* (Shimizu-Saito et al., 1997). HSCs spontaneously *trans*-differentiate to an activated state when cultured in vitro on plastic dishes (Maher and McGuire, 1990). They also undergo activation in intact liver subjected to injury by bile duct ligation (BDL) (Lotersztajn et al., 2005). We recently showed that both *MAT2A* and *MAT2B* mRNA and the MATα2 and MATβ proteins were induced during in vitro and in vivo rat HSC activation (Ramani et al., 2010). Despite the increase in the subunit expression, the activity of MATII dropped during HSC activation. This is consistent with other reports showing a decrease in the activity of MATII in *trans*-differentiated HSCs from carbon tetrachloride-treated rat liver (Shimizu-Saito et al., 1997). HSC *trans*-differentiation led to a drop in intracellular AdoMet levels and global DNA hypomethylation (Ramani et al., 2010). It appears that a lower AdoMet level in activated HSCs favors growth and *trans*-differentiation. Exogenous AdoMet treatment has been reported by several groups to inhibit HSC activation, and carbon tetrachloride–induced fibrosis (Nieto and Cederbaum, 2005). Silencing the *MAT2A* gene inhibited HSC activation as judged by a decrease in activation markers, α-SMA and collagen (Ramani et al., 2010), and overexpression of *MAT2A* in quiescent rat HSCs raised α-SMA and inhibited the expression of a marker of HSC quiescence, peroxisome proliferator–activated receptor γ (PPAR-γ) (Ramani and Tomasi, 2012). Silencing *MAT2A* depleted the existing AdoMet pools in activated HSCs, and this drastic drop inhibited proliferation and promoted apoptosis (Ramani et al., 2010). The findings point toward the important role of *MAT2A* in maintaining a physiological level of AdoMet necessary for entry into the cell cycle.

As with *MAT2A*, silencing *MAT2B* in activated HSCs also inhibits *trans*-differentiation, but the mechanism appears to be independent of changes in AdoMet levels. We have shown that *MAT2B* favors induction of survival signaling pathways, ERK and PI3-K (Ramani et al., 2010), which are known to positively influence HSC activation during liver fibrogenesis (Marra et al., 1997, 1999).

MECHANISMS OF *MAT2A* AND *MAT2B* DEREGULATION DURING HSC ACTIVATION

Our recent work addresses the question of how *MAT2A* and *MAT2B* are deregulated during HSC activation. We have shown that in quiescent rat HSCs, the *MAT2A* gene is transcriptionally controlled by binding of the nuclear transcription factor, PPAR-γ to putative PPAR response elements (PPRE) in the *MAT2A* promoter (Ramani and Tomasi, 2012). Decrease in PPAR-γ expression and activity during HSC activation is an important factor contributing to the myofibroblastic state (Hazra et al., 2004), and we have shown that there is substantially less PPAR-γ binding to the *MAT2A* PPREs in activated HSCs. Lack of PPAR-γ binding allows another PPAR, PPARβ to bind to *MAT2A* PPREs and promote *MAT2A* transcription (Ramani and Tomasi, 2012). PPARβ is known to positively contribute to HSC activation and proliferation (Hellemans et al., 2003). In myofibroblastic human HSCs, the control of *MAT2A* appears to be different from that in rat HSCs. Human HSCs do not exhibit transcriptional upregulation of *MAT2A* during myofibroblastic *trans*-differentiation (Ramani et al., unpublished observations, 2013). However, the MATα2 protein is induced in activated HSCs. The reason for this protein induction is the post-translational stabilization of MATα2 by phosphorylation in *trans*-differentiated human HSCs versus quiescent cells (Ramani et al., unpublished observations, 2013).

MAT2B appears to be both transcriptionally and post-translationally regulated in human HSCs. The promoter activity and mRNA level of the *MAT2B-V1* (but not *MAT2B-V2*) is induced during HSC activation, and the MATβ subunit, like MATα2, is post-translationally stabilized by phosphorylation. Certain phosphorylation events in MATα2 and MATβ play a role in promoting HSC activation (Ramani et al., unpublished observations, 2013). Mechanistic insight on how these modifications influences HSC *trans*-differentiation remains to be elucidated.

SUMMARY AND FUTURE DIRECTIONS

MAT genes are essential for the biosynthesis of AdoMet, the principal biological methyl donor. The *MAT1A* gene is a marker of adult, differentiated liver, whereas *MAT2A* and *MAT2B* are expressed in extrahepatic tissues and in fetal liver. Liver injury is associated with changes in MAT expression. Although *MAT1A* is silenced under this condition, *MAT2A* and *MAT2B* are upregulated. Hence, in the de-differentiated liver, *MAT1A* is replaced by *MAT2A* and *MAT2B*. This is further associated with dramatic changes in AdoMet homeostasis leading to oxidative and genotoxic stress, de-regulated lipid and carbohydrate metabolism, and alterations in cell growth pathways. In HCC, mechanisms known to downregulate *MAT1A* are hypermethylation of its promoter and coding regions, post-transcriptional destabilization of its mRNA and microRNA-mediated downregulation. *MAT2A* induction occurs by promoter hypomethylation, histone acetylation, transcriptional induction, post-transcriptional mRNA stabilization, and growth factor–mediated induction. *MAT2B* is transcriptionally induced via growth factor signaling and by induction of *cis*-acting elements in its promoter. In liver cirrhosis, *MAT1A* is transcriptionally suppressed by promoter hypermethylation and MATI/III enzymes are inactivated by oxidative and nitrosative stress. *MAT2A* is induced in fibrotic livers of rats. *MAT2A* and *MAT2B* are also induced in activated rat HSCs from injured liver. Transcriptional mechanisms negatively control *MAT2A* expression in quiescent rat HSCs, and alteration in key transcription factors allows *MAT2A* induction in HSCs from injured liver. In myofibroblastic human HSCs, *MAT2A*- and *MAT2B*-encoded proteins are post-translationally stabilized. Based on the above research, it is clear that a relevant future direction is to identify novel molecules that could interact with MAT proteins and be used to either block MATII or induce MATI/III in the damaged liver. Recently, it was reported that fluorinated *N,N*-dialkylaminostilbenes, called FIDAS agents, act as anticancer drugs for colorectal cancer. The mode of action of these agents is by their exclusive and direct binding to the active site of the MATII enzyme (Zhang et al., 2013). These studies provide the direction to examine therapeutic molecules targeting MATII in HCC and fibrosis. Designing drugs that could block HSC activation by interfering with *MAT2A* and *MAT2B* expression and/or protein stability may be a reasonable way of treating the fibrotic liver. More studies on crystal structures and interactions of MAT proteins are required to establish their use as therapeutic targets for liver disease.

ACKNOWLEDGMENTS

This work was supported by NIH grants R00AA017774 (K.R.) and R01DK51719 (S.C.L.).

REFERENCES

Antic, D., Keene, J.D. 1997. Embryonic lethal abnormal visual RNA-binding proteins involved in growth, differentiation, and posttranscriptional gene expression. *Am. J. Hum. Genet.* 61:273–78.

Avila, M.A., Berasain, C., Torres, L. et al. 2000. Reduced mRNA abundance of the main enzymes involved in methionine metabolism in human liver cirrhosis and hepatocellular carcinoma. *J. Hepatol.* 33:907–14.

Avila, M.A., Mingorance, J., Martínez-Chantar, M.L., Casado, M., Martín-Sanz, P., Bascá, L. et al. 1997. Regulation of rat liver S-adenosylmethionine synthetase during septic shock: Role of nitric oxide. *Hepatology* 25:391–6.

Bartel, D.P. 2004. MicroRNAs: Genomics, biogenesis, mechanism, and function. *Cell* 116:281–97.

Burt, A.D. 1993. Cellular and molecular aspects of hepatic fibrosis. *J. Pathol.* 70:105–14.

Cai, J., Mao, Z., Hwang, J.J., Lu, S.C. 1998. Differential expression of methionine adenosyl-transferase genes influences the rate of growth of human hepatocellular carcinoma cells. *Cancer Res.* 58:1444–50.

Cai, J., Sun, W.M., Hwang, J.J., Stain, S.C., Lu, S.C. 1996. Changes in S-adenosylmethionine synthetase in human liver cancer: Molecular characterization and significance. *Hepatology* 24:1090–97.

Calvisi, D.F., Pinna, F., Meloni, F., Ladu, S., Pellegrino, R., Sini, M. et al. 2008. Dual-specificity phosphatase 1 ubiquitination in extracellular signal-regulated kinase-mediated control of growth in human hepatocellular carcinoma. *Cancer Res.* 68:4192–200.

Calvisi, D.F., Simile, M.M., Ladu, S., Pellegrino, R., De Murtas, V., Pinna, F. et al. 2007. Altered methionine metabolism and global DNA methylation in liver cancer: Relationship with genomic instability and prognosis. *Int. J. Cancer* 121:2410–20.

Cano, A., Buqué, X., Martínez-Uña, M., Aurrekoetxea, I., Menor, A., García-Rodríguez, J.L. et al. 2011. Methionine adenosyltransferase 1A gene deletion disrupts hepatic very low-density lipoprotein assembly in mice. *Hepatology* 54:1975–86.

Cederbaum, A.I. 2010. Hepatoprotective effects of S-adenosyl-L-methionine against alcohol- and cytochrome P450 2E1-induced liver injury. *World J. Gastroenterol.* 16:1366–76.

Chawla, R.K., Lewis, F.W., Kutner, M.H., Batek, D.M., Roy, R.G.B., Rudman, D. 1984. Plasma cysteine, cystine, and glutathione in cirrhosis. *Gastroenterology* 87:770–6.

Clarke, S.G. 2006. Inhibition of mammalian protein methyltransferases by 5′-methylthio-adenosine (MTA): A mechanism of action of dietary SAMe? *Enzymes* 24:467–93.

Corrales, F., Cabrero, C., Pajares, M.A., Ortiz, P., Martin-Duce, A., Mato, J.M. 1990. Inactivation and dissociation of S-adenosylmethionine synthetase by modification of sulfhydryl groups and its possible occurrence in cirrhosis. *Hepatology* 11:216–22.

Corrales, F., Gimenez, L, Alvarez, L., Caballeria, M.A., Pajares, M.A., Andreu, J. 1992. S-Adenosylmethionine treatment prevents carbon tetrachloride induced S-adenosyl-methionine synthetase inactivation and attenuates liver injury. *Hepatology* 16:1022–7.

Corrales, F., Ochoa, P., Rivas, C., Martin-Lomas, M., Mato, J.M., Pajares, M.A. 1991. Inhibition of glutathione synthesis in the liver leads to S-adenosyl-L-methionine synthetase reduction. *Hepatology* 14:528–33.

Dai, C.X., Gao, Q., Qiu, S.J., Ju, M.J., Cai, M.Y., Xu, Y.F. et al. 2009. Hypoxia-inducible factor-1 alpha, in association with inflammation, angiogenesis and MYC, is a critical prognostic factor in patients with HCC after surgery. *BMC Cancer* 9:418.

Ding, W., Mouzaki, M., You, H., Laird, J.C., Mato, J., Lu, S.C. et al. 2009. CD133+ liver cancer stem cells from methionine adenosyl transferase 1A-deficient mice demonstrate resistance to transforming growth factor (TGF)-beta-induced apoptosis. *Hepatology* 49:1277–86.

Eden, A., Gaudet, F., Waghmare, A., Jaenisch, R. 2003. Chromosomal instability and tumors promoted by DNA hypomethylation. *Science* 300:455.

Fan, X.C., Steitz, J.A. 1998. Overexpression of HuR, a nuclear-cytoplasmic shuttling protein, increases the in vivo stability of ARE-containing mRNAs. *EMBO J.* 17:3448–60.

Fang, H.L., Lai, J.J., Lin, W.L., Lin, W.C. 2007 A fermented substance from Aspergillus phoenicis reduces liver fibrosis induced by carbon tetrachloride in rats. *Biosci. Biotechnol. Biochem.* 71:1154–61.

Finkelstein, J.D. 1990. Methionine metabolism in mammals. *J. Nutr. Biochem.* 1:228–37.

Frau, M., Tomasi, M.L., Simile, M.M., Demartis, M.I., Salis, F., Latte, G. et al. 2012. Role of transcriptional and posttranscriptional regulation of methionine adenosyltransferases in liver cancer progression. *Hepatology* 56:165–75.

Gaull, G.E., Tallan, H.H., Lonsdale, D., Przyrembel, H., Schaffner, F., Von Bassewitz, D.B. 1981. Hypermethioninemia associated with methionine adenosyltransferase deficiency: Clinical, morphologic, and biochemical observations on four patients. *J. Pediatr.* 98:734–41.

Gil, B., Casado, M., Pajares, M.A., Bosca, L., Mato, J.M., Martin-Sanz, P., Alvarez, L. 1996. Differential expression pattern of S-adenosylmethionine synthetase isoenzymes during rat liver development. *Hepatology*, 24:876–81.

González, B., Garrido, F., Ortega, R., Martínez-Júlvez, M., Revilla-Guarinos, A., Pérez-Pertejo, Y. et al. 2012. NADP+ binding to the regulatory subunit of methionine adenosyltransferase II increases intersubunit binding affinity in the hetero-trimer. *PLoS One.* 7:e50329.

Hagen, R.M., Rodriguez-Cuenca, S., Vidal-Puig, A. 2010. An allostatic control of membrane lipid composition by SREBP1. *FEBS Lett.* 584:2689–98.

Halim, A.B., LeGros, L., Geller, A., Kotb, M. 1999. Expression and functional interaction of the catalytic and regulatory subunits of human methionine adenosyltransferase in mammalian cells. *J. Biol. Chem.* 274:29720–25.

Hazra, S., Xiong, S., Wang, J., Rippe, R.A., Krishna, V., Chatterjee, K. et al. 2004. Peroxisome proliferator–activated receptor gamma induces a phenotypic switch from activated to quiescent hepatic stellate cells. *J. Biol. Chem.* 279:11392–401.

Hellemans, K., Michalik, L., Dittie, A., Knorr, A., Rombouts, K., De Jong, J. et al. 2003. Peroxisome proliferator–activated receptor-beta signaling contributes to enhanced proliferation of hepatic stellate cells. *Gastroenterology* 124:184–201.

Horikawa, S., Tsukada, K. 1992. Molecular cloning and developmental expression of a human kidney S-adenosylmethionine synthetase. *FEBS Lett.* 312:37–41.

Huang, J.S., Chao, C.C., Su, T.L., Yeh, S.H., Chen, D.S., Chen, C.T. et al. 2004. Diverse cellular transformation capability of overexpressed genes in human hepatocellular carcinoma. *Biochem. Biophys. Res. Commun.* 315:950–8.

Jelnes, P., Santoni-Rugiu, E., Rasmussen, M., Friis, S.L., Nielsen, J.H., Tygstrup, N. et al. 2007. Remarkable heterogeneity displayed by oval cells in rat and mouse models of stem cell-mediated liver regeneration. *Hepatology* 45:1462–70.

Kaplowitz, N. 1981. The importance and regulation of hepatic glutathione. *Yale J. Biol. Med.* 54:497–502.

Katoh, Y., Ikura, T., Hoshikawa, Y., Tashiro, S., Ito, T., Ohta, M. et al. 2011. Methionine adenosyltransferase II serves as a transcriptional corepressor of Maf oncoproteins. *Mol. Cell* 41:554–66.

Kinsell, L.W., Harper, H.A., Barton, H.C., Hutchin, M.E., Hess, J.R. 1948. Studies in methionine and sulfur metabolism. I. The fate of intravenously administered methionine, in Normal individuals and in patients with liver damage. *J. Clin. Invest.* 27:677–88.

Ko, K.S., Tomasi, M.L., Iglesias-Ara, A., French, B.A., French, S.W., Ramani, K. et al. 2010. Liver-specific deletion of prohibitin 1 results in spontaneous liver injury, fibrosis, and hepatocellular carcinoma in mice. *Hepatology* 52:2096–108.

Kotb, M., Mudd, S.H., Mato, J.M., Geller, A.M., Kredich, N.M., Chou, J.Y. et al. 1997. Consensus nomenclature for the mammalian methionine adenosyltransferase genes and gene products. *Trends Genet.* 13:51–2.

Koturbash, I., Melnyk, S., James, S.J., Beland, F.A., Pogribny, I.P. 2013. Role of epigenetic and miR-22 and miR-29b alterations in the downregulation of *MAT1A* and Mthfr genes in early preneoplastic livers in rats induced by 2-acetylaminofluorene. *Mol. Carcinog.* 52:318–27.

Latasa, M.U., Boukaba, A., Garcia-Trevijano, E.R., Torres, L., Rodriguez, J.L., Caballeria, J. et al. 2001. Hepatocyte growth factor induces *MAT2A* expression and histone acetylation in rat hepatocytes: Role in liver regeneration. *FASEB J.*15:1248–50.

Li, J., Ramani, K., Sun, Z., Zee, C., Grant, E.G., Yang, H. et al. 2010. Forced expression of methionine adenosyltransferase 1A in human hepatoma cells suppresses in vivo tumorigenicity in mice. *Am. J. Pathol.* 176:2456–66.

Lieber, C.S., Casini, A., DeCarli, L.M., Kim, C.I., Lowe, N., Sasaki, R. et al. 1990. S-Adenosyl-L-methionine attenuates alcohol-induced liver injury in the baboon. *Hepatology* 11:165–72.

Lieber, C.S., Packer, L. 2002. S-Adenosylmethionine: Molecular, biological, and clinical aspects-an introduction. *Am. J. Clin. Nutr.* 76:1148S–50S.

Lin, Y.W., Chuang, S.M., Yang, J.L. 2003. ERK1/2 achieves sustained activation by stimulating MAPK phosphatase-1 degradation via the ubiquitin-proteasome pathway. *J. Biol. Chem.* 278:21534–41.

Liu, Q., Liu, L., Zhao, Y., Zhang, J., Wang, D., Chen, J. et al. 2011. Hypoxia induces genomic DNA demethylation through the activation of HIF-1a and transcriptional upregulation of *MAT2A* in hepatoma cells. *Mol. Cancer. Ther.* 10:1113–23.

Lotersztajn, S., Julien, B., Clerc, F.T., Grenard, P., Mallat, A.H. 2005. Hepatic fibrosis: Molecular mechanisms and drug targets. *Annu. Rev. Pharmacol. Toxicol.* 45:605–28.

Lu, S.C. 2013. Glutathione synthesis. *Biochim. Biophys. Acta* 1830:3143–53.

Lu, S.C., Alvarez, L., Huang, Z.Z., Chen, L., An, W., Corrales, F.J. 2001. Methionine adenosyltransferase 1 A knockout mice are predisposed to liver injury and exhibit increased expression of genes involved in proliferation. *Proc. Natl. Acad. Sci. USA* 98:5560–65.

Lu, S.C, Gukovsky, I., Lugea, A., Reyes, C.N., Huang, Z.Z., Chen, L. et al. 2003. Role of S-adenosylmethionine in two experimental models of pancreatitis. *FASEB J.* 17:56–8.

Lu, S.C., Mato, J.M. 2012. S-Adenosylmethionine in liver health, injury, and cancer. *Physiol. Rev.* 92:1515–42.

Maher, J.J., McGuire, R.F. 1990. Extracellular matrix gene expression increases preferentially in rat lipocytes and sinusoidal endothelial cells during hepatic fibrosis in vivo. *J. Clin. Invest.* 86:1641–8.

Marra, F., Arrighi, M.C., Fazi, M., Caligiuri, A., Pinzani, M., Romanelli, R.G. et al. 1999. Extracellular signal-regulated kinase activation differentially regulates platelet-derived growth factor's actions in hepatic stellate cells, and is induced by in vivo liver injury in the rat. *Hepatology* 30:951–8.

Marra, F., Gentilini, A., Pinzani, M., Choudhury, G.G., Parola, M., Herbst, H. et al. 1997. Phosphatidylinositol 3-kinase is required for platelet-derived growth factor's actions on hepatic stellate cells. *Gastroenterology* 112:1297–306.

Martín-Duce, A., Ortiz, P., Cabrero, C., Mato, J.M. 1988. S-Adenosyl-L-methionine synthetase and phospholipid methyltransferase are inhibited in human cirrhosis. *Hepatology* 8:65–8.

Martínez-Chantar, M.L., Corrales, F.J., Martínez-Cruz, L.A., García-Trevijano, E.R., Huang, Z.Z., Chen, L. et al. 2002a. Spontaneous oxidative stress and liver tumors in mice lacking methionine adenosyltransferase 1A. *FASEB J.* 16:1292–4.

Martínez-Chantar, M.L., Garcia-Trevijano, E.R., Latasa, M.U., Martin-Duce, A., Fortes, P., Caballeria, J. et al. 2003. Methionine adenosyltransferase II beta subunit gene expression provides a proliferative advantage in human hepatoma. *Gastroenterology* 124:940–8.

Martínez-Chantar, M.L., García-Trevijano, E.R., Latasa, M.U., Pérez-Mato, I., Sánchez del Pino, M.M., Corrales, F.J. et al. 2002b. Importance of a deficiency in S-adenosyl-L-methionine synthesis in the pathogenesis of liver injury. *Am. J. Clin. Nutr.* 76:1177S–82S.

Martínez-Chantar, M.L., Vázquez-Chantada, M., Garnacho-Echevarria, M., Latasa, M.U., Varela-Rey, M., Dotor, J. et al. 2006. S-Adenosylmethionine regulates cytoplasmic HuR via AMP-activated kinase. *Gastroenterology* 131:223–32.

Martínez-López, N., Varela-Rey, M., Fernández-Ramos, D., Woodhoo, A., Vázquez-Chantada, M., Embade, N. et al. 2010. Activation of LKB1-Akt pathway independent of phosphoinositide 3-kinase plays a critical role in the proliferation of hepatocellular carcinoma from nonalcoholic steatohepatitis. *Hepatology* 52:1621–31.

Mato, J.M., Alvarez, L., Ortiz, P., Pajares, M.A. 1997. S-Adenosylmethionine synthesis: Molecular mechanisms and clinical implications. *Pharmacol Ther.* 73:265–80.

Mato, J.M, Corrales, F.J., Lu, S.C, Avila, M.A. 2002. S-Adenosylmethionine: A control switch that regulates liver function. *FASEB J.* 16:15–26.

Mol, C.D., Hosfield, D.J., Tainer, J.A. 2000. Abasic site recognition by two apurinic/apyrimidinic endonuclease families in DNA base excision repair: The 3′ ends justify the means. *Mutat. Res.* 460:211–29.

Moschos, S.J., Mo, Y.Y. 2006. Role of SUMO/Ubc9 in DNA damage repair and tumorigenesis. *J. Mol. Histol.* 37:309–19.

Nieto, N., Cederbaum, A.I. 2005. S-Adenosylmethionine blocks collagen I production by preventing transforming growth factor induction of the *COL1A2* promoter. *J. Biol. Chem.* 280:30963–74.

Pajares, M.A., Duran, C., Corrales, F., Mato, J.M. 1994. Protein kinase C phosphorylation of rat liver methionine adenosyltransferase: Dissociation and product of an active monomer. *Biochem. J.* 303:949–55.

Paneda, C., Gorospe, I., Herrera, B., Nakamura, T., Fabregat, I., Varela-Nieto, I. 2002. Liver cell proliferation requires methionine adenosyltransferase 2A mRNA upregulation. *Hepatology* 35:1381–91.

Peng, H., Dara, L., Li, T.W., Zheng, Y., Yang, H., Tomasi, L.M. et al. 2013. Methionine adenosyltransferase 2B-GIT1 interplay activates MEK1-ERK1/2 to induce growth in human liver and colon cancer. *Hepatology* 57:2299–313.

Perez-Mato, I., Castro, C., Ruiz, F.A., Corrales, F.J., Mato, J.M. 1999. Methionine adenosyltransferase S-nitrosylation is regulated by the basic and acidic amino acids surrounding the target thiol. *J. Biol. Chem.* 274:17075–79.

Ramana, C.V., Boldogh, I., Izumi, T., Mitra, S. 1998. Activation of apurinic/apyrimidinic endonuclease in human cells by reactive oxygen species and its correlation with their adaptive response to genotoxicity of free radicals. *Proc. Natl. Acad. Sci. USA* 95:5061–6.

Ramani, K., Donoyan, S., Park, S., Tomasi, M.L. 2013. Post-translational stabilization of methionine adenosyltransferases $\alpha2$ and β during human hepatic stellate cell *trans*-differentiation. Manuscript submitted to *J. Biol. Chem.*

Ramani, K., Tomasi, M.L. 2012. Transcriptional regulation of methionine adenosyltransferase 2A by peroxisome proliferator–activated receptors in rat hepatic stellate cells. *Hepatology* 55:1942–53.

Ramani, K., Yang, H., Kuhlenkamp, J., Tomasi, L., Tsukamoto, H., Mato, J.M. et al. 2010. Changes in the Expression of Methionine Adenosyltransferase Genes and S-adenosylmethionine Homeostasis during Hepatic Stellate Cell Activation. *Hepatology* 51:986–95.

Ramani, K., Yang, H., Xia, M., Iglesias Ara, A., Mato, J.M., Lu, S.C. 2008. Leptin's mitogenic effect in human liver cancer cells requires induction of both methionine adenosyltransferase 2A and 2β. *Hepatology* 47:521–31.

Reytor, E., Perez-Miguelsanz, J., Alvarez, L., Perez-Sala, D., Pajares, MA. 2009. Conformational signals in the C-terminal domain of methionine adenosyltransferase I/ III determine its nucleocytoplasmic distribution. *FASEB J.* 23:3347–60.

Roberts, P.J., Der, C.J. 2007. Targeting the Raf-MEK-ERK mitogen-activated protein kinase cascade for the treatment of cancer. *Oncogene* 26:3291–310.

Rodríguez, J.L., Boukaba, A., Sandoval, J., Georgieva, E.I., Latasa, M.U., García-Trevijano, E.R. et al. 2007. Transcription of the *MAT2A* gene, coding for methionine adenosyl-transferase, is upregulated by E2F and Sp1 at a chromatin level during proliferation of liver cells. *Int. J. Biochem. Cell Biol.* 39:842–50.

Romanenko, A.M., Kinoshita, A., Wanibuchi, H., Wei, M., Zaparin, W.K., Vinnichenko, W.I. et al. 2006. Involvement of ubiquitination and sumoylation in bladder lesions induced by persistent long-term low dose ionizing radiation in humans. *J. Urol.* 175:739–43.

Rountree, C.B., Senadheera, S., Mato, J.M., Crooks, G.M. Lu, S.C. 2008. Expansion of liver cancer stem cells during aging in methionine adenosyltransferase 1A-deficient mice. *Hepatology* 47:1288–97.

Ruiz, F., Corrales, F.J., Miqueo, C. Mato, J.M. 1998. Nitric oxide inactivates rat hepatic methi-onine adenosyltransferase in vivo by S-nitrosylation. *Hepatology* 28:1051–7.

Santamaría, E., Avila, M.A., Latasa, M.U., Rubio, A., Martín-Duce, A., Lu, S.C. et al. 2003. Functional proteomics of non-alcoholic *stea*tohepatitis: Mitochondrial proteins as tar-gets of S-adenosylmethionine. *Proc. Natl. Acad. Sci. USA* 100:3065–70.

Saxena, N.K., Sharma, D., Ding, X., Lin, S., Marra, F., Merlin, D. et al. 2007. Concomitant acti-vation of the JAK/STAT, PI3K/AKT, and ERK signaling is involved in leptin-mediated promotion of invasion and migration of hepatocellular carcinoma cells. *Cancer Res.* 67:2497–507.

Schröder, M. 2010. Human DEAD-box protein 3 has multiple functions in gene regulation and cell cycle control and is a prime target for viral manipulation. *Biochem. Pharmacol.* 79:297–306.

Schröder, P.C., Fernández-Irigoyen, J., Bigaud, E., Serna, A., Renández-Alcoceba, R., Lu, S.C. et al. 2012. Proteomic analysis of human hepatoma cells expressing methionine adeno-syltransferase I/III: Characterization of DDX3X as a target of S-adenosylmethionine. *J. Proteomics* 75:2855–68.

Schwabe, R.F., Brenner, D.A. 2006. Mechanisms of liver injury. I. TNF-alpha-induced liver injury: Role of IKK, JNK, and ROS pathways. *Am. J. Physiol. Gastrointest. Liver Physiol.* 290:G583–9.

Shimizu-Saito, K., Horikawa, S., Kojima, N., Shiga, J., Senoo, H., Tsukada, K. 1997. Differential expression of S-adenosylmethionine synthetase isozymes in different cell types of rat liver. *Hepatology* 26:424–31.

Stramentinoli, G., Pezzoli, C., Galli-Kienle, M. 1979. Protective role of S-adenosyl-l-methionine against acetaminophen induced mortality and hepatotoxicity in mice. *Biochem. Pharmacol.* 28:3567–71.

Sullivan, D.M., Hoffman, J.L. 1983. Fractionation and kinetic properties of rat liver and kid-ney methionine adenosyltransferase isozymes. *Biochemistry* 22:1636–41.

Suzuki, Y., Imai, K., Takai, K., Hanai, T., Hayashi, H., Naiki, T. et al. 2013. Hepatocellular carcinoma patients with increased oxidative stress levels are prone to recurrence after curative treatment: A prospective case series study using the d-ROM test. *J. Cancer Res. Clin. Oncol.* 139:845–52.

Tomasi, M.L., Iglesias-Ara, A., Yang, H., Ramani, K., Feo, F., Pascale, M.R. et al. 2009. S-Adenosylmethionine regulates apurinic/apyrimidinic endonuclease 1 stability: Impli-cation in hepatocarcinogenesis. *Gastroenterology* 136:1025–36.

Tomasi, M.L., Li, T.W., Li, M., Mato, J.M., Lu, S.C. 2012a. Inhibition of human methionine adenosyltransferase 1A transcription by coding region methylation. *J. Cell. Physiol.* 227:1583–91.

Tomasi, M.L., Ramani, K., Lopitz-Otsoa, F., Rodriguez, M.S., Li, T.W., Ko, K. et al. 2010. S-Adenosylmethionine regulates dual-specificity mitogen-activated protein kinase phosphatase expression in mouse and human hepatocytes. *Hepatology* 51:2152–61.

Tomasi, M.L., Ryoo, M., Skay, A., Tomasi, I., Giordano, P., Mato, J.M. et al. 2013. Polyamine and methionine adenosyltransferase 2A crosstalk in human colon and liver cancer. *Exp. Cell. Res.* 319:1902–11.

Tomasi, M.L., Tomasi, I., Ramani, K., Pascale, R.M., Xu, J., Giordano, P. et al. 2012b. S-Adenosyl methionine regulates ubiquitin-conjugating enzyme 9 protein expression and sumoylation in murine liver and human cancers. *Hepatology* 56:982–93.

Tonks, N.K., Neel, B.G. 1996. From form to function: Signaling by protein tyrosine phosphatases. *Cell.* 87:365–8.

Torres, L., Avila, M.A., Carretero, M.V., Latasa, M.U., Caballería, J., López-Rodas, G. 2000. Liver-specific methionine adenosyltransferase *MAT1A* gene expression is associated with a specific pattern of promoter methylation and histone acetylation: Implications for *MAT1A* silencing during transformation. *FASEB J.* 14:95–102.

Vázquez-Chantada, M., Ariz, U., Varela-Rey, M., Embade, N., Martínez-Lopez, N., Fernández-Ramos, D. et al. 2009. Evidence for an LKB1/AMPK/eNOS cascade regulated by HGF, S-adenosylmethionine and NO in hepatocyte proliferation. *Hepatology* 49:608–17.

Vázquez-Chantada, M., Fernandez-Ramos, D., Embade, N., Martınez-Lopez, N., Varela-Rey, M., Woodhoo, A. et al. 2010. HuR/methyl-HuR and AUF1 regulate the MAT expressed during liver proliferation, differentiation, and carcinogenesis. *Gastroenterology* 138:1943–53.

Walker, A.K., Jacobs, R.L., Watts, J.L., Rottiers, V., Jiang, K., Finnegan, D.M. et al. 2011. A conserved SREBP-1/phosphatidylcholine feedback circuit regulates lipogenesis in metazoans. *Cell* 147:840–52.

Wullaert, A., Van Loo, G., Heyninck, K., Beyaert, R. 2007. Hepatic tumor necrosis factor signaling and nuclear factor-kappaB: Effects on liver homeostasis and beyond. *Endocr. Rev.* 28:365–86.

Xia, M., Chen, Y., Wang, L.C., Zandi, E., Yang, H., Bemanian, S. et al. 2010. Novel function and intracellular localization of methionine adenosyltransferase 2beta splicing variants. *J. Biol. Chem.* 285:20015–21.

Yang, H., Ara, A.I., Magilnick, N., Xia, M., Ramani, K., Chen, H. et al. 2008. Expression pattern, regulation, and functions of methionine adenosyltransferase 2beta splicing variants in hepatoma cells. *Gastroenterology* 134:281–91.

Yang, H., Huang, Z.Z., Zeng, Z.H., Chen, C.J., Selby, R.R., Lu, S.C. 2001a. Role of promoter methylation in increased methionine adenosyltransferase 2A expression in human liver cancer. *Am. J. Physiol. Gastrointest. Liver Physiol.* 280:G184–90.

Yang, H., Huang, Z.Z., Zeng, Z.H., Chen, C.J., Wang, J.H., Lu, S.C. 2001b. The role of c-Myb and Sp1 in the upregulation of methionine adenosyltransferase 2A gene expression in human hepatocellular carcinoma. *FASEB J.* 15:1507–16.

Yang, H., Sadda, M.R., Yu, V., Zeng, Y., Lee, T.D., Ou, X.P. et al. 2003. Induction of human methionine adenosyltransferase 2A expression by tumor necrosis factor alpha: Role of NF-κB and AP-1. *J. Biol. Chem.* 278:50887–96.

Yang, H., Zheng, Y., Li, T.W., Peng, H., Fernandez Ramos, D., Martínez-Chantar, M.L. et al. 2013a. Methionine adenosyltransferase 2B, HuR and Sirtuin 1 crosstalk impacts on resveratrol's effect on apoptosis and growth in liver cancer cells. *J. Biol. Chem.* [Epub ahead of print] PubMed PMID:23814050.

Yang, H., Cho, M.E., Li, T.W., Peng, H., Ko, K.S., Mato, J.M. et al. 2013b. MicroRNAs regulate methionine adenosyltransferase 1A expression in hepatocellular carcinoma. *J. Clin. Invest.* 123:285–98.

Zeng, Z., Huang, Z.Z., Chen, C., Yang, H., Mao, Z., Lu, S.C. 2000. Cloning and functional characterization of the 5′-flanking region of human methionine adenosyltransferase 1A gene. *Biochem. J.* 346:475–82.

Zhang, W., Sviripa, V., Chen, X., Shi, J., Yu, T., Hamza, A. et al. 2013. Fluorinated N,N-dialkylaminostilbenes repress colon cancer by targeting methionine S-adenosyltransferase 2A. *ACS Chem. Biol.* 8:796–803.

7 Role and Modulation of Nitric Oxide in the Cirrhotic Liver

Jordi Gracia-Sancho, Juan Carlos García-Pagán, and Jaime Bosch

CONTENTS

NITRIC OXIDE BIOCHEMISTRY

NITRIC OXIDE BIOSYNTHESIS

Nitric oxide (NO) is synthesized by nitric oxide synthase (NOS) through a complex set of redox reactions involving molecular oxygen and L-arginine as substrates, NADPH as electron donor, and flavin-adenine dinucleotide, flavin mononucleotide, tetrahydrobiopterin (BH_4), heme, and calmodulin as cofactors (Sessa, 1994). Three major isoforms of NOS have been described: neuronal NOS (NOS1 or nNOS), inducible NOS (NOS2 or iNOS), and endothelial NOS (NOS3 or eNOS).

Neuronal NOS, located in nervous tissue from both central and peripheral nervous systems, is activated by depolarization of nerve endings and mainly facilitates cell communication (Zhou and Zhu, 2009).

Inducible NOS can be expressed in a variety of cell types including vascular smooth muscle cells, hepatic stellate cells, macrophages, and hepatocytes in response to inflammatory cytokines and bacterial products. iNOS activity is Ca^{2+}-independent, and once activated, it produces large amounts of NO (Forstermann and Sessa, 2012).

Endothelial NOS is not only expressed in the endothelium but also in a variety of cells such as neurons, myocytes, and hepatocytes. This isoform synthesizes low amounts of NO for short periods in response to molecular (endogenous and exogenous) or biomechanical stimuli. eNOS activity is required to maintain circulatory homeostasis, also within the liver (Moncada and Higgs, 2006).

To note, two more recently described isoforms of NOS enlarge the NO synthases family. The mitochondrial NOS (mtNOS) may play an essential role regulating this organelle functions (Brookes, 2004), and the bacterial NOS (bNOS) that may confer bacterial protection against oxidative stress and antibiotics (Sudhamsu and Crane, 2009).

NO CHEMISTRY

Physical–chemical properties of NO make this gas an ideal biotransmitter for transient paracrine and autocrine signals. Indeed, NO has a short half-life (around 1 s) and a large diffusion coefficient, allowing it to freely penetrate cellular membranes. However, and considering that NO is an unstable free radical, many chemical interactions may limit its diffusion. As an example, NO can react with the superoxide anion (O_2^-), oxygen (O_2), and hemoproteins such as hemoglobin, myoglobin, and certain cytochromes. In fact, NO interaction with the prosthetic heme moiety group of the soluble guanylate cyclase activates the conversion of guanosine $5'$-triphosphate (GTP) to cyclic guanosine $3'$–$5'$-monophosphate (cGMP), ultimately inducing vasodilation. In addition, NO may be autooxidised by oxygen to generate reactive intermediates, generally termed reactive oxygen species, which promote many pathophysiologically damaging reactions such as nitrosation, nitration, lipid peroxidation, and DNA strand breaks (Beckman and Koppenol, 1996).

In conclusion, effective NO levels (from here on termed NO bioavailability) within a specific cellular environment is not only determined by the rate of synthesis but also by the rate of undesired reactivity and decomposition.

CIRRHOTIC PORTAL HYPERTENSION

Portal hypertension is a very frequent and severe complication of chronic liver disease. Its consequences, which include bleeding from gastroesophageal varices, ascites, hepatorenal syndrome, spontaneous bacterial peritonitis, hepatopulmonary syndrome, hyperkinetic syndrome, and hepatic encephalopathy, represent the first non-neoplastic cause of death and liver transplantation in patients with chronic liver disease (Bosch et al., 1992; Groszmann, 1994; Bosch and Garcia-Pagan, 2000; Iwakiri and Groszmann, 2006; Bosch et al., 2008; Garcia-Pagan et al., 2012). Moreover, it is associated with an increased risk of hepatocellular carcinoma development and with an increased mortality (Befeler and Di Bisceglie, 2002).

During the last three decades, different research groups have devoted their efforts to better understand the pathophysiology of portal hypertension, clearly demonstrating that an increase in the intrahepatic vascular resistance (IVR), due both to marked structural changes in the liver circulation and to the deregulation of hepatic cells phenotype, represents the primary factor in the development of portal hypertension. Secondary to the increased IVR, a progressive splanchnic vasodilatation that increments portal blood flow further aggravates portal hypertension and its complications. Additionally, development of intrahepatic shunts interferes with metabolic and O_2 exchange between the sinusoidal blood and the hepatocytes, further deteriorating liver function.

INCREASED IVR IN CIRRHOSIS

As mentioned, a significant increment in IVR results in portal hypertension development. Much of the increased IVR is due to the architectural distortions originated by the chronic liver tissue damage due to a variety of injuries (chronic viral infection, toxic-induced, autoimmune, and metabolic), together with the reiterative activation of the wound healing reaction (Pinzani et al., 2011). Moreover, a significant deregulation of the hepatic cells phenotype further contributes to raise the hepatic resistance. This dynamic and reversible component of IVR was first described by Bhathal and Grossmann in 1985 (Bathal and Grossmann, 1985) and may represent up to 30%–40% of the total increase of IVR in cirrhosis. Hepatic cells influencing the hepatic vascular tone involve sinusoidal and extrasinusoidal elements, and mainly include liver sinusoidal endothelial cells (LSEC), Kupffer cells (KC), and contractile cells (hepatic stellate cells [HSC], myofibroblasts, and vascular smooth muscle cells) (Smedsrod et al., 1994; Pinzani and Gentilini, 1999; DeLeve, 2007).

HEPATIC ENDOTHELIAL DYSFUNCTION IN CIRRHOSIS

In healthy conditions, the hepatic endothelium is able to produce vasodilatory molecules to prevent or attenuate an increase in IVR in response to increments in blood volume, blood pressure, or vasoconstrictors. However, in cirrhosis there is an impairment in the endothelial-mediated vasodilatation, a phenomenon known as endothelial dysfunction (Albillos et al., 1995; Gupta et al., 1998; Rockey and Chung, 1998; Cahill et al., 2001; Bosch et al., 2010; Iwakiri, 2012). Indeed, the cirrhotic vascular bed cannot accommodate elevations of portal flow resulting in marked increases in portal pressure (Bosch et al., 1992). In experimental models of cirrhosis, hepatic endothelial dysfunction gives rise to an impaired vasodilatory response to the endothelial-selective vasodilator acetylcholine (Gupta et al., 1998), which is used to quantify the degree of endothelial dysfunction.

Liver endothelial dysfunction in cirrhosis has been attributed to increased generation of vasoconstrictors (mainly cyclooxygenase 1–derived thromboxane A2 and probably also prostaglandin H2), and importantly to reduced bioavailability of NO (Rockey and Weisiger, 1996; Shah et al., 1997; Gupta et al., 1998; Graupera et al., 2003; Gracia-Sancho et al., 2007; Anegawa et al., 2008).

ENDOGENOUS DOWNREGULATION OF NO BIOAVAILABILITY IN THE CIRRHOTIC LIVER

Nitric oxide plays a variety of roles within the hepatic sinusoid, being the activation of the soluble guanylate cyclase (sGC), the most important in maintaining a correct vascular tone. Once activated, sGC leads to cGMP generation, activation of the cGMP-dependent protein kinase, phosphorylation of proteins involved in Ca^{2+} homeostasis, decrease in intracellular Ca^{2+} concentration, relaxation of contractile elements, and finally vasodilatation (Wiest and Groszmann, 2002). Thus, regulation of hepatic vascular tone in normal conditions is tightly dependent on the NO bio-availability that counterbalances the effects of systemic and local vasoconstrictors.

In addition, activation of sGC in HSC by endothelial-derived NO is key to preserve HSC phenotype and avoid their activation (Marrone et al., 2013). Indeed, situations with downregulation in hepatic endothelial NO bioavailability lead to deregulation of HSC, which become proliferative, pro-fibrotic, and pro-vasoconstrictive (DeLeve et al., 2008; Marrone et al., 2013).

Hepatic NO bioavailability in cirrhosis is markedly diminished. Two main mech-anisms provoke low NO content: (1) insufficient NO production and (2) O_2-mediated NO scavenging.

Reduced NO production in cirrhotic LSEC is due to diverse deregulations in the eNOS system. First, inefficient eNOS mRNA translation (and/or eNOS mRNA insta-bility) has been described in experimental models of cirrhosis, but its underlying mechanisms have not yet appropriately studied (Gracia-Sancho et al., 2011). Second, hepatic eNOS protein expression seems to be unaltered, or even reduced, in cirrhosis (Zimmermann et al., 1996; Rockey and Chung, 1998; Shah et al., 1999a; Gracia-Sancho et al., 2011), but its enzymatic activity is markedly diminished (Rockey and Chung, 1998; Shah et al., 1999a). Third, several post-translational regulations that reduce eNOS activity have been described in cirrhotic livers (Rockey and Chung, 1998; Shah et al., 1999a, b, 2001; Liu et al., 2002, 2005; Laleman et al., 2005; Matei et al., 2006, 2008; Rosado et al., 2012).

eNOS protein post-translational deactivation results from decreased interac-tion with calmodulin, AKT, and BH_4, and increased caveolin 1, RhoA, asymmetric dimethylarginine (ADMA), and COX-derived vasoconstrictor prostanoids (Shah et al., 1999a, b, 2001; Rockey and Chung, 1998; Liu et al., 2002, 2005; Laleman et al., 2005; Matei et al., 2006, 2008; Rosado et al., 2012).

Caveolins are the main component of cellular caveolae membranes and act as scaffolding proteins interacting with several molecular pathways. Indeed, caveolin 1 negatively interacts with eNOS pathway, inhibiting its binding capability with the stimulatory protein calmodulin (Fleming and Busse, 2003). Interestingly, cirrhotic livers exhibit elevated levels of caveolin 1, increased eNOS–caveolin 1 interaction and reduced calmodulin levels (Shah et al., 2001; Hendrickson et al., 2003).

Akt, a serine/threonine protein kinase, upregulates eNOS activity phosphorylat-ing specific activator sites (Dimmeler et al., 1999). In cirrhosis, hepatic Akt levels and Akt-dependent eNOS phosphrylation are reduced (Morales-Ruiz et al., 2003; Abraldes et al., 2007). One of the mechanisms for reduced Akt phosphorylation within the cirrhotic liver relates to increased endothelin 1–mediated activation of G-protein–coupled receptor kinase 2 (GRK-2), which directly interacts and inhibits Akt (Liu et al., 2005).

BH_4 is an essential cofactor of eNOS that is reduced in livers with cirrhosis (Matei et al., 2006, 2008). BH_4 serves as catalyst of eNOS activity facilitating the electron transfer necessary for NO production. In situations of low BH_4 availability, eNOS becomes "uncoupled," and instead of producing NO, it synthesizes the radical oxygen species superoxide (O_2^-), which can interact with NO further diminishing NO bioavailability (Gracia-Sancho et al., 2008).

ADMA has been shown to inhibit NO production by competing with L-arginine as substrate of eNOS (Fleming and Busse, 2003); interestingly, cirrhotic animals exhibit increased hepatic ADMA expression in comparison to controls (Laleman et al., 2005). Recent data demonstrated that hepatic ADMA levels correlate with HVPG in cirrhotic patients (Vizzutti et al., 2007), further suggesting its role in the pathophysiology of portal hypertension.

As stated, COX-derived vasoconstrictor prostanoids significantly aggravate portal hypertensive syndrome in cirrhosis because of their constrictive properties. However, recent data from Rosado and colleagues demonstrated that elevated COX activity in cirrhotic livers also negatively affects eNOS activity, inducing a marked reduction in hepatic NO bioavailability (Rosado et al., 2012). Thus, strategies aimed at blocking COX activity may also improve NO levels, which may foster ameliorate portal hypertension.

The second main mechanism influencing hepatic NO bioavailability in cirrhosis is the accumulation of oxidative stress within the liver. It has been demonstrated that the superoxide radical (O_2^-) avidly reacts with NO to form a new radical oxygen species termed peroxynitrite ($ONOO^-$), thus reducing NO levels and overall increasing oxidative stress (Huie and Padmaja, 1993). Importantly, this chemical reactivity has been demonstrated within the cirrhotic liver. In fact, we demonstrated that cirrhotic livers exhibit elevated levels of O_2^-, which result from increased activity of COX and xanthine oxidase as well as reduced superoxide dismutase (SOD) activity and increased expression of nitrotyrosinated proteins, which are surrogate markers of $ONOO^-$ levels (Gracia-Sancho et al., 2008). In addition, this study also demonstrated that in vitro deregulation of healthy endothelial cells by increasing intracellular levels of oxidative stress using two different pharmacological strategies results in marked diminution of endothelial NO levels (Gracia-Sancho et al., 2008). These findings opened the rationale to use antioxidants as potential treatment to increase hepatic NO bioavailability, and ultimately to ameliorate portal hypertension.

NO MODULATION AS THERAPEUTIC STRATEGY FOR PORTAL HYPERTENSION

Amelioration of NO levels within the cirrhotic liver probably represents the most challenging venture that liver vascular research teams have faced. Considering the underlying mechanisms of low NO levels in the cirrhotic liver, therapeutic strategies will be described depending on their molecular target.

EXOGENOUS NO ADMINISTRATION

The first attempt to improve NO bioavailability was the exogenous administration of NO donors. Administration of nitrates, such as isosorbide-5-mononitrate, has been shown to decrease portal pressure. However, a major concern with the use of these drugs in patients with advanced cirrhosis is that, by reducing arterial blood pressure, they may promote the activation of endogenous vasoactive systems that finally may lead to water and sodium retention (Bosch et al., 2010). NCX-1000, a NO-releasing derivative of the ursodeoxycolic acid, was designed to selectively release NO in the intrahepatic circulation, and consequently reduce portal pressure without adverse effects on the systemic and splanchnic circulation. Experimental studies were promising (Fiorucci et al., 2003); however, data from a study with cirrhotic patients indicated that NCX-1000 did not reduce basal HVPG, and it decreased hepatic blood flow and systolic blood pressure (Berzigotti et al., 2010). Inefficacy of NCX-1000 at the bedside was attributed to poor bioavailability and to the lack of specific intrahepatic vasodilatory effect (Berzigotti et al., 2010).

The search of an effective way to specifically supplement NO within the liver, thus reducing portal pressure without affecting systemic circulation, is still necessary. Importantly, recent experimental data from our group demonstrated that exogenous administration of NO to cirrhotic LSEC not only improves the bioavailability of this vasodilator but also inhibits the activity and release of COX-derived vasoconstrictor prostanoids (Rosado et al., 2012), thus further reinforcing the importance of developing a hepatic-selective NO donor.

ALTERED eNOS ACTIVITY

Considering the profound deregulation that the endothelial NO synthase suffers during cirrhosis progression, therapeutic approaches should be designed to improve NO production by LSEC rather that increasing NO levels from external sources. This prompted us to first propose in 2004 the use of statins as a new therapeutic option to improve LSEC phenotype and liver circulation in cirrhosis, without affecting other vascular territories (Zafra et al., 2004). The molecular mechanisms of this groundbreaking study were latterly unraveled in experimental models of cirrhosis demonstrating that statins significantly upregulate NO production by, at least, two different means: (1) upregulating Akt-dependent eNOS activation (Abraldes et al., 2007; Trebicka et al., 2007) and (2) inducing eNOS mRNA expression through the activation of the transcription factor Kruppel-like factor 2 (KLF2) (Gracia-Sancho et al., 2010; Marrone et al., 2013). Moreover, a recent study from our team demonstrated that liver endothelial phenotype amelioration achieved by statins treatment paracrinally improves HSC phenotype (Marrone et al., 2013). Interestingly, this last beneficial effect of statins was dependent on the integrity of the endothelial KLF2-NO-cGMP molecular axis and may explain the favorable effects on liver fibrosis observed after a semichronic administration of statins to animals with cirrhosis (Marrone et al., 2013).

Tetrahydrobipterin (BH$_4$) is an essential cofactor for the adequate generation of NO by NOS enzymes. If adequate quantities of BH4 are not present, production of NO is decreased. Studies from our laboratory have shown that in cirrhotic livers there is a deficiency in BH$_4$, which is associated with decreased NOS activity and NO bioavailability. In cirrhotic animals, administration of BH$_4$ increased hepatic NOS activity and cGMP levels and significantly reduced portal pressure (Matei et al., 2006, 2008). Amelioration in portal hypertension was associated with normalization of arterial pressure. These data support the concept that BH_4 supplementation may represent a new and effective therapeutic strategy for portal hypertension.

Other experimental strategies aimed at improving endothelial NO synthesis have been based on overexpressing NOS infecting the liver with adenovirus codifying for eNOS (Shah et al., 2000; Van de Casteele et al., 2002) and nNOS (Yu et al., 2000) or activating endogenous NOS through administration of a constitutively active Akt adenoviral construct (Morales-Ruiz et al., 2003). Obvious controversial issues regarding use of adenovirus in humans raised, and still need additional investigations.

ANTIOXIDANT STRATEGIES

Oxidative stress markedly contributes to reduce NO bioavailability in cirrhotic livers; thus, antioxidant therapies able to remove hepatic O_2^- may represent new therapeutic strategies to ameliorate hepatic vascular tone in cirrhosis. In fact, experimental studies using adenovirus of SOD (Lavina et al., 2009), exogenous administration of recombinant SOD (Guillaume et al., 2013), acetylcysteine (Yang et al., 2008), vitamin E (Yang et al., 2012), and resveratrol (Di Pascoli et al., 2013) have shown beneficial effects on cirrhotic portal hypertension due to their capability to reduce intrahepatic O_2^- and concomitantly increase NO bioavailability. Indeed, very recent data obtained in experimental models of portal hypertension demonstrated that 2-week administration of resveratrol (a polyphenol found in variety of foods) induces a 15% reduction in portal pressure, without modification in systemic hemodynamics, and very importantly, it is associated with a marked regression in liver fibrosis (Di Pascoli et al., 2013). Clinical application of resveratrol, or other activators of its underlying molecular mechanisms, to ameliorate cirrhosis and portal hypertension require further investigations.

The hepatic beneficial effects of other antioxidants have also been validated in cirrhotic patients and demonstrate that exogenous administration of vitamin C (Hernandez-Guerra et al., 2006) or high-antioxidant aliments like black chocolate (De Gottardi et al., 2012) significantly ameliorate portal hypertensive syndrome, thus proposing nutritional supplementation of cirrhotic patients with antioxidants as a novel and easy-to-accomplish therapeutic strategy.

CONCLUSIONS

Liver cirrhosis, and its main complication portal hypertension, represents a serious unsolved clinical problem worldwide, with more than 170,000 deaths per year in Europe (Blachier et al., 2013). Reduced intrahepatic levels of nitric oxide significantly contribute to the development and perpetuation of portal hypertension and therefore represent an obvious and theoretically ideal therapeutic target. Antioxidant therapies able to diminish intrahepatic oxidative stress-mediated scavenge of nitric oxide, together with statins that upregulate the KLF2-eNOS molecular axis, are the most promising translational approaches to effectively increase hepatic nitric oxide bioavailability, reduce vascular tone, and, overall, improve portal hypertension syndrome. Nearby results from ongoing clinical trials will validate these hypotheses.

REFERENCES

Abraldes, J. G., A. Rodriguez-Vilarrupla, M. Graupera, C. Zafra, H. Garcia-Caldero, J. C. Garcia-Pagan, and J. Bosch. 2007. Simvastatin treatment improves liver sinusoidal endothelial dysfunction in CCl(4) cirrhotic rats. *J. Hepatol.* 46:1040–1046.

Albillos, A., I. Rossi, G. Cacho, M. V. Martinez, I. Millan, L. Abreu, C. Barrios, and P. Escartin. 1995. Enhanced endothelium-dependent vasodilation in patients with cirrhosis. *Am. J. Physiol.* 268:G459–G464.

Anegawa, G., H. Kawanaka, D. Yoshida, K. Konishi, S. Yamaguchi, N. Kinjo, A. Taketomi, M. Hashizume, H. Shimokawa, and Y. Maehara. 2008. Defective endothelial nitric oxide synthase signaling is mediated by rho-kinase activation in rats with secondary biliary cirrhosis. *Hepatology* 47:966–977.

Bathal, P. S. and H. J. Grossmann. 1985. Reduction of the increased portal vascular resistance of the isolated perfused cirrhotic rat liver by vasodilators. *J. Hepatol.* 1:325–329.

Beckman, J. S. and W. H. Koppenol. 1996. Nitric oxide, superoxide, and peroxynitrite: The good, the bad, and ugly. *Am. J. Physiol.* 271:C1424–C1437.

Befeler, A. S. and A. M. Di Bisceglie. 2002. Hepatocellular carcinoma: Diagnosis and treatment. *Gastroenterology* 122:1609–1619.

Berzigotti, A., P. Bellot, G. A. De, J. C. Garcia-Pagan, C. Gagnon, J. Spenard, and J. Bosch. 2010. NCX-1000, a nitric oxide-releasing derivative of UDCA, does not decrease portal pressure in patients with cirrhosis: Results of a randomized, double-blind, dose-escalating study. *Am. J. Gastroenterol.* 105:1094–1101.

Blachier M., H. Leleu, M. Peck-Radosavljevic, D. C. Valla, and F.Roudot-Thoraval. 2013. The burden of liver disease in Europe: A review of available epidemiological data. *J Hepatol.* 58(3):593-608. doi: 10.1016/j.jhep.2012.12.005.

Bosch, J., J. G. Abraldes, A. Berzigotti, and J. C. Garcia-Pagan. 2008. Portal hypertension and gastrointestinal bleeding. *Semin. Liver Dis.* 28:3–25.

Bosch, J., J. G. Abraldes, M. Fernandez, and J. C. Garcia-Pagan. 2010. Hepatic endothelial dysfunction and abnormal angiogenesis: New targets in the treatment of portal hypertension. *J. Hepatol.* 53:558–567.

Bosch, J. and J. C. Garcia-Pagan. 2000. Complications of cirrhosis. I. Portal hypertension. *J. Hepatol.* 32:141–156.

Bosch, J., P. Pizcueta, F. Feu, M. Fernandez, and J. C. Garcia-Pagan. 1992. Pathophysiology of portal hypertension. *Gastroenterol. Clin. North Am.* 21:1–14.

Brookes, P. S. 2004. Mitochondrial nitric oxide synthase. *Mitochondrion.* 3:187–204.

Cahill, P. A., E. M. Redmond, and J. V. Sitzmann. 2001. Endothelial dysfunction in cirrhosis and portal hypertension. *Pharmacol. Ther.* 89:273–293.

De Gottardi, A., A. Berzigotti, S. Seijo, M. D'Amico, W. Thormann, J. G. Abraldes, J. C. Garcia-Pagan, and J. Bosch. 2012. Postprandial effects of dark chocolate on portal hypertension in patients with cirrhosis: Results of a phase 2, double-blind, randomized controlled trial. *Am. J. Clin. Nutr.* 96:584–590.

DeLeve, L. D. 2007. Hepatic microvasculature in liver injury. *Semin. Liver Dis.* 27:390–400.

DeLeve, L. D., X. Wang, and Y. Guo. 2008. Sinusoidal endothelial cells prevent rat stellate cell activation and promote reversion to quiescence. *Hepatology* 48:920–930.

Di Pascoli M., M. Divi, A. Rodriguez-Vilarrupla, E. Rosado, J. Gracia-Sancho, M. Vilaseca, J. Bosch, and J. C. Garcia-Pagan. 2013. Resveratrol improves intrahepatic endothelial dysfunction and reduces hepatic fibrosis and portal pressure in cirrhotic rats. *J. Hepatol.* 58:904–910.

Dimmeler, S., I. Fleming, B. Fisslthaler, C. Hermann, R. Busse, and A. M. Zeiher. 1999. Activation of nitric oxide synthase in endothelial cells by Akt-dependent phosphorylation. *Nature* 399:601–605.

Fiorucci, S., E. Antonelli, V. Brancaleone, L. Sanpaolo, S. Orlandi, E. Distrutti, G. Acuto, C. Clerici, M. Baldoni, S. P. Del, and A. Morelli. 2003. NCX-1000, a nitric oxide-releasing derivative of ursodeoxycholic acid, ameliorates portal hypertension and lowers norepinephrine-induced intrahepatic resistance in the isolated and perfused rat liver. *J. Hepatol.* 39:932–939.

Fleming, I. and R. Busse. 2003. Molecular mechanisms involved in the regulation of the endothelial nitric oxide synthase. *Am. J. Physiol. Regul. Integr. Comp. Physiol.* 284:R1–12.

Forstermann, U. and W. C. Sessa. 2012. Nitric oxide synthases: Regulation and function. *Eur. Heart J.* 33:829–837d.

Garcia-Pagan, J. C., J. Gracia-Sancho, and J. Bosch. 2012. Functional aspects on the pathophysiology of portal hypertension in cirrhosis. *J. Hepatol.* 57:458–461.

Gracia-Sancho, J., B. Lavina, A. Rodriguez-Vilarrupla, H. Garcia-Caldero, J. Bosch, and J. C. Garcia-Pagan. 2007. Enhanced vasoconstrictor prostanoid production by sinusoidal endothelial cells increases portal perfusion pressure in cirrhotic rat livers. *J. Hepatol.* 47:220–227.

Gracia-Sancho, J., B. Lavina, A. Rodriguez-Vilarrupla, H. Garcia-Caldero, M. Fernandez, J. Bosch, and J. C. Garcia-Pagan. 2008. Increased oxidative stress in cirrhotic rat livers: A potential mechanism contributing to reduced nitric oxide bioavailability. *Hepatology* 47:1248–1256.

Gracia-Sancho, J., L. Russo, H. Garcia-Caldero, J. C. Garcia-Pagan, G. Garcia-Cardena, and J. Bosch. 2011. Endothelial expression of transcription factor Kruppel-like factor 2 and its vasoprotective target genes in the normal and cirrhotic rat liver. *Gut.* 60:517–524.

Gracia-Sancho, J., G. Villarreal, Jr., Y. Zhang, and G. Garcia-Cardena. 2010. Activation of SIRT1 by resveratrol induces KLF2 expression conferring an endothelial vasoprotective phenotype. *Cardiovasc. Res.* 85:514–519.

Graupera, M., J. C. Garcia-Pagan, J. G. Abraldes, C. Peralta, M. Bragulat, H. Corominola, J. Bosch, and J. Rodes. 2003. Cyclooxygenase-derived products modulate the increased intrahepatic resistance of cirrhotic rat livers. *Hepatology* 37:172–181.

Groszmann, R. J. 1994. Hyperdynamic circulation of liver disease 40 years later: Pathophysiology and clinical consequences. *Hepatology* 20:1359–1363.

Guillaume, M., A. Rodriguez-Vilarrupla, J. Gracia-Sancho, E. Rosado, A. Mancini, J. Bosch, and J. C. Garcia-Pagan. 2013. Recombinant human manganese superoxide dismutase reduces liver fibrosis and portal pressure in CCl_4-cirrhotic rats. *J. Hepatol.* 58:240–246.

Gupta, T. K., M. Toruner, M. K. Chung, and R. J. Groszmann. 1998. Endothelial dysfunction and decreased production of nitric oxide in the intrahepatic microcirculation of cirrhotic rats. *Hepatology* 28:926–931.

Hendrickson, H., S. Chatterjee, S. Cao, M. M. Ruiz, W. C. Sessa, and V. Shah. 2003. Influence of caveolin on constitutively activated recombinant eNOS: Insights into eNOS dysfunction in BDL rat liver. *Am. J. Physiol. Gastrointest. Liver Physiol.* 285:G652–G660.

Hernandez-Guerra, M., J. C. Garcia-Pagan, J. Turnes, P. Bellot, R. Deulofeu, J. G. Abraldes, and J. Bosch. 2006. Ascorbic acid improves the intrahepatic endothelial dysfunction of patients with cirrhosis and portal hypertension. *Hepatology.* 43:485–491.

Huie, R. E. and S. Padmaja. 1993. The reaction of NO with superoxide. *Free Radic. Res. Commun.* 18:195–199.

Iwakiri, Y. 2012. Endothelial dysfunction in the regulation of cirrhosis and portal hypertension. *Liver Int.* 32:199–213.

Iwakiri, Y. and R. J. Groszmann. 2006. The hyperdynamic circulation of chronic liver diseases: From the patient to the molecule. *Hepatology* 43:S121–S131.

Laleman, W., A. Omasta, M. Van de Casteele, M. Zeegers, I. Vander Elst, L. Van Landeghem, T. Severi, J. van Pelt, T. Roskams, J. Fevery, and F. Nevens. 2005. A role for asymmetric dimethylarginine in the pathophysiology of portal hypertension in rats with biliary cirrhosis. *Hepatology.* 42:1382–1390.

Lavina, B., J. Gracia-Sancho, A. Rodriguez-Vilarrupla, Y. Chu, D. D. Heistad, J. Bosch, and J. C. Garcia-Pagan. 2009. Superoxide dismutase gene transfer reduces portal pressure in CCl4 cirrhotic rats with portal hypertension. *Gut* 58:118–125.

Liu, S., C. R. Reynolds, J. Huang, and D. C. Rockey. 2002. The role of Akt in sinusoidal endothelial cell production of nitric oxide: Implications for the pathogenesis of portal hypertension. *Hepatology* 36:229A.

Liu, S. L., R. T. Premont, C. D. Kontos, S. K. Zhu, and D. C. Rockey. 2005. A crucial role for GRK2 in regulation of endothelial cell nitric oxide synthase function in portal hypertension. *Nature Medicine* 11:952–958.

Marrone, G., L. Russo, E. Rosado, D. Hide, G. Garcia-Cardena, J. C. Garcia-Pagan, J. Bosch, and J. Gracia-Sancho. 2013. The transcription factor KLF2 mediates hepatic endothelial protection and paracrine endothelial-stellate cell deactivation induced by statins. *J. Hepatol.* 58:98–103.

Matei, V., A. Rodriguez-Vilarrupla, R. Deulofeu, D. Colomer, M. Fernandez, J. Bosch, and J. C. Garcia-Pagan. 2006. The eNOS cofactor tetrahydrobiopterin improves endothelial dysfunction in livers of rats with CCl4 cirrhosis. *Hepatology* 44:44–52.

Matei, V., A. Rodriguez-Vilarrupla, R. Deulofeu, H. Garcia-Caldero, M. Fernandez, J. Bosch, and J. C. Garcia-Pagan. 2008. Three-day tetrahydrobiopterin therapy increases in vivo hepatic NOS activity and reduces portal pressure in CCl4 cirrhotic rats. *J. Hepatol.* 49:192–197.

Moncada, S. and E. A. Higgs. 2006. Nitric oxide and the vascular endothelium. *Handb. Exp. Pharmacol.* 213–254.

Morales-Ruiz, M., P. Cejudo-Martín, G. Fernandez-Varo, S. Tugues, J. Ros, P. Angeli, F. Rivera, V. Arroyo, J. Rodes, W. C. Sessa, and W. Jimenez. 2003. Transduction of the liver with activated Akt normalizes portal pressure in cirrhotic rats. *Gastroenterology* 125:522–531.

Pinzani, M. and P. Gentilini. 1999. Biology of hepatic stellate cells and their possible relevance in the pathogenesis of portal hypertension in cirrhosis. *Semin. Liver Dis.* 19:397–410.

Pinzani, M., M. Rosselli, and M. Zuckermann. 2011. Liver cirrhosis. *Best. Pract. Res. Clin. Gastroenterol.* 25:281–290.

Rockey, D. C. and J. J. Chung. 1998. Reduced nitric oxide production by endothelial cells in cirrhotic rat liver: Endothelial dysfunction in portal hypertension. *Gastroenterology* 114:344–351.

Rockey, D. C. and R. A. Weisiger. 1996. Endothelin induced contractility of stellate cells from normal and cirrhotic rat liver: Implications for regulation of portal pressure and resistance. *Hepatology* 24:233–240.

Rosado, E., A. Rodriguez-Vilarrupla, J. Gracia-Sancho, M. Monclus, J. Bosch, and J. C. Garcia-Pagan. 2012. Interaction between NO and COX pathways modulating hepatic endothelial cells from control and cirrhotic rats. *J. Cell Mol. Med.* 16:2461–2470.

Sessa, W. C. 1994. The nitric oxide synthase family of proteins. *J. Vasc. Res.* 31:131–143.

Shah, V., S. Cao, H. Hendrickson, J. Yao, and Z. S. Katusic. 2001. Regulation of hepatic eNOS by caveolin and calmodulin after bile duct ligation in rats. *Am. J. Physiol. Gastrointest. Liver Physiol.* 280:G1209–G1216.

Shah, V., A. F. Chen, S. Cao, H. Hendrickson, D. Weiler, L. Smith, J. Yao, and Z. S. Katusic. 2000. Gene transfer of recombinant endothelial nitric oxide synthase to liver in vivo and in vitro. *Am. J. Physiol. Gastrointest. Liver Physiol.* 279:G1023–G1030.

Shah, V., F. G. Haddad, G. Garcia-Cardena, J. A. Frangos, A. Mennone, R. J. Groszmann, and W. C. Sessa. 1997. Liver sinusoidal endothelial cells are responsible for nitric oxide modulation of resistance in the hepatic sinusoids. *J. Clin. Invest.* 100:2923–2930.

Shah, V., M. Toruner, F. Haddad, G. Cadelina, A. Papapetropoulos, K. Choo, W. C. Sessa, and R. J. Groszmann. 1999a. Impaired endothelial nitric oxide synthase activity associated with enhanced caveolin binding in experimental cirrhosis in the rat. *Gastroenterology* 117:1222–1228.

Shah, V., R. Wiest, G. Garcia-Cardena, G. Cadelina, R. J. Groszmann, and W. C. Sessa. 1999b. Hsp90 regulation of endothelial nitric oxide synthase contributes to vascular control in portal hypertension. *Am. J. Physiol.* 277:G463–G468.

Smedsrod, B., P. J. De Bleser, F. Braet, P. Lovisetti, K. Vanderkerken, E. Wisse, and A. Geerts. 1994. Cell biology of liver endothelial and Kupffer cells. *Gut.* 35:1509–1516.

Sudhamsu, J. and B. R. Crane. 2009. Bacterial nitric oxide synthases: What are they good for? *Trends Microbiol.* 17:212–218.

Trebicka, J., M. Hennenberg, W. Laleman, N. Shelest, E. Biecker, M. Schepke, F. Nevens, T. Sauerbruch, and J. Heller. 2007. Atorvastatin lowers portal pressure in cirrhotic rats by inhibition of RhoA/Rho-kinase and activation of endothelial nitric oxide synthase. *Hepatology* 46:242–253.

Van de Casteele, M., A. Omasta, S. Janssens, T. Roskams, V. Desmet, F. Nevens, and J. Fevery. 2002. In vivo gene transfer of endothelial nitric oxide synthase decreases portal pressure in anaesthetised carbon tetrachloride cirrhotic rats. *Gut.* 51:440–445.

Vizzutti, F., R. G. Romanelli, U. Arena, L. Rega, M. Brogi, C. Calabresi, E. Masini, R. Tarquini, M. Zipoli, V. Boddi, F. Marra, G. Laffi, and M. Pinzani. 2007. ADMA correlates with portal pressure in patients with compensated cirrhosis. *Eur. J. Clin. Invest.* 37:509–515.

Wiest, R. and R. J. Groszmann. 2002. The paradox of nitric oxide in cirrhosis and portal hypertension: Too much, not enough. *Hepatology* 35:478–491.

Yang, Y. Y., K. C. Lee, Y. T. Huang, Y. W. Wang, M. C. Hou, F. Y. Lee, H. C. Lin, and S. D. Lee. 2008. Effects of N-acetylcysteine administration in hepatic microcirculation of rats with biliary cirrhosis. *J. Hepatol.* 49:25–33.

Yang, Y. Y., T. Y. Lee, Y. T. Huang, C. C. Chan, Y. C. Yeh, F. Y. Lee, S. D. Lee, and H. C. Lin. 2012. Asymmetric dimethylarginine (ADMA) determines the improvement of hepatic endothelial dysfunction by vitamin E in cirrhotic rats. *Liver Int.* 32:48–57.

Yu, Q., R. Shao, H. S. Qian, S. E. George, and D. C. Rockey. 2000. Gene transfer of the neuronal NO synthase isoform to cirrhotic rat liver ameliorates portal hypertension. *J. Clin. Invest.* 105:741–748.

Zafra, C., J. G. Abraldes, J. Turnes, A. Berzigotti, M. Fernandez, J. C. Garca-Pagan, J. Rodes, and J. Bosch. 2004. Simvastatin enhances hepatic nitric oxide production and decreases the hepatic vascular tone in patients with cirrhosis. *Gastroenterology* 126:749–755.

Zhou, L. and D. Y. Zhu. 2009. Neuronal nitric oxide synthase: Structure, subcellular localization, regulation, and clinical implications. *Nitric Oxide.* 20:223–230.

Zimmermann, H., P. Kurzen, W. Klossner, E. L. Renner, and U. Marti. 1996. Decreased constitutive hepatic nitric oxide synthase expression in secondary biliary fibrosis and its changes after Roux-en-Y choledocho-jejunostomy in the rat. *J. Hepatol.* 25:567–573.

8 Role of Mitochondria in Alcoholic Liver Disease and Nonalcoholic Fatty Liver Disease

Nicole Rubin, Ho Leung, Jacob E. Valk,
Stephen M. Wertheimer, and Derick Han

CONTENTS

INTRODUCTION

Fat accumulation in the liver (steatosis) is associated with alcohol consumption, obesity, and many metabolic disorders [1,2]. Cases of fatty liver have been dramatically increasing in the United States due in part to increasing rates of obesity and metabolic syndromes. Although fat accumulation in the liver is considered somewhat benign, it can dramatically and unpredictably progress to more serious conditions such as steatohepatitis (fatty liver and inflammation) and in severe cases, cirrhosis (fibrosis of liver and extensive hepatocyte death) [1,2]. Liver diseases associated with steatosis are generally divided into two broad categories: alcoholic liver disease (ALD) and nonalcoholic fatty liver disease (NAFLD). As the name suggests, ALD is associated with chronic alcohol intake, which triggers steatosis. NAFLD, meanwhile, is associated with obesity and metabolic disorders. Although the causes of ALD and NAFLD are different, the two liver pathologies share many biochemical and histological similarities.

The factors mediating the pathogenesis of ALD and NAFLD have not been completely characterized, but mitochondrial dysfunction has been traditionally considered an important and early event in disease development [3–5]. This hypothesis arose from observations of changes in mitochondrial morphology, increased mitochondrial reactive oxygen species generation, increased mtDNA damage, and declines in mitochondrial respiration in various steatosis animals models (i.e., chronic alcohol feeding, high-fat diet [HFD], methionine–choline-deficient [MCD] diet) [5–8]. However, do these findings conclusively suggest that mitochondrial dysfunction is a central feature of steatosis? There are key issues such as variations in animal models and methodological considerations that suggest mitochondrial dysfunction may be an incomplete assessment of mitochondrial changes that accompany ALD and NAFLD. Our recent work with alcohol-fed mice suggests that mitochondrial adaptation and remodeling may be the predominant mitochondrial alterations that occur during steatosis [9]. Mitochondria are very dynamic organelles that undergo many types of alterations (i.e., fusion-fission changes, respiratory complex remodeling, morphological changes, etc.) that help cells adapt to stress and metabolic changes [10,11]. It is clear that steatosis caused by alcohol and other metabolic stresses cause mitochondrial injury and damage. However, following mitochondrial injury, mitochondrial adaptation and remodeling will occur, which is only beginning to be explored. In this chapter, we review the alterations that occur in mitochondria during ALD and NAFLD. The question of whether mitochondrial dysfunction or mitochondrial remodeling is central to ALD or NAFLD will be examined.

ALCOHOLIC LIVER DISEASE

ROLE OF MITOCHONDRIA IN ALCOHOL METABOLISM IN THE LIVER

ALD remains an important clinical problem in the United States, affecting more than 2 million people and causing more than 15,000 deaths annually. The liver is the major site of alcohol metabolism and thus the major site of alcohol-induced injury. Alcohol is primarily metabolized by two enzymes in the liver: alcohol dehydrogenase

(ADH) in the cytoplasm and aldehyde dehydrogenase 2 (ALDH2) in mitochondria (reactions 1 and 2).

$$\text{Ethanol} + NAD^+ + H^+ \leftrightarrow \text{acetaldehyde} + NADH \quad \text{catalyzed by ADH} \quad (1)$$

$$\text{Acetaldehyde} + NAD^+ + H^+ \leftrightarrow \text{acetate} + NADH \quad \text{catalyzed by ALDH2} \quad (2)$$

Cytochrome p450 2E1 isoform (CYP2E1) is also upregulated by chronic alcohol feeding; however, this pathway mainly becomes significant when alcohol levels are very high [12]. Both ADH and ALDH2 are kinetically limited by NAD^+ levels, which are dependent on mitochondrial respiration to oxidize NADH to NAD^+ [13–15]. ADH and ALDH2 levels have not been observed to change with alcohol feeding in rats [15–17]. This suggests that mitochondrial respiration is extremely important in alcohol metabolism to regenerate NAD^+ needed for alcohol metabolism by ADH and ALDH2 in the liver (Figure 8.1).

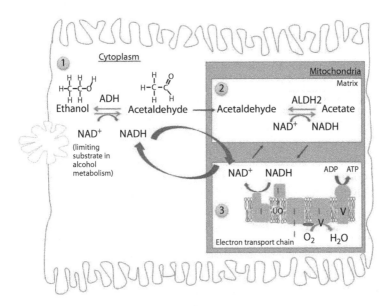

FIGURE 8.1 Role of mitochondria in alcohol metabolism in the liver. The metabolism of alcohol in the liver is dependent on three pathways: (1) the conversion of alcohol to acetaldehyde by ADH, which occurs in the cytoplasm and is rate limited by NAD^+; (2) the conversion of acetaldehyde to acetate by ALDH2, which occurs in the mitochondrial matrix and is rate limited by NAD^+; and (3) mitochondrial respiration, which oxidizes NADH to regenerate NAD^+ for alcohol metabolism, which occurs in the mitochondrial inner membrane. An important rate determining step in alcohol metabolism is mitochondrial respiration to regenerate NAD^+.

It is also well established animals adapt to alcohol feeding by developing an enhanced ability to metabolize alcohol in liver [16–18]. Even one dose of alcohol is known to enhance alcohol metabolism in the liver [19]. Acute adaptation of liver to alcohol is associated with a "hypermetabolic state," which is characterized by a rapid increase in oxygen uptake by the liver following alcohol intake [13,18,20]. The hypermetabolic state and the associated increase in oxygen consumption are believed to occur because of increased mitochondrial respiration needed to regenerate NAD^+ for alcohol metabolism [13]. However, direct evidence that enhanced mitochondrial respiration underlies the hypermetabolic state has not been established. Chronic alcohol feeding is associated with enhanced oxygen consumption in the liver, but again, the direct role of mitochondria in this process has not been firmly established.

MITOCHONDRIAL DYSFUNCTION PARADIGM OF ALD

Given the importance of mitochondria in alcohol metabolism and its possible role in the hypermetabolic state, it is somewhat surprising that alcohol feeding has been reported to cause mitochondria dysfunction in the liver. In fact, the notion of mitochondrial dysfunction being central to ALD has become an important dogma in ALD. Central to the mitochondrial dysfunction hypothesis has been the observation that chronic alcohol feeding (Lieber-DeCarli oral diet) to rats causes a decline in mitochondria respiration (state III: respiration in presences of substrates and ADP) and a decline in the respiratory control ratio (RCR; state III/state IV) in isolated liver mitochondria [7,21,22]. A decline in the RCR suggests uncoupling of mitochondria, which would reduce ATP production by the respiratory chain. The decline in mitochondrial respiration in the liver has been associated with decreases in ribosome activity and synthesis of respiratory complex proteins in the liver of rats orally fed with alcohol [23,24]. These findings suggest that alcohol feeding reduces the bioenergetic activity of mitochondria and its ability to produce ATP in hepatocytes of rats.

In addition to changes in mitochondrial respiration in the liver, many other mitochondrial changes have been reported following alcohol feeding in rats. Alcohol feeding has been suggested to enhance mitochondrial reactive oxygen species (ROS) generation in cultured primary hepatocytes. Using the redox dye 2′,7′-dichlorofluorescin (DCFH), it has been shown that alcohol increases 2′,7′-dichlorofluorescein (DCF; oxidation product of DCFH) fluorescence in isolated hepatocytes suggesting enhanced ROS generation [25]. Work with mitochondrial inhibitors such as antimycin has led to the suggestion that complexes I and III in the respiratory chain are responsible for mitochondrial ROS generation following alcohol treatment [6]. Overall, there is extensive evidence of oxidative stress with alcohol feeding including increased lipid peroxidation and oxidation of mitochondrial DNA (mtDNA) [26]. Bolus doses of alcohol have been shown to cause degradation of mtDNA in the liver, likely due to mtDNA damage [27]. Alcohol feeding has also been shown to cause a selective decrease in mitochondrial glutathione (GSH) [28]. The decrease in mitochondrial GSH has been attributed to an alcohol-induced accumulation of cholesterol in mitochondrial membranes, which interferes with GSH transport into mitochondria [29]. Mitochondria lack the enzymes needed to synthesize GSH and are therefore dependent on GSH transport and import to sustain its GSH pool [30]. Several studies have demonstrated that alcohol feeding increases post-translational redox modifications to mitochondrial proteins [31,32]. Post-translational redox changes can alter protein activity and have been suggested to play a role in mitochondrial dysfunction [33]. Finally, mitochondria from alcohol-fed rats are morphologically variable, often with abnormal morphologies [34]. These findings, taken together, have led to the belief that mitochondrial dysfunction in the liver plays an important role in the pathogenesis of ALD.

REASSESSMENT OF MITOCHONDRIAL CHANGES IN ALD

Although the evidence is compelling that mitochondrial dysfunction occurs with chronic alcohol intake, there are many problems and discrepancies to state that mitochondrial dysfunction is a universal feature of ALD. It is clear that chronic alcohol feeding is a major stress to hepatocytes that causes some oxidative damage and injury to mitochondria and the liver overall. However, oxidative damage and injury does not necessarily mean mitochondrial dysfunction is central in ALD. There are several issues regarding methodology and animal models that have led us to question the mitochondrial dysfunction paradigm in ALD.

Variations in Mitochondrial Changes among Different Alcohol Models

The decline in mitochondrial respiration in the liver following alcohol feeding to rats has been central to the mitochondrial dysfunction hypothesis. However, these data have been primarily obtained from studies using the oral Lieber-DeCarli alcohol diet in rats [7,21,22]. Decline in mitochondrial respiration is not seen in all animal alcohol models and is unknown in different models of alcohol delivery. Alcohol has been traditionally provided to mice and rats using the Lieber-DeCarli oral diet or intragastric infusion. The Lieber-DeCarli oral diet is a commonly used model to deliver alcohol to animals but it produces only a mild form of liver injury, primarily fatty liver (steatosis) in mice and rats. This is largely due to the fact the animals will not consume large amounts of alcohol [35]. The intragastric alcohol infusion model, meanwhile, produces more severe liver injury with some pathophysiological features such as fibrosis and inflammation observed in alcoholic humans because alcohol is force fed to mice and rats using a pump [36,37]. It had been assumed that intragastric alcohol feeding of rats will also lead to a greater decline in mitochondrial respiration due to greater liver injury; however, this notion remains untested. Recently, we reported that chronic alcohol feeding (both intragastric or oral) to mice enhances state III mitochondrial respiration in the liver [9]. Intragastric alcohol feeding, which produces more injury, was more effective in enhancing mitochondrial respiration than oral alcohol feeding. Intragastric alcohol feeding caused an almost 2-fold increase in state III respiration, whereas oral alcohol feeding enhanced mitochondria respiration in the liver by ~30%. The increase in mitochondrial respiration following alcohol feeding was associated with increases in both proteins that compose the respiratory complexes and increased levels of mitochondrial pyridine nucleotides (NADH, NAD^+). The observations that alcohol feeding increases state III respiration and protein levels in the respiratory complexes are in stark contrast to previous data reported in rats. It is becoming clear that mice and rats respond differently to alcohol in many ways other than mitochondrial changes. Mice are more sensitive to alcohol-induced injury and have lower expression of betaine homocysteine methyltransferase (BHMT), which is important in detoxifying homocysteine [38]. It is interesting that mitochondrial respiration declines do not correlate with liver injury caused by alcohol. Mice, in which liver mitochondrial respiration increases with oral alcohol feeding, usually have higher ALT levels (~50–90 U/L) than rats (~40–60), in which liver mitochondria respiration dramatically declines. Why liver mitochondria of mice and rats respond so differently to alcohol remains unclear. However, our data with mice clearly suggests that ALD is not always associated with mitochondrial dysfunction.

The important question that remains is which animal model, the rat or the mouse, is relevant in alcoholic patients. Humans represent a genetically diverse population, and it is possible that some people may respond to alcohol with mitochondrial changes seen in rats, whereas others to changes seen in mice. An important work by Lieber showed that baboons given alcohol orally have declines in mitochondrial respiration similarly seen in rats [39]. Mitochondrial respiration and activities of respiratory complex proteins (succinate dehydrogenase [complex II], cytochrome oxidase [complex IV], etc.) declined in the liver of baboons. Meanwhile, in liver biopsies of patients with ALD, no changes in activities of succinate dehydrogenase and cytochrome oxidase were observed [40]. In fact, the enzyme activity of many mitochondrial matrix proteins (i.e., glutamate dehydrogenase, malate dehydrogenase, and aspartate aminotransferase) were greatly enhanced in ALD patients, leading the authors to suggest that some mitochondrial adaptation was occurring. Clearly, more studies are needed in patients to fully understand the extent of mitochondrial changes that occur in the liver with ALD. However, a decline in mitochondrial respiration in the liver is unlikely to be a universal event and could vary depending on the genetic makeup of patients.

Mitochondrial ROS Generation following Alcohol Feeding

Mitochondria are major sources of ROS in cells [41,42]. The electron transport chain, mainly complexes I and III, releases superoxide both toward the intermembrane, which can diffuse from mitochondria via VDAC [43,44], and toward the matrix, where Mn-SOD converts most superoxide to H_2O_2 [45]. Mitochondria are thus the major sources of superoxide and H_2O_2 in cells. Chronic alcohol feeding is associated with enhanced oxidative stress and increased ROS in the liver. Many biomarkers of oxidative stress have been shown to increase in the liver with alcohol feeding in rats and mice [27,46]. In addition, antioxidants (vitamin E, coenzyme Q, etc.) and Mn-SOD treatment have been shown to reduce alcohol-induced injury in the liver [26,27,47]. Since mitochondria are major sources of ROS in cells and alcohol feeding is known to alter mitochondrial function, it is reasonable to assume enhanced mitochondrial ROS generation is associated with ALD. However, more experimental data are required to truly determine if mitochondrial ROS generation in the liver is enhanced with alcohol feeding. The early and important works of Bailey and Cunningham suggested that alcohol treatment to primary hepatocytes enhances mitochondrial ROS generation [6,25]. However, these findings are problematic because they utilized DCFH as the method for measuring ROS. Later works have clearly established that DCFH is a poor and nonspecific marker for ROS measurement [48–51]. Many factors, such as redox status, iron, and antioxidants can affect DCF fluorescence independent of ROS generation. In some cases, DCFH can redox cycle and enhance ROS generation in cells. Due to the short lifetime of most ROS, their detection in biology systems is very difficult and prone to artifact. Even newer, more specific dyes such as hydroethidine have some issues of nonspecificity and require HPLC to be a specific measure of superoxide production [52,53]. The mitochondrial respiratory chain may be the major source of ROS following alcohol treatment, but alcohol feeding is also known to upregulate CYP2E1, which can also be major sources of superoxide in cells. Further research using newer and more specific techniques to measure ROS are needed to determine the changes in mitochondrial ROS generation that occur in the liver with alcohol feeding.

Mitochondria as the Final Target of JNK-Induced Apoptosis in ALD

Although it remains in question whether mitochondrial bioenergetic changes and ROS generation play an important role in ALD, mitochondria are likely to play an important role in apoptosis that occurs with ALD. Mitochondria plays a central role in apoptosis in many pathologies because they house key apoptotic proteins such as cytochrome c and AIF. In addition, mitochondria have been shown to be targets of many pro-apoptotic proteins such c-Jun N-terminal kinase (JNK) [54–56]. Liver injury during ALD is associated with a low level of hepatocyte apoptosis, which is likely triggered by tumor necrosis factor (TNF) α and mediated by JNK [48]. TNF is a pluripotent cytokine that has been shown to play a key role in various liver diseases including ALD. TNF knockout mice have been shown to be more protected from liver injury caused by chronic alcohol feeding than control mice [57,58]. Hepatocytes are normally resistant to TNF, but stresses such as ROS and GSH depletion can sensitize hepatocytes to TNF-induced apoptosis [48,59,60]. TNF-induced apoptosis involves sustained JNK activation and translocation to mitochondria to induce mitochondrial permeability transition (MPT), important in triggering apoptosis or necrosis in cells following various stresses [56]. JNK normally resides in the cytoplasm; however upon activation, JNK has been shown to translocate to mitochondria and regulate various mitochondrial functions including MPT. Thus, ALD likely involves TNF-induced JNK activation and translocation to mitochondria that triggers MPT. JNK inhibitor treatment has been shown to reduce alcohol-induced liver injury in mice [61].

NONALCOHOLIC FATTY LIVER DISEASE

Pathology of NAFLD

Although alcohol is the main cause of fatty liver disease, nonalcoholic fatty liver disease, which occurs in patients who consume less than 40 g of alcohol a day, is a growing epidemic for the industrialized world [1,2]. Largely associated with type II diabetes and metabolic syndrome, both growing in prevalence, NAFLD has become one of the many associated health consequences of the high-fat, high-carbohydrate diets of the westernized world. Excessive accumulation of fatty acid droplets in the hepatic cells characterizes hepatic steatosis, although steatosis of other organs such as the heart may also be associated with these syndromes. The leading risk factor for developing NAFLD is obesity. Obesity in individuals can initiate the pathogenesis of metabolic syndrome and type II diabetes, which are both often associated with this disease. However, NAFLD can arise in patients for various reasons. This can include drug-related hepatic steatosis, which occurs in patients on long-term regimens of certain classes of drugs, toxins, or other factors (excluding alcohol-related liver injury). With obesity as a major risk factor, unsurprisingly, type II diabetes is also often associated with NAFLD. Insulin resistance is universally associated with NAFLD. Obesity is the major risk factor for developing type II diabetes and, thus, may either be pivotal in the progression of NAFLD in conjunction with diabetes or may complement the development of diabetes through NAFLD. As in a pathological positive-feedback loop, high levels of circulating insulin, the very mechanism to counteract insulin resistance, will increase fatty acid synthesis in the liver. Although steatosis may be a somewhat benign condition, 10%–20% of steatosis patients can progress to nonalcoholic steatohepatitis (NASH), which is characterized by necro-inflammation and some fibrosis. NASH patients are at risk of developing cirrhosis and requiring liver transplants.

ANIMAL MODELS FOR NAFLD AND NASH

Many animal models of steatosis have been developed, but models that represent the pathogenesis of NASH have not been fully developed. No animal model truly presents all the clinical manifestations of human NASH patients. In mice, many mutants that exemplify obesity and NAFLD have been developed. These include the various mutants with impaired leptin synthesis, *ob/ob* mice, or impaired leptin receptors, *db/db* mouse and *fa/fa* mice. Because of the relationship of obesity with NAFLD, mice that can develop obesity are useful in studying hepatic steatosis. Unfortunately, these mice fail to progress to NASH and leave much to be addressed in the process of pathogenesis. Furthermore, they highlight the yet unclear possible differences in the development of NAFLD in humans. The amenability of the mouse embryo to manipulation has led to numerous transgenic models that can be highly manipulatable to obtain temporal or tissue specificity and a snapshot of the entire process of NAFLD. In an attempt to replicate the human conditions leading to NAFLD, various models of diet-induced hepatic steatosis, such as the "Western" diet, have been developed. These models of high-fat and/or high-glucose better replicate the scenario for the majority of humans that have NAFLD. In a model consisting of 10–50 weeks of 45%–60% calories from saturated fat, pathology included slight inflammation and slight fibrosis. An alternative dietary model is the MCD diet. This model fails to represent a clinically relevant scenario for developing hepatic steatosis, as most patient cases of NAFLD are not due to a diet deficient in methionine and choline. However, this model though dissimilar in it pathogenesis of NAFLD, it has histological similarities that make it a useful model. In the MCD model, there is decreased hepatic lipid export and hepatic steatosis ensues. In addition to the lipid accumulation in hepatocytes, histologically, there is necro-inflammation and fibrosis, with some similar histopathology to humans.

Mitochondrial Alterations Associated with NAFLD and NASH

The relationship between mitochondria and steatosis in the liver is complicated and multifaceted. Mitochondria are the major sites of fatty acid metabolism (β-oxidation); thus, the inhibition of mitochondrial function can lead to the accumulation of fatty acids in hepatocytes. Many drugs that inhibit β-oxidation and/or mitochondrial respiration can induce steatosis in hepatocytes by decreasing lipid degradation pathways [5,62]. These observations regarding drug-induced steatosis and some initial observations that mitochondrial respiration is impaired in some steatosis-induced dietary have led to the idea that mitochondrial dysfunction is central to NAFLD, as similarly suggested for ALD. Although it is true that certain drugs can induce steatosis by inhibiting mitochondrial function, steatosis caused by mitochondrial dysfunction may be limited to a handful of mitochondria-interfering drugs and toxins. It is unlikely that steatosis-associated obesity or metabolic syndrome are caused by the inhibition of β-oxidation in mitochondria. Rather, in many cases, β-oxidation is enhanced in mitochondria as an adaptation to excess accumulation of lipids due to enhanced fatty acid synthesis or excess fatty acids in diet. NALFD induced by diet or obesity have a wide range of mitochondrial changes (both positive and negative), as seen in ALD animal models. Thus, it remains uncertain if mitochondrial dysfunction plays a central role on NAFLD, except in a few examples (drug-induced steatosis). In the next section, we will examine the major mitochondrial changes that have been observed with NAFLD and NASH in animal models and in patients.

Mitochondrial Bioenergetic Changes Associated with Steatosis

Like mitochondrial alterations observed in ALD animal models, there is a great variability in mitochondrial changes in NAFLD models. It should be noted that changes in mitochondrial respiration is dynamic and can change with time. In rats fed an MCD diet, there is initially an increase in mitochondrial respiration in the liver, which declines to near-normal levels over time [8]. In rats fed a HFD, little change in mitochondrial respiration, except a decrease in β-oxidation was observed with 8 weeks' feeding [63]. In mice, one study reported that A/J mice upregulated oxidative phosphorylation genes and had increased mitochondrial respiration (states 2, 3, and 4) in the liver following a HFD [64]. These mice also had increased mitochondrial uncoupling after 10 days on a HFD. The same study observed little changes in liver mitochondria in C57BL/6 mice fed a HFD. Meanwhile, another study found that feeding C57BL/6 mice a HFD caused a decline in mitochondrial respiration (state III) in the liver, which corresponds with decreased levels of proteins in the respiratory complexes [3]. In *ob/ob* mice (obesity model), complex I activity was observed to decline, however, activity of other complexes were not altered [65]. In another study, it was observed that injection of leptin in *ob/ob* mice, which caused weight loss, caused a decline in mitochondria respiration, mass, and protein levels [66]. This study suggests that mitochondrial respiration and mass are related to obesity, with higher mitochondria number and respiration occurring when greater obesity and steatosis occurs. This is in agreement with our ongoing work suggesting that weight gain in *ob/ob* mice increases mitochondrial mass and bioenergetic activity in the liver (unpublished results).

Mitochondrial dysfunction has been suspected in NASH patients because they display decreased ATP resynthesis rates following fructose challenge, which transiently depletes hepatic ATP. Although these data suggest that ATP resynthesis, which occurs primarily in mitochondria, is altered in NASH patients, it only indirectly suggests that mitochondrial bioenergetic activity is altered in the liver. Direct measurement of mitochondrial activity in patients show mixed results regarding the type of changes that occur. In NASH patients, one study reported that the activities of respiratory complexes were significantly decreased (complex I, 37%; II, 41.5%; III, 29.4%; IV, 37.5%; V, 37.6%) in the liver [67]. Conversely, another study measuring mitochondrial respiration in NASH patients using cybrids observed no noticeable changes in mitochondrial respiration [68]. In this study, however, abnormal mitochondrial morphology was observed, which has also been seen in some animal models of NAFLD. Finally, another study observed in NASH patients an enhancement of β-oxidation in the liver, even in the presence of significant oxidative and nitrosative stress [69]. There are clearly many mitochondrial alterations in the liver of NASH patients, but more studies are needed to understand the extent of these changes and their importance in the disease.

Mitochondria as Sources of ROS in NAFLD

As observed in ALD, NAFLD is associated with an increase in many biomarkers of oxidative stress such as lipid peroxidation products, mtDNA oxidation, and upregulation of antioxidants enzymes such as superoxide dismutase [5,70]. Enhanced mitochondrial ROS generation is likely to play a major role in liver injury in drug-induced steatosis; however, it remains to be determined whether mitochondrial ROS is increased in other forms of NAFLD. Surprisingly, CYP2E1 is also upregulated in the liver in some NAFLD animal models. The function of CYP2E1 in NAFLD is unclear, unlike in ALD where CYP2E1 plays an important role in alcohol metabolism. Oxidative stress observed in NAFLD, therefore, could originate to a large extent from CYP2E1, rather than from the mitochondrial respiratory chain.

Mitochondria as the Final Target of JNK-Induced Apoptosis in NAFLD

Fatty acids are injurious to hepatocytes and can induce lipotoxicity, general associated with JNK-induced apoptosis [71]. Because of the toxicity of fatty acids, its storage as triacylglycerols in lipid droplets in the liver has been suggested to be a protective mechanism [72]. Palmitate treatment to primary hepatocytes will induce apoptosis that can be inhibited by treatment with JNK inhibitors [71]. It is also likely that JNK translocation to mitochondria is important in mediating hepatocyte death caused by fatty acids, as seen in TNF-induced apoptosis. Although JNK seems central in mediating lipotoxicity in cultured hepatocytes, the role of JNK in animal models is more complicated. JNK1 appears to have an important role in promoting steatosis and insulin resistance induced by HFD, whereas JNK 2 appears to have a protective role and prevent hepatocyte cell death and mitochondrial-dependent death pathways [73]. The discrepancy of JNK being injurious to mitochondria in cultured hepatocytes, while protecting the mitochondria (JNK 2) in an animal steatosis model requires further investigation.

MITOCHONDRIAL DYSFUNCTION OR MITOCHONDRIAL ADAPTATION IN ALD AND NAFLD?

Although the paradigm of mitochondria dysfunction in ALD and NAFLD has been widely accepted, it may represent an incomplete or inaccurate picture of mitochondrial dynamics in the liver. It is clear that mitochondria are altered and damaged to some extent in various ALD and NAFLD disease models. However, dysfunction implies an impairment of function, and in many animal models, mitochondrial function is often enhanced suggesting an adaptive response. Clearly, there are some variations depending on type of steatosis induced. In drug-induced steatosis, drugs directly inhibit mitochondria function to promote steatosis and liver injury [5,62]. However, overall we would argue that "mitochondrial remodeling or adaptation" rather than "mitochondrial dysfunction" better characterizes the changes that occur in liver mitochondria in ALD and NAFLD. In recent years, the dynamic and adaptive nature of mitochondria has become better understood and appreciated. Mitochondria undergo many types of alterations in response to stress or metabolic changes to adapt to the needs of the cell. For example, the energy demand of acute or chronic exercise has been shown to cause mitochondrial biogenesis and remodeling (i.e., increased components of the mitochondria respiratory chain and proteins involved in β-oxidation) in skeletal muscle [74–76]. Liver mitochondria, like muscle mitochondria, can adapt and alter in response to stress and metabolic changes. Mitochondrial adaptation is likely the predominant early mitochondrial changes observed in most models of ALD and NAFLD.

MITOCHONDRIAL DYNAMICS AND ADAPTATION

Mitochondrial biogenesis and remodeling is mediated through peroxisome proliferator–activated receptor γ coactivator 1α (PGC-1α), the master regulator of mitochondria, in most cells. PGC-1α knockout mice have decreased levels of many key mitochondrial proteins (i.e., cytochrome c, ATP synthase, cytochrome oxidase [COX]) [77,78], while overexpression of PGC-1α promotes mitochondrial biogenesis [79]. PGC-1α is a co-activator and does not bind DNA directly but acts through protein–protein interactions with key transcription factors to promote transcription of mitochondrial genes. PGC-1α has been shown to bind and activate many transcription factors including nuclear respiratory factor 1 (NRF-1), which transcribes subunits of all five respiratory complexes [80]. Both NRF-1 and PGC-1α are upregulated by exercise to mediate mitochondria biogenesis and remodeling [74,81]. HFD has also been shown to upregulate PGC-1α in muscle [82]. The half-life of PGC-1α in cells is extremely short (~2 h), allowing cells to dynamically control protein expression of PGC-1α to regulate mitochondria biogenesis according to the needs of the cell [79]. In rats fed with alcohol (Lieber-DeCarli diet), PGC-1α proteins levels remained unchanged, although the protein was found to be acetylated [83]. In contrast, we and another study [9,84] observed in mice fed with alcohol, PGC-1α levels were increased in a time-dependent manner with alcohol feeding.

A different type of mitochondrial dynamic adaptation involves morphological changes due to alteration in mitochondrial fusion–fission rates. Mitochondria constantly undergo fusion–fission to exchange mtDNA, proteins, and other constituents [85,86]. Stress can dramatically alter fusion–fission rates and consequently mitochondrial morphology [10]. In embryonic fibroblasts, starvation causes a decrease in mitochondrial fission to produce elongated mitochondria that are more resistant to mitophagy (mitochondrial autophagy) and have greater cristae surface area, thereby greater mitochondrial respiration [87]. Mitochondrial fusion and fission are primarily controlled by four highly conserved GTPases: mitofusins (MFN1 and MFN2) in mitochondrial outer membranes promote fusion; optic atrophy (OPA1) in the inner membranes (IMM) promotes fusion; and dynamin-related protein1 (DRP1) from the cytoplasm regulates fission [85]. Phosphorylation of DRP1 by PKA at serine 637 has been shown to sequester DRP1 in the cytoplasm and inhibit its translocation to mitochondria that promotes fission [88]. Mitochondrial fusion–fission has been also shown to modulate cell death [85,88]. Could some of the mitochondrial morphology changes observed in various liver steatosis model be an adaptive response that alters mitochondrial bioenergetic activity as seen in serum deprived cells? Mitochondrial morphology and its relation to bioenergetic activity are just beginning to be explored in the liver.

Mitochondrial Dysfunction or Mitochondrial Adaptation in ALD

It is likely many mitochondrial alterations observed in various steatosis models are adaptations to metabolic stress. In some steatosis models and in NASH patients, mitochondrial β-oxidation has been observed to increase. The enhanced β-oxidation is likely an important adaptive response in hepatocytes to help enhance fatty acid degradation. In mice fed with alcohol, we believe enhanced mitochondrial respiration in the liver is an adaptation to improve alcohol metabolism by increasing regeneration of NAD^+, the limiting substrate for alcohol metabolism [9]. In support of this idea, we observed that isolated liver mitochondria from alcohol-fed mice have greater acetaldehyde-driven mitochondrial respiration and acetaldehyde metabolism than control mice. Although these mitochondrial alterations are more evident as adaptation because mitochondrial function increases, could declines in mitochondrial respiration be adaptive responses?

The observation that oral alcohol feeding to rats causes a decline in mitochondrial respiration has been central to the mitochondrial dysfunction hypothesis in ALD. We would argue a decline in respiratory complex proteins and mitochondrial respiration do not signal mitochondrial dysfunctional. Instead, it could be a normal adaptation of the liver to metabolic changes and stress. Several arguments can be made that a decline in mitochondrial respiration is an adaptive response rather than a sign of dysfunction. As previously mentioned, proteins in the mitochondrial respiratory chain can increase in liver and muscle when energy or metabolic demand is high. Conversely, could decline in respiratory proteins and consequent decline in respiration be an adaptive change when energy demands are low? Alcohol feeding is associated with excess energy intake. Thus, it is possible that the liver may downregulate mitochondrial respiration and proteins as a response to the excess energy. Rats have been shown to have excess mitochondrial respiratory capacity and thus have excessive levels of mitochondrial respiratory proteins [89]. The decline in mitochondrial respiration in rat liver has always been difficult to reconcile with the observation of increased oxygen consumption (hypermetabolic state) in the liver of rats fed with alcohol. Enhanced oxygen consumption by the liver is seen with acute alcohol feeding and chronic alcohol feeding. In liver slices from chronic alcohol-fed rats, oxygen consumption is greater than control in the presence of alcohol [16,90]. If mitochondrial respiration is suppressed, how is oxygen consumption increased? Upregulation of CYP2E1 in the liver could, at least in part, potentially increase oxygen uptake by the liver. If CYP2E1 is partially responsible for the enhanced oxygen uptake seen with chronic alcohol feeding, then it could be argued that mitochondrial proteins in the liver are downregulated in response to the upregulation of CYP2E1. It is also possible that liver mitochondria in rats remodel such that many mitochondrial respiration pathways are downregulated (i.e., succinate driven respiration), whereas other mitochondrial respiration pathways may be upregulated (i.e., glycerol phosphate driven respiration). We are presently investigating this hypothesis that liver mitochondria in rats adapt in different ways such that mitochondrial respiration through complexes I and II is downregulated, but respiration through other pathways such as glycerol phosphate dehydrogenase II is upregulated.

Another factor that is commonly cited as evidence of mitochondrial dysfunction is the decline in RCR, which suggests mitochondrial uncoupling in the liver. In many ALD and NAFLD models, mitochondrial uncoupling has been observed, even in cases where mitochondrial respiration is enhanced. Mitochondrial uncoupling reduces the ATP production capacity of mitochondria. Uncoupling of mitochondria, besides the decline in ATP production, is not necessarily a negative phenomenon. In fact, mitochondrial uncoupling can have positive effects, such as decreased mitochondrial ROS generation due to shorter half-life of ubisemiquinone, the radical responsible for ROS generation in complex III [91]. ALD and NAFLD are diseases with excess energy, where ATP levels are likely in excess. Under these conditions of energy excess, the uncoupling of mitochondria may be an adaption to rapidly regenerate NAD^+ needed for alcohol metabolism and β-oxidation while generating less ATP and less ROS. Mitochondrial uncoupling is regulated by the family of uncoupling proteins (UCPs) and further research is needed to understand the possible relationship between UCP and steatosis in the liver.

MODEL OF MITOCHONDRIAL ADAPTATION IN ALD AND NAFLD

Mitochondrial adaption may be the major response observed in many steatosis models. However, this is not to say that mitochondrial adaptation and dysfunction are mutually exclusive. In fact, some mitochondrial changes such as enhanced mitochondrial respiration may, in the long term, have negative consequences that promote liver injury. For example, it is possible that the enhanced mitochondrial respiration with alcohol feeding in mice is associated with increased ROS generation, which could damage the liver in the long run. Although enhanced mitochondrial ROS generation has not been definitely established in steatosis model, enhanced mitochondrial respiration is likely to generate greater superoxide as a side reaction. It is for this reason mitochondrial uncoupling may be occurring with steatosis. Our model is based on the concept that mitochondria are dynamic and help the liver adapt to chronic alcohol intake (Figure 8.2). Alcohol intake causes mitochondrial remodeling and

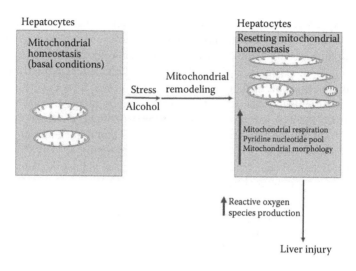

FIGURE 8.2 Model of mitochondrial remodeling and adaptation in the liver. Mitochondrial homeostasis is reset in the liver by metabolic stresses such as alcohol. The resetting of mitochondrial homeostasis helps the liver adapt, but can also have negative consequences that promote liver injury on the long term.

resetting of mitochondrial homeostasis in the liver to adapt to metabolic changes. Mitochondrial remodeling and adaptation are likely the major mitochondrial alterations observed during the early and middle stages of steatosis. Long-term resetting of mitochondrial homeostasis may have some negative consequences, such as increased mitochondrial ROS generation that may ultimately promote liver injury.

SUMMARY

Although mitochondrial dysfunction has been a widely accepted dogma in ALD and NAFLD, we would argue that this view is a very incomplete and poor description of mitochondrial dynamics that occur in the liver. Mitochondrial injury and damage occur in most animal models of steatosis; however, following injury, mitochondria remodel to help the liver adapt. Mitochondrial remodeling and adaptation are likely important mechanisms for the liver to deal with metabolic stresses such as alcohol or HFD.

REFERENCES

1. Altamirano J, and Bataller R. Alcoholic liver disease: Pathogenesis and new targets for therapy. *Nat Rev Gastroenterol Hepatol.* 2011;8:491–501.
2. Scaglioni F, Ciccia S, Marino M, Bedogni G, and Bellentani S. ASH and NASH. *Dig Dis.* 2011;29:202–10.
3. Mantena SK, King AL, Andringa KK, Eccleston HB, and Bailey SM. Mitochondrial dysfunction and oxidative stress in the pathogenesis of alcohol- and obesity-induced fatty liver diseases. *Free Radic Biol Med.* 2008;44:1259–72.

4. Hoek JB, Cahill A, and Pastorino JG. Alcohol and mitochondria: A dysfunctional relationship. *Gastroenterology.* 2002;122:2049–63.

5. Pessayre D, Berson A, Fromenty B, and Mansouri A. Mitochondria in steatohepatitis. *Semin Liver Dis.* 2001;21:57–69.

6. Bailey SM, Pietsch EC, and Cunningham CC. Ethanol stimulates the production of reactive oxygen species at mitochondrial complexes I and III. *Free Radic Biol Med.* 1999;27:891–900.

7. Spach PI, and Cunningham CC. Control of state 3 respiration in liver mitochondria from rats subjected to chronic ethanol consumption. *Biochim Biophys Acta.* 1987;894:460–7.

8. Serviddio G, Bellanti F, Tamborra R, Rollo T, Romano AD, Giudetti AM, Capitanio N, Petrella A, Vendemiale G, and Altomare E. Alterations of hepatic ATP homeostasis and respiratory chain during development of non-alcoholic steatohepatitis in a rodent model. *Eur J Clin Invest.* 2008;38:245–52.

9. Han D, Ybanez MD, Johnson HS, McDonald JN, Mesropyan L, Sancheti H, Martin G, Martin A, Lim AM, Dara L et al. Dynamic adaptation of liver mitochondria to chronic alcohol feeding in mice: Biogenesis, remodeling, and functional alterations. *J Biol Chem.* 2012;287:42165–79.

10. Han D, Dara L, Win S, Than TA, Yuan L, Abbasi SQ, Liu ZX, and Kaplowitz N. Regulation of drug-induced liver injury by signal transduction pathways: Critical role of mitochondria. *Trends Pharmacol Sci.* 2013;34:243–53.

11. Liesa M, and Shirihai OS. Mitochondrial dynamics in the regulation of nutrient utilization and energy expenditure. *Cell Metab.* 2013;17:491–506.

12. Teschke R, Hasumura Y, and Lieber CS. Hepatic microsomal alcohol-oxidizing system. Affinity for methanol, ethanol, propanol, and butanol. *J Biol Chem.* 1975;250:7397–404.

13. Israel Y, and Orrego H. Hypermetabolic state and hypoxic liver damage. *Recent Dev Alcohol.* 1984;2:119–33.

14. Videla L, and Israel Y. Factors that modify the metabolism of ethanol in rat liver and adaptive changes produced by its chronic administration. *Biochem J.* 1970;118:275–81.

15. Hasumura Y, Teschke R, and Lieber CS. Characteristics of acetaldehyde oxidation in rat liver mitochondria. *J Biol Chem.* 1976;251:4908–13.

16. Videla L, Bernstein J, and Israel Y. Metabolic alterations produced in the liver by chronic ethanol administration. Increased oxidative capacity. *Biochem J.* 1973;134:507–14.

17. Tobon F, and Mezey E. Effect of ethanol administration on hepatic ethanol and drug-metabolizing enzymes and on rates of ethanol degradation. *J Lab Clin Med.* 1971;77:110–21.

18. Israel Y, Kalant H, Orrego H, Khanna JM, Videla L, and Phillips JM. Experimental alcohol-induced hepatic necrosis: Suppression by propylthiouracil. *Proc Natl Acad Sci USA.* 1975;72:1137–41.

19. Thurman RG, Paschal D, Abu-Murad C, Pekkanen L, Bradford BU, Bullock K, and Glassman E. Swift increase in alcohol metabolism (SIAM) in the mouse: Comparison of the effect of short-term ethanol treatment on ethanol elimination in four inbred strains. *J Pharmacol Exp Ther.* 1982;223:45–9.

20. Bradford BU, and Rusyn I. Swift increase in alcohol metabolism (SIAM): Understanding the phenomenon of hypermetabolism in liver. *Alcohol.* 2005;35:13–7.

21. Cederbaum AI, Lieber CS, and Rubin E. Effects of chronic ethanol treatment of mitochondrial functions damage to coupling site I. *Arch Biochem Biophys.* 1974;165:560–9.

22. Bernstein JD, and Penniall R. Effects of chronic ethanol treatment upon rat liver mitochondria. *Biochem Pharmacol.* 1978;27:2337–42.

23. Cunningham CC, Coleman WB, and Spach PI. The effects of chronic ethanol consumption on hepatic mitochondrial energy metabolism. *Alcohol Alcohol.* 1990;25:127–36.

24. Venkatraman A, Landar A, Davis AJ, Chamlee L, Sanderson T, Kim H, Page G, Pompilius M, Ballinger S, Darley-Usmar V et al. Modification of the mitochondrial

proteome in response to the stress of ethanol-dependent hepatotoxicity. *J Biol Chem.* 2004;279:22092–101.

25. Bailey SM, and Cunningham CC. Contribution of mitochondria to oxidative stress associated with alcoholic liver disease. *Free Radic Biol Med.* 2002;32:11–6.
26. Arteel GE. Oxidants and antioxidants in alcohol-induced liver disease. *Gastroenterology.* 2003;124:778–90.
27. Mansouri A, Demeilliers C, Amsellem S, Pessayre D, and Fromenty B. Acute ethanol administration oxidatively damages and depletes mitochondrial dna in mouse liver, brain, heart, and skeletal muscles: Protective effects of antioxidants. *J Pharmacol Exp Ther.* 2001;298:737–43.
28. Colell A, Garcia-Ruiz C, Morales A, Ballesta A, Ookhtens M, Rodes J, Kaplowitz N, and Fernandez-Checa JC. Transport of reduced glutathione in hepatic mitochondria and mitoplasts from ethanol-treated rats: Effect of membrane physical properties and S-adenosyl-L-methionine. *Hepatology.* 1997;26:699–708.
29. Fernandez-Checa JC, Kaplowitz N, Garcia-Ruiz C, and Colell A. Mitochondrial glutathione: Importance and transport. *Semin Liver Dis.* 1998;18:389–401.
30. Garcia J, Han D, Sancheti H, Yap LP, Kaplowitz N, and Cadenas E. Regulation of mitochondrial glutathione redox status and protein glutathionylation by respiratory substrates. *J Biol Chem.* 2010;285:39646–54.
31. Moon KH, Hood BL, Kim BJ, Hardwick JP, Conrads TP, Veenstra TD, and Song BJ. Inactivation of oxidized and S-nitrosylated mitochondrial proteins in alcoholic fatty liver of rats. *Hepatology.* 2006;44:1218–30.
32. Venkatraman A, Landar A, Davis AJ, Ulasova E, Page G, Murphy MP, Darley-Usmar V, and Bailey SM. Oxidative modification of hepatic mitochondria protein thiols: Effect of chronic alcohol consumption. *Am J Physiol Gastrointest Liver Physiol.* 2004;286:G521–7.
33. Han D, Hanawa N, Saberi B, and Kaplowitz N. Mechanisms of liver injury. III. Role of glutathione redox status in liver injury. *Am J Physiol Gastrointest Liver Physiol.* 2006;291:G1–7.
34. Arai M, Leo MA, Nakano M, Gordon ER, and Lieber CS. Biochemical and morphological alterations of baboon hepatic mitochondria after chronic ethanol consumption. *Hepatology.* 1984;4:165–74.
35. Arteel GE. Animal models of alcoholic liver disease. *Dig Dis.* 2010;28:729–36.
36. Tsukamoto H, French SW, Benson N, Delgado G, Rao GA, Larkin EC, and Largman C. Severe and progressive steatosis and focal necrosis in rat liver induced by continuous intragastric infusion of ethanol and low fat diet. *Hepatology.* 1985;5:224–32.
37. Tsukamoto H, Towner SJ, Ciofalo LM, and French SW. Ethanol-induced liver fibrosis in rats fed high fat diet. *Hepatology.* 1986;6:814–22.
38. Shinohara M, Ji C, and Kaplowitz N. Differences in betaine-homocysteine methyltransferase expression, endoplasmic reticulum stress response, and liver injury between alcohol-fed mice and rats. *Hepatology.* 2010;51:796–805.
39. Popper H, and Lieber CS. Histogenesis of alcoholic fibrosis and cirrhosis in the baboon. *Am J Pathol.* 1980;98:695–716.
40. Jenkins WJ, and Peters TJ. Mitochondrial enzyme activities in liver biopsies from patients with alcoholic liver disease. *Gut.* 1978;19:341–4.
41. Han D, Antunes F, Daneri F, and Cadenas E. Mitochondrial superoxide anion production and release into intermembrane space. *Methods Enzymol.* 2002;349:271–80.
42. Cadenas E, and Davies KJ. Mitochondrial free radical generation, oxidative stress, and aging. *Free Radic Biol Med.* 2000;29:222–30.
43. Han D, Antunes F, Canali R, Rettori D, and Cadenas E. Voltage-dependent anion channels control the release of the superoxide anion from mitochondria to cytosol. *J Biol Chem.* 2003;278:5557–63.

44. Han D, Williams E, and Cadenas E. Mitochondrial respiratory chain-dependent generation of superoxide anion and its release into the intermembrane space. *Biochem J.* 2001;353:411–6.

45. Han D, Canali R, Rettori D, and Kaplowitz N. Effect of glutathione depletion on sites and topology of superoxide and hydrogen peroxide production in mitochondria. *Mol Pharmacol.* 2003;64:1136–44.

46. Rouach H, Fataccioli V, Gentil M, French SW, Morimoto M, and Nordmann R. Effect of chronic ethanol feeding on lipid peroxidation and protein oxidation in relation to liver pathology. *Hepatology.* 1997;25:351–5.

47. Wheeler MD, Kono H, Yin M, Rusyn I, Froh M, Connor HD, Mason RP, Samulski RJ, and Thurman RG. Delivery of the Cu/Zn-superoxide dismutase gene with adenovirus reduces early alcohol-induced liver injury in rats. *Gastroenterology.* 2001;120:1241–50.

48. Han D, Ybanez MD, Ahmadi S, Yeh K, and Kaplowitz N. Redox regulation of tumor necrosis factor signaling. *Antioxid Redox Signal.* 2009;11:2245–63.

49. Bonini MG, Rota C, Tomasi A, and Mason RP. The oxidation of 2′,7′-dichlorofluorescin to reactive oxygen species: A self-fulfilling prophesy? *Free Radic Biol Med.* 2006;40:968–75.

50. Corda S, Laplace C, Vicaut E, and Duranteau J. Rapid reactive oxygen species production by mitochondria in endothelial cells exposed to tumor necrosis factor-alpha is mediated by ceramide. *Am J Respir Cell Mol Biol.* 2001;24:762–8.

51. Tampo Y, Kotamraju S, Chitambar CR, Kalivendi SV, Keszler A, Joseph J, and Kalyanaraman B. Oxidative stress-induced iron signaling is responsible for peroxide-dependent oxidation of dichlorodihydrofluorescein in endothelial cells: Role of transferrin receptor-dependent iron uptake in apoptosis. *Circ Res.* 2003;92:56–63.

52. Zielonka J, Hardy M, and Kalyanaraman B. HPLC study of oxidation products of hydroethidine in chemical and biological systems: Ramifications in superoxide measurements. *Free Radic Biol Med.* 2009;46:329–38.

53. Zielonka J, Srinivasan S, Hardy M, Ouari O, Lopez M, Vasquez-Vivar J, Avadhani NG, and Kalyanaraman B. Cytochrome c-mediated oxidation of hydroethidine and mitohydroethidine in mitochondria: Identification of homo- and heterodimers. *Free Radic Biol Med.* 2008;44:835–46.

54. Zhou Q, Lam PY, Han D, and Cadenas E. c-Jun N-terminal kinase regulates mitochondrial bioenergetics by modulating pyruvate dehydrogenase activity in primary cortical neurons. *J Neurochem.* 2008;104:325–35.

55. Hanawa N, Shinohara M, Saberi B, Gaarde WA, Han D, and Kaplowitz N. Role of JNK translocation to mitochondria leading to inhibition of mitochondria bioenergetics in acetaminophen-induced liver injury. *J Biol Chem.* 2008;283:13565–77.

56. Win S, Than TA, Han D, Petrovic LM, and Kaplowitz N. c-Jun N-terminal kinase (JNK)-dependent acute liver injury from acetaminophen or tumor necrosis factor (TNF) requires mitochondrial Sab protein expression in mice. *J Biol Chem.* 2011;286:35071–8.

57. Ji C, Deng Q, and Kaplowitz N. Role of TNF-alpha in ethanol-induced hyperhomocysteinemia and murine alcoholic liver injury. *Hepatology.* 2004;40:442–51.

58. Yin M, Wheeler MD, Kono H, Bradford BU, Gallucci RM, Luster MI, and Thurman RG. Essential role of tumor necrosis factor alpha in alcohol-induced liver injury in mice. *Gastroenterology.* 1999;117:942–52.

59. Han D, Hanawa N, Saberi B, and Kaplowitz N. Hydrogen peroxide and redox modulation sensitize primary mouse hepatocytes to TNF-induced apoptosis. *Free Radic Biol Med.* 2006;41:627–39.

60. Matsumaru K, Ji C, and Kaplowitz N. Mechanisms for sensitization to TNF-induced apoptosis by acute glutathione depletion in murine hepatocytes. *Hepatology.* 2003;37:1425–34.

61. Yang L, Wu D, Wang X, and Cederbaum AI. Cytochrome P4502E1, oxidative stress, JNK, and autophagy in acute alcohol-induced fatty liver. *Free Radic Biol Med.* 2012;53:1170–80.

62. Fromenty B, and Pessayre D. Inhibition of mitochondrial beta-oxidation as a mechanism of hepatotoxicity. *Pharmacol Ther.* 1995;67:101–54.

63. Flamment M, Rieusset J, Vidal H, Simard G, Malthiery Y, Fromenty B, and Ducluzeau PH. Regulation of hepatic mitochondrial metabolism in response to a high fat diet: A longitudinal study in rats. *J Physiol Biochem.* 2012.

64. Poussin C, Ibberson M, Hall D, Ding J, Soto J, Abel ED, and Thorens B. Oxidative phosphorylation flexibility in the liver of mice resistant to high-fat diet-induced hepatic steatosis. *Diabetes.* 2011;60:2216–24.

65. Finocchietto PV, Holod S, Barreyro F, Peralta JG, Alippe Y, Giovambattista A, Carreras MC, and Poderoso JJ. Defective leptin-AMP-dependent kinase pathway induces nitric oxide release and contributes to mitochondrial dysfunction and obesity in *ob/ob* mice. *Antioxid Redox Signal.* 2011;15:2395–406.

66. Singh A, Wirtz M, Parker N, Hogan M, Strahler J, Michailidis G, Schmidt S, Vidal-Puig A, Diano S, Andrews P et al. Leptin-mediated changes in hepatic mitochondrial metabolism, structure, and protein levels. *Proc Natl Acad Sci USA.* 2009;106:13100–5.

67. Perez-Carreras M, Del Hoyo P, Martin MA, Rubio JC, Martin A, Castellano G, Colina F, Arenas J, and Solis-Herruzo JA. Defective hepatic mitochondrial respiratory chain in patients with nonalcoholic steatohepatitis. *Hepatology.* 2003;38:999–1007.

68. Caldwell SH, Swerdlow RH, Khan EM, Iezzoni JC, Hespenheide EE, Parks JK, and Parker WD, Jr. Mitochondrial abnormalities in non-alcoholic steatohepatitis. *J Hepatol.* 1999;31:430–4.

69. Sanyal AJ, Campbell-Sargent C, Mirshahi F, Rizzo WB, Contos MJ, Sterling RK, Luketic VA, Shiffman ML, and Clore JN. Nonalcoholic steatohepatitis: Association of insulin resistance and mitochondrial abnormalities. *Gastroenterology.* 2001;120:1183–92.

70. Satapati S, Sunny NE, Kucejova B, Fu X, He TT, Mendez-Lucas A, Shelton JM, Perales JC, Browning JD, and Burgess SC. Elevated TCA cycle function in the pathology of diet-induced hepatic insulin resistance and fatty liver. *J Lipid Res.* 2012;53:1080–92.

71. Ibrahim SH, and Gores GJ. Who pulls the trigger: JNK activation in liver lipotoxicity? *J Hepatol.* 2012;56:17–9.

72. Yamaguchi K, Yang L, McCall S, Huang J, Yu XX, Pandey SK, Bhanot S, Monia BP, Li YX, and Diehl AM. Inhibiting triglyceride synthesis improves hepatic steatosis but exacerbates liver damage and fibrosis in obese mice with nonalcoholic steatohepatitis. *Hepatology.* 2007;45:1366–74.

73. Singh R, Wang Y, Xiang Y, Tanaka KE, Gaarde WA, and Czaja MJ. Differential effects of JNK1 and JNK2 inhibition on murine steatohepatitis and insulin resistance. *Hepatology.* 2009;49:87–96.

74. Baar K, Wende AR, Jones TE, Marison M, Nolte LA, Chen M, Kelly DP, and Holloszy JO. Adaptations of skeletal muscle to exercise: Rapid increase in the transcriptional coactivator PGC-1. *FASEB J.* 2002;16:1879–86.

75. Holloszy JO, and Booth FW. Biochemical adaptations to endurance exercise in muscle. *Annu Rev Physiol.* 1976;38:273–91.

76. Mole PA, Oscai LB, and Holloszy JO. Adaptation of muscle to exercise. Increase in levels of palmityl Coa synthetase, carnitine palmityltransferase, and palmityl Coa dehydrogenase, and in the capacity to oxidize fatty acids. *J Clin Invest.* 1971;50:2323–30.

77. Leone TC, Lehman JJ, Finck BN, Schaeffer PJ, Wende AR, Boudina S, Courtois M, Wozniak DF, Sambandam N, Bernal-Mizrachi C et al. PGC-1alpha deficiency causes multi-system energy metabolic derangements: Muscle dysfunction, abnormal weight control and hepatic steatosis. *PLoS Biol.* 2005;3:e101.

78. Lin J, Wu PH, Tarr PT, Lindenberg KS, St-Pierre J, Zhang CY, Mootha VK, Jager S, Vianna CR, Reznick RM et al. Defects in adaptive energy metabolism with CNS-linked hyperactivity in PGC-1alpha null mice. *Cell.* 2004;119:121–35.
79. Scarpulla RC. Transcriptional paradigms in mammalian mitochondrial biogenesis and function. *Physiol Rev.* 2008;88:611–38.
80. Scarpulla RC. Metabolic control of mitochondrial biogenesis through the PGC-1 family regulatory network. *Biochim Biophys Acta.* 2011;1813:1269–78.
81. Murakami T, Shimomura Y, Yoshimura A, Sokabe M, and Fujitsuka N. Induction of nuclear respiratory factor-1 expression by an acute bout of exercise in rat muscle. *Biochim Biophys Acta.* 1998;1381:113–22.
82. Garcia-Roves P, Huss JM, Han DH, Hancock CR, Iglesias-Gutierrez E, Chen M, and Holloszy JO. Raising plasma fatty acid concentration induces increased biogenesis of mitochondria in skeletal muscle. *Proc Natl Acad Sci USA.* 2007;104:10709–13.
83. Lieber CS, Leo MA, Wang X, and Decarli LM. Alcohol alters hepatic FoxO1, p53, and mitochondrial SIRT5 deacetylation function. *Biochem Biophys Res Commun.* 2008;373:246–52.
84. Oliva J, French BA, Li J, Bardag-Gorce F, Fu P, and French SW. Sirt1 is involved in energy metabolism: The role of chronic ethanol feeding and resveratrol. *Exp Mol Pathol.* 2008;85:155–9.
85. Otera H, and Mihara K. Molecular mechanisms and physiologic functions of mitochondrial dynamics. *J Biochem.* 2011;149:241–51.
86. Chan DC. Mitochondrial fusion and fission in mammals. *Annu Rev Cell Dev Biol.* 2006;22:79–99.
87. Gomes LC, Di Benedetto G, and Scorrano L. During autophagy mitochondria elongate, are spared from degradation and sustain cell viability. *Nat Cell Biol.* 2011;13:589–98.
88. Reddy PH, Reddy TP, Manczak M, Calkins MJ, Shirendeb U, and Mao P. Dynamin-related protein 1 and mitochondrial fragmentation in neurodegenerative diseases. *Brain Res Rev.* 2011;67:103–18.
89. Davey GP, Peuchen S, and Clark JB. Energy thresholds in brain mitochondria. Potential involvement in neurodegeneration. *J Biol Chem.* 1998;273:12753–7.
90. Israel Y, Kalant H, Khanna JM, Orrego H, Phillips MJ, and Stewart DJ. Ethanol metabolism, oxygen availability and alcohol induced liver damage. *Adv Exp Med Biol.* 1977;85A:343–58.
91. Cadenas E, and Boveris A. Enhancement of hydrogen peroxide formation by protophores and ionophores in antimycin-supplemented mitochondria. *Biochem J.* 1980;188:31–7.

Section III

*Nutrition Role in Liver
Protection and Damage*

9 Nutritional Induction of Nonalcoholic Fatty Liver Disease

Noga Budick-Harmelin, Michal Aharoni-Simon, and Zecharia Madar

CONTENTS

INTRODUCTION

Fatty liver disease has been shown to be affected by both hereditary and behavioral factors. Nutritional influences have been widely studied as contributors to nonalcoholic fatty liver disease (NAFLD), and findings of numerous studies indicate that nutritional intake is of major importance in emergence and development of this disorder. In this chapter, we review aspects of nutrition-related induction of fatty liver and discuss the mechanisms involved in their pathogenesis, as studied by relevant animal models and also among patients.

First reviewed is the induction of steatosis by overnutrition. This type of NAFLD is common in Western countries, typically associated with other features of the metabolic syndrome, such as obesity, insulin resistance, and hyperlipidemia. In this regard, the importance of Western lifestyle–related dietary habits in NAFLD pathogenesis is highlighted.

Other than increased caloric intake, the involvement of dietary components of the Western diet is reviewed. The impact of dietary fat content and composition is discussed, with focus on the effect and metabolic pathways of fats prevalent in the Western diet such as saturated fatty acids (SFA), *trans*-fat, and cholesterol. Thereafter, the mechanisms of carbohydrate-induced steatosis are presented and the contribution of increased carbohydrates consumption to NAFLD induction is described.

Finally, the induction of fatty liver by conditions of undernutrition is presented. The involvement of nutrients deficiencies including amino acids, carnitine, essential fatty acids (EFA), and lipotropic factors in fatty liver morbidity is underlined, and the induction of NAFLD by choline deficiency is reviewed.

INCREASED ENERGY INTAKE AND OBESITY: STEATOSIS CAUSED BY OVERNUTRITION

Overnutrition, which leads to lipid overload in nonadipose tissues, is a prominent cause of fat accumulation in the liver. In fact, fatty liver is widely regarded as the hepatic manifestation of the obesity-related metabolic syndrome, rather than an organ-specific pathology. Hence, increased energy intake and obesity are considered to represent major players in the pathophysiology of NAFLD (Figure 9.1).

Increased energy uptake directly supports hepatic fat accumulation by delivery of excess fat and carbohydrates to the liver, where they provoke lipogenic pathways (discussed below). In addition, indirect effect of increased energy intake is mediated

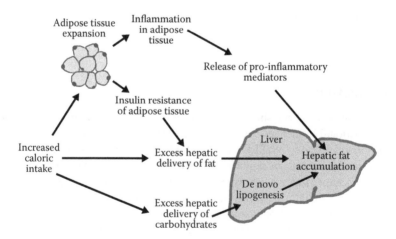

FIGURE 9.1   Pro-steatotic effects of overeating. Intrahepatic and extrahepatic pathways of steatosis induction by overnutrition.

via expansion of adipose tissue (Figure 9.1). When adipose tissue expands as result of obesity, it tends to become inflamed [1–3] and resistant to insulin-mediated suppression of lipolysis [4–8]. Thus, increased release of fatty acids (FA) from adipose tissue enhances nonesterified fatty acids (NEFA) pool in the serum, further potentiating uptake of free FA by the liver. Moreover, the secretion of proinflammatory cytokines from adipose tissue induces hepatic fat accumulation via modulation of adipokines release (reviewed in [9,10]). As evidence, increased macrophages counts in white adipose tissue is significantly associated with measurements of insulin resistance and with hepatic fibro-inflammatory lesions [11], indicating the relation between adipose inflammation and steatohepatitis among obese patients.

In accordance, human studies indicate that the risk for NAFLD and nonalcoholic steatohepatitis (NASH) is strongly associated with obesity and particularly with increased visceral adiposity deposits [12–15], which are able to release FA directly into the portal circulation. In fact, obesity was found to be the most reproducible risk factor for steatohepatitis severity [16]. Indeed, NASH patients are found to have higher caloric intake, compared with healthy subjects [17], and steatosis degree is significantly correlated to the caloric intake among NAFLD patients [18]. Furthermore, liver injury was shown to improve by simple caloric restriction in obese individuals [19], as well as among NASH patients [20]. Therefore, overnutrition leading to increased weight and, ultimately, obesity is recognized as primary driver of NAFLD.

Lessons Learned from Experimental Models of Overeating

Steatosis is induced by excess food intake of chow diet, without any manipulation of dietary composition, in some mutant rodents that spontaneously overeat, such as *ob/ob* mice [21], *db/db* mice [22], Zucker (*fa/fa*) rats [23], Otsuka Long-Evans Tokushima Fatty (OLETF) rats [24] KK-A^y mice [25], and *foz/foz* mice [26]. One might argue that this actually is the best experimental approach to studying steatohepatitis because it most closely resembles the natural progression of NAFLD observed among patients, accompanied by obesity and impaired glucose metabolism. Yet, this perception is somehow inaccurate because some of these genetic modifications cause broader phenotypic abnormalities than simple overeating, which questions their reliability as models of human pathology. A well-established case is *ob/ob* mice, in which the induction of steatosis by leptin deficiency is not mediated solely via change in food consumption (reviewed in [27,28]).

Still, the hyperphagic animals are useful for investigation of interaction between overconsumption of food and liver injury, as well as for evaluation of potential preventive interventions. For example, overexpression of adiponectin was shown to reduce dietary intake (per gram of body weight) and to significantly decrease steatosis in *ob/ob* mice [29]. Another interesting finding by Rector et al. [30] is that physical exercise limits the development of steatosis in hyperphagic OLETF rats, without decreasing food consumption (relative to body weight), probably by prompting hepatic oxidation of FA. These data are of greater relevance to clinical practice because, unlike in *ob/ob* mice, the metabolic derangements in OLETF rats are entirely attributable to the excess food intake [31]. Indeed, physical activity was shown to reduce steatosis in obese subjects, even in the absence of body weight reduction [32], supporting the recognition of sedentary lifestyle as independent determinant of NAFLD (further discussed in Chapter 11 of this book).

LIPID CONSUMPTION AS A DETERMINANT OF FATTY LIVER DISEASE

The strong association between increased food intake and fatty liver has prompted study of the contribution of specific macronutrients to the hepatic fat accumulation. Increased prevalence of NAFLD and NASH in the westernized societies [33] indicates the contribution of typical dietary components in determination of the morbidity and disease progression (Table 9.1). A key feature of the Western-style diets is high-fat content, which directly supports steatosis by promoting excess uptake of dietary lipids by hepatocytes (discussed in [27]).

In agreement with this, the percentage of fat in the diet was found to correlate significantly with liver fat content [34], and increased fat consumption is found among NASH patients, when compared with healthy controls [35]. Furthermore, intervention studies also indicate the influence of dietary fat content upon hepatic steatosis, which is increased by consumption of high-fat diet (HFD) and decreased by low-fat isocaloric diet [36].

Numerous studies were performed in animal models to reveal cellular pathways mediating the contribution of fat consumption to disease progression and aggravation of metabolic derangement in NAFLD. Nevertheless, the underlying mechanism is yet not fully understood. A possible mechanism by which HFD might promote hepatic inflammation is upregulation of nuclear factor κB (NF-κB) activity [37]. In support of this, hepatic fat accumulation and recruitment of macrophages and neutrophils induced by HFD is significantly decreased in absence of interleukin 6 (IL-6) and tumor necrosis factor receptor 1 (TNFR1) [38], both components of pathways activated in response to NF-κB induction. Moreover, liver-specific inhibition of NF-κB protected against inflammatory cytokines and macrophage-specific markers

TABLE 9.1
Characteristic Components of the Western Diet Associated with Obesity-Related NAFLD

Nutrient Overconsumed	Involvement in NAFLD Pathology
Saturated fat	Steatogenic,[a] highly lipotoxic, proinflammatory
Trans-fat	Steatogenic,[b] proinflammatory, fibrogenic(?)
Cholesterol	Pro-lipogenic,[b] proinflammatory, fibrogenic[c]
Simple sugars	Pro-lipogenic, proinflammatory[b,d]

[a] Particularly when consumed together with simple carbohydrates.
[b] Enhanced when consumed in setting of HFD.
[c] Mainly induced by cholate.
[d] In particular fructose.

expression and also eliminated development of insulin resistance in mice model of high-fat feeding [37]. Controversially, another work found that although blocking of hepatic NF-κB prevents HFD-induced insulin resistance, it exacerbates hepatic steatosis, inflammation, and apoptosis [39]. The effect was associated with downregulation of β-oxidation mediator peroxisome proliferator–activated receptor α (PPAR-α) and increased expression of lipogenic genes.

Another direction of investigation postulates that HFD promotes hepatic inflammation by sensitizing the liver to endotoxin-generated injury. This is indicated by hepatic upregulated expression of the macrophage scavenger receptor MARCO that is induced by HFD in mice [40]. This concept is in line with the well-recognized "two-hit" hypothesis, which proposes endotoxins as contributors to NASH development [41].

An additional mechanism by which HFD may promote NAFLD is by the induction of hepatic endoplasmic reticulum (ER) stress. High-fat feeding induces markers of ER stress in the liver [42], suggested as a mechanism for the development of insulin resistance. Hepatic ER stress response stimulates NAFLD progression and exacerbation by inducing lipogenesis, decreasing hepatic fat export, and triggering inflammatory and fibrotic processes (reviewed in [43]).

Lastly, since high fat consumption leads to obesity, certain pro-steatotic effects of HFDs can also be mediated by an extrahepatic influence, taking place in the expanded adipose tissue. Intriguing works indicate that apoptotic process in adipose tissue participates in induction of hepatic fat accumulation by HFD. This is demonstrated by alleviation of steatosis via inhibition of adipocyte apoptosis in models of high-fat feeding [44,45].

Dietary FA in Molecular Mechanisms of Hepatic Lipotoxicity

Dietary FA are delivered to the liver by lipoproteins or taken by the hepatocytes as NEFA after being "spilled over" from chylomicrons into the serum NEFA pool (which is also supplied by adipose tissue–derived FA) [46]. Within hepatocytes, FA can be oxidized in the mitochondria [47] by the cyclic degradation process of β-oxidation into acetyl-CoA units. However, when hepatocytes are overloaded with FA due to increased fat consumption, the rate of import exceeds the rate of catabolism and the capacity of β-oxidation pathway is surpassed. The increased availability of FA in the hepatocytes induces augmentation in FA esterification into triglycerides (TG), which are stored and create steatosis.

A considerable debate exists regarding whether fat accumulation per se is simply an "innocent bystander" to mechanisms of disease progression or that it plays causal role in NAFLD exacerbation [48]. Although TG accumulation can promote liver inflammation by potentiation of Kupffer cells (KC) activation [49], incorporation into TG is majorly postulated to be a protective mechanism against FA-mediated hepatotoxicity [50]. Still, being a nonadipose tissue, the capacity of the liver for lipid storage is limited. Therefore, accumulation of FA as TG beyond a certain limit that is tolerated by hepatocytes leads to diversion of these FA into cytotoxic pathways [51].

Hepatic lipotoxicity of FA is demonstrated by their ability to interfere with the cellular function by affecting several pathways (reviewed in [52]), which create difficulty in studying the distinctive effect of each specific signaling pathway. Within hepatocytes, FA are capable to support NAFLD progression by inducing proinflammatory gene expression [53–55] and apoptotic response [56–58] and also to promote metabolic aberration by interfering with insulin signaling [59–61]. In addition, FA are also capable of activating toll-like receptor 4 (TLR4)-dependent inflammatory signaling [62] and to promote inflammatory response [63] in macrophages. Therefore, high levels of free FA in the liver might support the transition of steatosis into NASH by promoting activation of KC, the liver resident macrophages.

Generation of reactive oxygen species (ROS) appears to underlie the FA-related cellular injury, inflammation, and fibrogenesis. A major route for generation of pro-oxidant ROS within liver cells is the oxidation of FA. Under physiological conditions, the main pathway for FA oxidation is β-oxidation in the mitochondria, which is acting in concert with the electron transport chain. In the fatty liver milieu, mitochondrial β-oxidative capacity becomes overwhelmed, and alternative cellular oxidation pathways are also activated (discussed in [27]). Hence, generation of ROS and cytotoxic metabolites is increased, contributing to cellular oxidative stress that might exceed the capacity of cellular antioxidant systems.

By interacting with biomolecules, ROS induce DNA damage and mediate apoptotic and inflammatory processes. In addition, increased ROS load in hepatocytes impairs the function of respiratory chain components [64], creating a vicious circle by sensitizing the liver to mitochondrial ROS formation. A pivotal mechanism in NASH development is lipid peroxidation, which is promoted by the disruptive redox balance in the setting of fat accumulation. Although lipid peroxidation levels are found to be minor in liver of healthy subjects, they are significantly increased in livers of subjects with fatty liver and even more in livers of NASH patients [65]. Lipid peroxidation may further promote steatosis due to their ability to inhibit lipoprotein secretion from hepatocytes [66]. In addition, research in animal model of NASH implies a role for lipid peroxidation in the mechanism of fibrogenic activation in the liver [67]. Hence, multiple mechanisms appear to mediate the lipotoxic effects of enhanced FA intake by the liver.

Evaluating the Effect of HFD by Increasing the Amount of Dietary Fat

To study the relation between increased fat intake and NAFLD, an impressive array of high-fat dietary animal models was developed and yielded a plethora of information. Steatosis is acquired in these models by supra-nutritional dietary regimens, enriched with fat. However, enormous variation exists between the pathophysiological results of different works, with regard to liver injury (steatosis degree, inflammation, and fibrosis) and to appearance of the associated morbidities (obesity and insulin resistance). Part of the inconsistency could arise from the diversity in dietary composition (fat content, fat source, and other nutrients) used in various studies, as well as from different experimental protocols (treatment duration, ad libitum versus force feeding) and difference in susceptibility of various species and strains of laboratory animals. Therefore, better understanding can be achieved by comparison between outcomes of various studies.

Fat content of high-fat murine regimen typically consists of 40%–70% of total calories. To describe the dependence between fat content of the diet and the pathophysiology induced, the results of different regimens should be compared with graduate increase of fat amount used.

Diets found around the low end of this spectrum (up to 45% calories from fat) are commonly used to induce obesity-related steatosis [44,68–70]. Yet, certain inconsistency exists, as some failed to report hepatic fat accumulation induced by these formulas [71]. Other works report that these formulas were sufficient to create steatosis accompanied by increased hepatic activation of inflammatory markers such as Jun N-terminal kinase (JNK), NF-κB, tumor necrosis factor α (TNF-α), and IL-6 [69, 72]. Of note is that in some cases, these "Western-style" high-fat formulations are also enriched with sucrose and cholesterol [44,72] or with *trans*-fatty acids (TFA) [70], which also play a role in fatty liver pathology (discussed below).

Using formulas with higher fat content (≈60% calories from fat), especially for treatment duration of several months, enables achieving obesity and markers of insulin resistance with a progressive biochemical and histological liver injury. This was demonstrated by significant features of inflammation, apoptosis [73], and even fibrotic changes [74,75]. Mechanistic investigations discovered that these injuries are associated with differential activation of intrahepatic JNK signaling cascades [73] and decreased PPAR-α expression [74]. It can be generalized that this group of models can better represent NASH phenotype in more advanced stage of human disease.

Using overfeeding of rats with a corn oil–based formula by total enteral nutrition (TEN), Baumgardner et al. have shown that the same trend of increase in liver pathology is kept also with increasing fat content in the diet up to 70% calories from fat [76]. In line with this, feeding rats a formula in which 71% of energy derived from fat allows to reproduce many key features of NASH already after 3 weeks [77]. The livers of treated animals were presented with substantial steatosis, inflammation, abnormal mitochondria, induction of cytochrome P450-2E1 (CYP2E1), increased oxidative stress, and collagen content, as well as evidence of insulin resistance. Of interest is that most injury measurements were significantly attenuated by restricting the consumption of the same HFD to two-thirds of the amount consumed ad libitum [77]. Similar injury is induced in rats fed a formula containing 77% of calories from fat via gavage for 6 weeks, along with reduced PPAR-α expression, which is indicative of impaired β-oxidation [78]. As discussed below, the type of lipids in the diet is also a determinant of pathological outcome. Therefore, it is important to note that it would be unsuitable to directly compare the results obtained in [76–78], using highly unsaturated FA-consisted formula, with those obtained by the works mentioned earlier in the text, that used SFA-based formulas.

In addition, due to their relative low melting point, these unsaturated fat diets are typically available in liquid formulation. Therefore, it is not uncommon that intragastric infusion is used for overfeeding animals with these diets [76,78]. The combined model of overfeeding with increased fat contact may better imitate the dietary habits of the Western lifestyle. The added effect of overfeeding above the effect of increased fat contact is well demonstrated by results of Ogasawara et al. [79]. In this study, overeating was induced in mice by administration of gold thioglucose (GTG), and then followed by HFD feeding (82% of calories from fat). Indeed, hyperphagic mice developed more severe NASH phenotype, with increased expression of inflammatory and fibrotic markers, accompanied by enhanced obesity and insulin resistance, when compared with high-fat–fed control animals.

The far end of the dietary fat content range is represented by the ketogenic diets, which contain very high fat content and are very low in carbohydrates. Ketogenic diets induce a unique metabolic state, which is incompletely defined, and much discrepancy exists between different works. A popular ketogenic regimen (95% of calories arise from fat with no carbohydrates) was shown to induce steatosis in mice [71] but still considered to cause only modest liver injury (discussed at [9]). However, a recent work using this regimen for longer duration, reports a unique pattern of hepatic fat accumulation, accompanied by hepatic macrophage accumulation and apoptotic markers with impaired glucose tolerance [70]. Noteworthy is the fact that in contrast to the "Western-style" HFD, the ketogenic diet evokes a significant weight loss in animals and, therefore, was criticized as less relevant to human NAFLD [80]. Interestingly, it appears that it is possible to achieve steatosis that is accompanied by weight gain in mice by increasing the protein content of the ketogenic regimen [81]. This finding demonstrates the involvement of different factors, other than fat content of the diet, in determining the pathophysiology in high-fat models.

It Is Not Only Fat Content: Other Effectors of Pathophysiology in Fat-Enriched Diets

As already mentioned, besides the level of fat consumed, other factors can affect the ability of enhanced fat consumption to induce fatty liver. A main determinant of NAFLD pathogenesis is the source and quality of the dietary lipids. Although all types of fat can contribute to NAFLD, the ability of different FA to induce steatosis varies according to the acyl-chain length, saturation level, and the presence of various carbohydrates in the diet (reviewed in [9]).

Considering the type of FA consumed, SFA appear to be highly relevant in NAFLD (Table 9.1). Human studies indicate a high intake of saturated fats among NASH patients [82], and that of all components of diet, percentage of hepatic fat is best correlated with the amount of saturated fat [34]. Intervention studies also imply that reduction of hepatic fat is connected to restriction of saturated fat intake [83]. These observations are explained by the pro-lipogenic effect of saturated fats [84,85], mediated by peroxisome proliferator–activated receptor γ coactivator 1β (PGC-1β) pathway [84]. On the contrary, saturated fats were also suggested to induce hepatic FA oxidation via peroxisome proliferator–activated receptor γ coactivator 1α (PGC-1α) activation [85] and to promote very-low-density lipoprotein (VLDL) secretion [84], thus reducing accumulation of TG in the liver. One suggested explanation for these seemingly contradictive effects is that the actual effect of saturated fat depends upon carbohydrate intake [9]. It is assumed that dietary saturated fat is a strong inducer of steatosis especially when it is consumed together with simple sugar. This can explain the lack of evidence for significant steatosis when feeding rats a high-saturated fat diet that contains no simple sugars [86], which enables avoiding the lipogenic impact of SFA by limiting the supply of substrates for lipogenesis. The strong association between saturated fat consumption and steatosis in humans [34] can be explained by the high content of SFA concomitant with simple sugars in the

Western diet. The sugars can supply lipogenic pathways activated by this fat, therefore masking beneficial ability of saturated fat to induce FA oxidation [9].

Direct comparisons between monounsaturated and saturated fat show that the former is more steatogenic both in vitro (N. Budick-Harmelin, unpublished data) [87,88] and in vivo [85]. In the absence of monounsaturated FA, the SFA less readily incorporate into TG, which explains the increased lipotoxic effects seen with free SFA [87,88]. Nevertheless, substantial liver injury can be induced in animals also by unsaturated FA–based dietary formulas [77]. In fact, when unsaturated fat is combined with simple monosaccharide and admitted by intragastric overfeeding protocol, a formula with 37% of calories from fat is sufficient to achieve prominent NASH pathology with hepatic fibrosis and insulin resistance [89].

Additional characteristic of the Western diet, which was comprehensively studied in rodent models, is high content of *trans*-fat (Table 9.1). Using a model of Western diet and sedentary behavior, it was shown that *trans*-fats promote hepatic steatosis and liver injury [90], probably due to their ability to induce lipogenic genes expression in the liver [84,91]. Interestingly, the deleterious role played by TFA appears in the context of high-fat–fed animals [91,92] but is not significant when *trans*-fats are consumed in absence of increased fat intake [91]. In addition, TFA also support inflammatory activation, as demonstrated by their ability to induce inflammatory cells infiltration [91], expression of hepatic interleukin–1β (IL–1β) [92], and hepatic inflammation [93] in vivo and to modulate the immune function of isolated KC [91]. Conflict still exists regarding ability [91] or disability [92] of *trans*-fat to induce fibrotic changes. Data from intervention studies in human is limited and does not necessarily support a role for TFA in hepatic fat accumulation [94].

Beyond the effect of macronutrients composition itself, experience gained using animal models indicates that species, strain, and sex of animals can impact the effect of high-fat dietary regimen. This probably reflects, at least to some level, the existence of heterogeneity in susceptibility level among human subpopulations. Comparing different species is somewhat complex, but yet it seems that rabbits are quite vulnerable to high-fat feeding and develop advanced NASH phenotype, with features of cirrhosis-closed fibrosis, in response to long treatment [95]. Substantial differences exist also among strains (reviewed in [96]). For example, C57BL/6 mice appear to be more sensitive to HFD-induced steatosis than 129S6/SvEvTac mice, possibly due to greater activation of lipogenic gene array mediated by increased sterol regulatory element-binding protein 1c (SREBP-1c) response [97]. Analysis of strain and sex-related effects, demonstrated greater tendency to develop steatosis in response to HFD in BALB/c male mice in comparison to C57BL/6J male mice, and also in comparison to BALB/c female mice [98].

SIGNIFICANCE OF CHOLESTEROL INTAKE IN NAFLD

Dietary cholesterol consumption is also considered to contribute to formation and deterioration of NAFLD (Table 9.1). This concept is supported by superabundant cholesterol intake found among NASH patients [82]. In vivo treatment with atherogenic diet (enriched with cholesterol and sometimes also with cholate) induces marked steatosis in mice [99,100], rats [101], and rabbits [102] within a few weeks. Besides the predictable increase in cholesterol content in fatty livers [99,100], treated animals were presented with hepatic histology reminiscent of progressive NASH, including inflammatory and fibrotic changes, accompanied by markers of oxidative stress [99–102].

Differential effects of cholesterol-enriched diet upon hepatic pathways of FA synthesis and TG accumulation were reported. Upregulation of lipogenic genes expression and downregulation of FA oxidation-related genes was noticed in response to atherogenic diet after 6 weeks and significant increase in hepatic TG was measured after 24 weeks by Matsuzawa et al. [99]. Another work that examined the effect of long-term high-cholesterol (HC) feeding, reports decrease in expression level of FA synthase and decrease in TG content at 55 weeks' time point [100]. This result can be explained by the high carbohydrate content of control diet used in this study, which might shift the expression reference level [100]. However, since lipogenic genes tend to decrease back to basal expression levels after 24 weeks also in the study of Matsuzawa et al. the results may actually reflect the time course of pathology development in this model. Nonetheless, conflicting data arise from another study that found decreased hepatic TG levels in response to 3-week feeding of atherogenic diet alone or in combination with HFD [103]. Upregulation of cholesterol synthesis–associated enzymes in the liver of NAFLD patients [104] supports the recent proposal that surplus cholesterol contributes to synthesis of FA by activation of LXRα-SREBP-1c pathway in hepatocytes (discussed in [105]).

Dietary cholesterol represents an important risk factor also for NAFLD progression, because an atherogenic diet induces genes related to inflammation and fibrogenesis in the liver [99]. Examination of the distinct contribution of each dietary component of the atherogenic diet indicates that while cholesterol is required for induction of genes involved in acute inflammation, the induction of hepatic fibrosis is attributed more to cholate consumption [103]. Cholesterol also promotes KC-mediated inflammatory activation in the liver and influences the development of insulin and glucose intolerance (discussed in [106]). In addition, hepatocytes from short-term atherogenic diet-fed rats exhibit cellular susceptibility to Fas- and lipopolysaccharide-mediated injury in vivo as well as to TNF-mediated apoptosis in vitro [107]. The findings also indicate a critical role of mitochondrial cholesterol loading in the hepatocellular sensitization to TNF [107].

However, when compared with human steatosis, the disease induced in animals by HC feeding seems to develop in different metabolic context. Although one study reported weight gain induced by HC diet in rats [101], NAFLD induced by HC was not accompanied by obesity in mice [99,100,102], and was associated with increased systemic insulin sensitivity [99]. Therefore, it is questionable whether HC-fed animals can be used as models for typical NAFLD/NASH in humans.

Interestingly, when high-fat component was added to the atherogenic diet, the development of histopathological features was accelerated, hepatic insulin resistance appeared, and genes of antioxidant enzymes were downregulated [99]. Other works that analyzed the effect of atherogenic and HFD separately or together show that cholesterol and fat induce distinct sets of gene expression [103] and that addition of cholesterol to HFD potentiates hepatic TG accumulation [108]. Thus, it is conceivable that combining HFD with atherogenic diet creates a better replicate of human NASH with relevant human metabolic parameters.

Intriguing notion, connecting increased cholesterol consumption with fatty liver disease among nonobese individuals, is proposed by the group of Enjoji and colleagues [105]. Manifestation of liver injury without obesity or insulin resistance, observed in atherogenic diet-fed models, resembles the phenomenon commonly seen among nonobese NASH patients. The contribution of nutritional factors to the NAFLD in this subpopulation of individuals is poorly understood. Yet, dietary cholesterol intake was found to be significantly higher among nonobese NAFLD patients, when compared with control subjects as well as with obese patients [109]. In agreement, expression of genes associated with cholesterol sensing and cholesterol esterification was increased in the liver of NAFLD patients, and to a greater extent in the liver of nonobese patients [104]. The overwork of hepatocytes, resulting in overload of cholesterol in tissues is suggested to explain the absence of hypercholesterolemia, despite overconsumption of cholesterol, among nonobese NAFLD patients [105]. These findings brought to suggest not only control of dietary cholesterol intake, but even pharmaceutical inhibition of cholesterol absorption as beneficial treatment strategy in nonobese NAFLD patients [110].

CONTRIBUTION OF DIETARY CARBOHYDRATES TO HEPATIC LIPOGENESIS

Other than dietary lipids, dietary carbohydrates arriving to the liver can promote hepatic steatosis by providing precursors for synthesis of new FA by de novo lipogenesis (DNL). Quantitative metabolic data collected in NAFLD patients document that 26% of liver TG were derived from DNL, indicating that DNL contribute roughly one-fourth of FA accumulated in the fatty liver [46]. The significance of carbohydrates is reinforced due to the worldwide increase in consumption of sweetened food products throughout the last decades, paralleling prevalence of obesity, and metabolic syndrome. Of major importance is the widespread intake of high-fructose corn syrup, commonly used as a sweetener of soft drinks, juices, canned foods, candies, and baked goods in the westernized world.

Human dietary studies indicate the involvement of dietary carbohydrates, and particularly simple sugars, in the pathophysiology of fatty liver (Table 9.1). Evaluation performed among subjects with NAFLD indicates significant relation between the percentage of steatosis and carbohydrate consumption [18], suggesting that reduction of dietary carbohydrates may help to reduce liver fat in NAFLD. This is also supported by a study that examined the dietary composition among obese individuals, and reports association between carbohydrates intake and higher odds of hepatic inflammation [111]. Interestingly, as negative correlation found between the percentages of calories from carbohydrates and from fat, higher fat intake was unexpectedly associated with lower odds of hepatic inflammation in this study population.

In addition, DNL is found to be markedly increased in NAFLD patients in comparison to control subjects [112]. Findings from current intervention studies also support an immediate role for DNL in the pathogenesis of NAFLD. Addition of simple carbohydrates to the dietary consumption of overweight subjects resulted in significant increase in DNL and in liver fat content already after 3 weeks [113]. Likewise, greater decrease in steatosis was achieved among NAFLD patients by 2 weeks of dietary carbohydrate restriction than by a low-calorie diet [114].

When carbohydrate intake is increased, the glucose supply to the liver is enhanced, resulting in activation of the transcription factor carbohydrate response element-binding protein (ChREBP) and lipogenesis induction in the hepatocytes [115,116]. Carbohydrates also increase circulating insulin levels, which induce activation of the transcription factor SREBP-1c, which act in synergy with ChREBP to induce hepatic lipogenic gene expression (reviewed in [117]). The lipogenic effect of SREBP-1c is demonstrated by its overexpression, which results in lipogenic genes expression and hepatic TG accumulation in transgenic mice [118]. SREBP-1c is also induced by fat consumption and, therefore, can mediate DNL in response to high-fat feeding [97]. However, studies in mice with liver-specific knockout of stearoyl-CoA desaturase 1 (SCD1), which is a downstream target of SREBP-1c, reveal that SCD1 expression is required for induction of steatosis by high-carbohydrates, but not by HFD [119].

Increased synergistic activation of hepatic lipogenesis can be triggered by ChREBP and SREBP-1c among NAFLD patients with related morbidity of insulin resistance, in which both glucose and insulin are high in the circulation (discussed in [120]). Interestingly, NAFLD patients who are also diagnosed with the metabolic syndrome show greater histological severity as well as higher carbohydrates intake, in comparison to NAFLD patients without diagnosis of the metabolic syndrome [121]. This finding led the authors to suggest a role of increased carbohydrates consumption in development of NAFLD-related morbidities.

INDUCTION OF STEATOSIS BY SUCROSE- AND FRUCTOSE-ENRICHED DIETS

Supplementation of diet with excessive portion of carbohydrates creates models of NAFLD by acquired increased DNL. Increase in the relative part of carbohydrates in the diet obviously decrease the relative part of fat and, therefore, different high-energy regimens can be graded according to their relative carbohydrate and fat content [9] to understand the effect of various dietary compositions. In addition, the use of strictly controlled dietary interventions, which is not possible in human studies, allows comparing the effect of different carbohydrates.

Sucrose can provoke steatosis and obesity simply by supplementing it to the drinking water of rats for 8 weeks [122]. Feeding a low-fat high-sucrose dietary regimen for the same period also results in steatotic phenotype in mice [58]. Other features of human NAFLD were also recapitulated in this study, including obesity and insulin resistance, but steatohepatitis was not reported. The high-sucrose diet was also associated with increased Fas expression and the sensitivity to activation of apoptotic signaling [58]. The development of steatosis, liver injury, and insulin resistance by high-sucrose diet was demonstrated to be mediated via activation of the lysosomal cysteine protease cathepsin B (CTSB) and by TNFR1 signaling in this model [55]. High-sucrose diet is also implied to promote apoptosis of natural killer T (NKT) cells because it induces reduction of NKT cells numbers in the liver [123].

Various other studies were using monosaccharides instead of sucrose to enrich the diet with carbohydrates to create model of greater liver injury. Findings in animals indicate that fructose is stronger inducer of hepatic lipid accumulation than other dietary sugars, and hence, experimental models of fructose-enriched diet are widely used as good models of fatty liver. This may be attributable to the unique metabolic properties of fructose and its rapid utilization by the liver [124]. In agreement with this notion, higher steatosis and inflammation grades are seen in rats fed high-fructose diet then in rats fed high-sucrose diet for 5 weeks [125]. By comparing the effects of sucrose-, glucose-, and fructose-sweetened water, Bergheim et al. also show that hepatic lipid accumulation and markers of oxidative stress and inflammatory process in the liver were significantly higher in mice consuming fructose [122]. Steatosis can be induced in rodents by high-fructose consumption via feeding of modified formulation [125,126] or supplementation of drinking water [122,127,128], but conflicting results exist regarding the ability of fructose to induce [127] or not induce [122,125,126] the accompanied adiposity that is common in human patients. This discrepancy might be explained by the use of different experimental designs that differ in fructose dosage, treatment times, and animal species.

Large-scale epidemiological studies associate NAFLD with excessive dietary fructose (measured by consumption of fructose-containing beverages) [129,130] and higher fructose consumption correlates with fibrosis severity among NASH patients [131]. Data from intervention studies are more limited and more difficult to conclude. Six days of high-fructose consumption led to stimulation of hepatic DNL and induced hepatic insulin resistance [132]. Yet, a longer treatment (4 weeks) with fructose overfeeding did not increase hepatic lipid content in healthy individuals [133]. Suggested explanation for the absence of steatosis after longer exposure is adaptive increase in TG secretion from the liver as VLDL [133]. However, differences in manipulation protocol may also explain the inconsistency, due to double dosage of supplementation in the former study (3 g fructose versus 1.5 g fructose per kilogram of body weight per day).

Beyond the ability of fructose to induce steatosis by increasing DNL, a growing body of evidence indicates the involvement of fructose in multiple cellular pathways that lead to inflammatory activation (reviewed in [134]). Fructose consumption induces expressions of proinflammatory cytokines (reported in [135]) [122], neutrophils infiltration [122], nitric oxide (NO) production [128], and lipid peroxidation [122,128] in the liver of treated animals. Intriguingly, portal endotoxemia is evident in fructose-fed animals [122], and the fructose-induced steatosis is markedly attenuated by concomitant treatment with antibiotics [122] and in TLR4-knockout mice [136]. These findings, together with absence of obesity in many steatotic high-fructose models [122,125,126], support the proposed hypothesis of fructose as inducer of the proinflammatory "second hit" in pathogenesis of NAFLD [134]. The suggested mechanism is that fructose increases the intestinal translocation of endotoxin and therefore promotes development of NASH [122].

MODELING THE WESTERN DIET: COMBINING HIGH CARBOHYDRATES WITH HIGH FAT

In an effort to gain better insight into the global effect of the sugar- and fat-enriched Western diet upon NAFLD induction in the correct pathological context, animal models that combine high carbohydrate with high fat have been developed. Experimental formulas typically contain a mixture of both carbohydrates and fats and, therefore, as mentioned earlier, steatosis tend to be amplified by increasing the relative content of simple sugar regardless of the fat composition of the diet [9]. Indeed, simultaneous consumption of high fructose and high fat for 8 weeks can induce apparent phenotypes of the metabolic syndrome in mice, including obesity, insulin resistance, and hepatic manifestations of steatosis with induction of proinflammatory and lipogenic genes [137].

Kohli et al. investigated the additive effect of high carbohydrate in HFD model (58% calories from fat, mostly medium-chain *trans*-fats) by supplementation of sucrose and fructose to drinking water of treated mice for a period of 16 weeks [138]. The results indicate development of hepatic steatosis, inflammation, and apoptosis, accompanied by obesity and insulin resistance in all high-fat–fed animals, compared with chow-fed mice. However, mice treated with high-carbohydrate diets in addition to HFD had higher hepatic oxidative stress, more monocyte infiltration into the liver, and significantly more fibrosis compared with the animals treated with HFD alone. Therefore, the consumption of high carbohydrate together with the HFD allowed achieving a more advanced NASH phenotype with fibrotic changes. Likewise, combined high sucrose and HFD resulted in greater reduction of hepatic NKT cells numbers, then each of these diets alone [123]. This result is obtained although the absolute contents of sucrose and fat in the combined regimen are lower than contents of each of these components in the high-sucrose diet and HFD, respectively. Hence, an additive detrimental effect of sucrose and high dietary fat on NKT cell population is suggested.

Hence, much data strengthens the case for adding carbohydrates to high-fat animal models of fatty liver to promote disease severity. Yet, inconsistent results arise from another work, indicating a decrease in hepatic steatosis and inflammation scores by addition of high fat content to fructose-enriched dietary regimen [125]. Treatment with HFD alone also resulted in greater concentrations of hepatic TG then the combined high-fat, high-fructose diet [125]. Of note is that the fat content of HFD in this study was low relative to other high-fat models (comprising 39% of total calories).

Finally, a more complex model combines HFD (*trans*-fat–enriched) with high-fructose supplementation and restricted physical activity to model the American lifestyle–induced obesity syndrome (ALIOS) in mice [90]. Investigating the roles of individual components of this diet indicates that the addition of fructose promoted food consumption, obesity, and impaired insulin sensitivity but did not worsen liver injury of steatotic animals in this model. Further studies are required to address the effects of fat composition and dietary carbohydrates on relevant metabolic parameters in the integrated context of Western diet.

STEATOSIS INDUCED BY UNDERNUTRITION AND NUTRITIONAL DEFICIENCIES

In addition to high dietary intake, which induces obesity-related fatty liver, steatosis can result from certain states of undernutrition and nutritional deficiencies (summarized in Table 9.2). In this regard, the most severe nutritional state related to steatosis is protein–calorie malnutrition. Fatty liver is observed in kwashiorkor, a

TABLE 9.2

Nutritional Deficiencies Related to NAFLD

Deficiency	Mechanism(s) of Hepatic Fat Accumulation
Inadequate protein consumption[a]	↑ FA supply to the liver
Carnitine deficiency	↓ Hepatic FA oxidation
n-3 FA deficiency	↓ Hepatic FA oxidation, ↑ hepatic lipogenesis
Lipotropes deficiency	↓ Hepatic fat export

[a] Without carbohydrate deficiency.

condition of protein–energy malnutrition, in which the protein supply is inadequate while carbohydrate–calorie intake is sufficient or in excess (reviewed in [139]). When protein malnutrition predominant the deficiency in total calories, steatosis may result due to increased NEFA supply to the liver from the periphery, as high circulating levels of FA are demonstrated in this metabolic state.

Another plausible contributor to the development of steatosis among malnourished individuals is nutrient deficiencies. Nutrient deficiencies have also been implicated in steatosis developed as complication in individuals receiving total parenteral nutrition (TPN), in which hepatic lipid accumulation is very prevalent sequelae [140]. TPN-related steatosis is commonly accompanied by insulin resistance and high circulating levels of TG and NEFA, hence somehow resembling obesity-related NAFLD. Yet, the hepatic fat accumulation is not necessarily associated only to caloric imbalances, as many evidence indicate improvement in steatosis by correction of nutritional deficiencies in TPN-supported patients (reviewed in [139]). The role of some of these deficient nutrients in NAFLD will be presented herein shortly.

Deprived protein intake may lead to carnitine deficiency, which is characteristic of impaired nutritional conditions such as kwashiorkor and long-term TPN (discussed in [139]). The major dietary sources of carnitine are meat and dairy products, and it can also be biosynthesized from the essential amino acids lysine and methionine. Carnitine is an essential cofactor of FA transportation into the mitochondria for β-oxidation (Table 9.2), and accordingly, hepatic fat accumulation is observed in animal models of systemic carnitine deprivation [141,142].

Insufficient consumption of EFA is another nutritional cause of steatosis. EFA deficiency may donate to pathogenesis of steatosis in conditions such as malnutrition and TPN (discussed in [139]), and steatosis develops quickly in animal models of EFA deficiency [143,144]. Lower hepatic levels of polyunsaturated fatty acids (PUFA) were also found in overnutrition-related NASH patients [145]; thus, inadequate consumption of PUFA may also exist in obesity-related NAFLD. Interestingly, a dietary pattern of decreased PUFA consumption was found among nonobese NAFLD patients when compared with obese patients [109] and among nonobese NASH patients compared with healthy controls [82]. The effect of PUFA can be mediated by their influence on membrane fluidity, and hence upon membrane-dependent processes. Moreover, PUFA, particularly those of the n-3 family, play pivotal roles as "fuel partitioners" in hepatocytes, exerting their beneficial effects by directly influencing gene expression pattern to induce FA oxidation and simultaneously inhibit lipid synthesis (reviewed in [146]) (Table 9.2).

An additional important group of essential nutrients in prevention of NAFLD consist of methyl donors, including choline, methionine, folic acid, and vitamin B12, collectively referred to as lipotropes. Lipotropes participate, as precursors and cofactors, in cellular biosynthesis of phosphatidylcholine, which is a necessary component of functional VLDL [147]. Hence, lipotrope deficiencies may impair the mechanism of fat export from hepatocytes, leading to steatosis (Table 9.2). Conflicting data arise with some reports indicate that vitamin B12 and folate levels are decreased in NAFLD as well as with disease severity [148], whereas others found that they are not affected [149]. Both vitamin B12 and folate are involved in the reaction of biosynthesis of methionine from homocysteine and, therefore, they are both crucial for homocysteine removal. Indeed, increased homocysteine levels are significantly associated with NAFLD and even suggested as a potential diagnostic tool [148]. Derangements in lipotropes status are also common among patients receiving long-term TPN [150]. Authors suggest that the imbalanced delivery of these factors during long-term TPN may lead to choline deficiency [150]. Indeed, diminished choline levels in long-term TPN are corrected by simultaneous supplementation with lecithin or with choline for several weeks, together with amelioration of steatosis [151,152].

These findings are in line with human studies demonstrating that choline deprivation leads to fatty liver and hepatic damage, which led to the recognition of choline as an essential nutrient [153–155]. Choline is consumed from variety of foods, with high concentrations in beef and chicken livers, eggs, and wheat germ [156]. Other than the dietary source, choline is generated by de novo biosynthesis of phosphatidylcholine in the liver, which modulates the dietary requirements of choline. This reaction is catalyzed by phosphatidylethanolamine-N-methyltransferase (PEMT) enzyme, which uses S-adenosylmethionine to form a new choline moiety [153], and differences in PEMT activity have been suggested to modulate dietary requirement of choline in different genders or ages [153,155]. In support of this, a common genetic polymorphism in the *PEMT* gene as well as estrogen levels, which induces PEMT activation, affects the susceptibility of animals and humans to hepatic damage during low-choline diet [155,157–161].

CHOLINE-DEFICIENT DIETS AS MODELS OF FATTY LIVER DISEASE

The observation that choline deficiency in human diets induces fatty liver and hepatic damage led to the establishment of choline-deficient (CD) animal models for NAFLD and NASH. Unlike experimental models of overnutrition that induce steatosis by increasing hepatic fat import or synthesis, fat accumulation in CD models results from hepatic failure to export fat. Four variations of CD diets have been established: CD, choline-deficient L-amino acid (CDAA), methionine–choline-deficient (MCD), and choline-deficient ethionine-supplemented (CDE) diets. Feeding rodents with each one of these diets induces fat accumulation in the liver, which further develops into fibrosis, cirrhosis, and carcinoma with morphological phenotypes that resembles human NAFLD [162–164]. However, histopathological and pathophysiological differences exist between these models.

Feeding rodents with CD diet induces accumulation of VLDL in hepatocytes [162,164] and significant increase in hepatic TG and cholesterol [163]. The lipids accumulate in the form of both macrovesicular and microvesicular steatosis, eventually filling up the entire hepatocyte [165]. Fat accumulation induced by CD diet is also accompanied by obesity, dyslipidemia, and insulin resistance [163], suggesting that the CD diet is a suitable model of human disease. The progressive hepatic damage in this model is reflected by increased lipid peroxidation and DNA damage, elevated TNF-α levels, and an increase in plasma transaminases levels [163,166,167]. Steatosis and hepatic damage increase progressively through the first 7–12 weeks of the CD diet, when signs of liver fibrosis and hyperplastic foci also appear [163,167]. Massive fibrosis and cirrhosis are observed after 40 weeks on the diet [166] and hepatocellular carcinoma (HCC) at week 52 [168].

Another formula with the same overall composition as the CD diet is the CDAA diet, in which the proteins are replaced with equivalent and corresponding mixture of L-amino acids to avoid unpredicted contamination of choline in the protein sources of semipurified diets [167]. Rats fed with CD or CDAA diets gain weight in a similar manner [169], but the development of steatosis and hepatic damage is accelerated in CDAA-fed rats. Steatosis is demonstrated already following 2 weeks on CDAA diet, and it is followed by fibrosis at week 8, cirrhosis at week 16 and HCC at week 50 [166,167,169]. CDAA induces HCC in mice as well, although no significant difference is found in the weight of CDAA-fed compared with control-fed mice [170].

The progressive development of liver tumors, with histopathological similarities to human HCC, established the CDAA diet as an animal model for this neoplasia [171], although the underlying mechanism of this model is not fully revealed yet. Several studies suggested involvement of inflammatory response, due to recruitment of macrophages [172], palmitic acid–regulated KC activation [173], and IL-1β release by KC [174]. Other findings imply the participation of gut microflora that regulates choline absorption and disease progression [165,175]. Suppression of liver gluconeogenesis due to downregulation of PGC-1α protein levels was also postulated [176], as well as redox status modulating disease progression and hepatic recovery form CDAA-induced damage [175,177]. An important role of NO is also demonstrated in the progression of liver fibrosis in mice and rats that were fed the CDAA diet [178, 179] but has no effect on tumor development [178].

Since choline, methionine, and folate metabolism interact at the point where homocysteine is converted to methionine [153], liver injury is increased when adequate levels of folate and methionine are lacking during a CD diet [162,180,181]. Accordingly, a MCD diet is widely used as a model of steatohepatitis. Feeding a MCD diet induces hepatic fat accumulation in rodents by inhibiting VLDL secretion, as well as by increasing FA uptake and influencing gene expression [182,183]. In a MCD diet, steatohepatitis and hepatic damage occurs earlier than in the other forms of the CD diets, with evidence of oxidative stress and inflammation following 3 weeks of diet, and markers of fibrosis following 5–7 weeks in rats [163]. In mice, evidence of fibrosis appears after 2 weeks [184]. This is accompanied by hepatic insulin resistance that involves JNK1 activation [170,185,186], inflammasome and caspase 1 activation in KC [187], and reduced β-oxidation [188]. Additional factors that may induce the transition from steatosis to steatohepatitis is NO, by inducing the formation of microvesicular steatosis and increasing oxidative stress in MCD diet-fed mice (M. Aharoni-Simon, unpublished data) and by inhibiting hepatocytes proliferation [189,190].

In a CDE diet, which results in less severe phenotype in comparison to MCD, 0.15% ethionine (a metabolic antagonist of methionine) is supplemented to a CD diet [191–194]. In mice, steatosis level is maximal (with more than 80% parenchymal steatosis measured) following 2 weeks of CDE feeding, and declines gradually thereafter [191,194] (Figure 9.2). This is accompanied by an increased levels of liver cytokines, infiltration of progenitor oval cells, increased oxidative stress and decreased liver mitochondrial content [176,191–193]. Feeding rodents with CDE or CDAA diets results in impaired PGC-1α activity and gluconeogenesis [176,191,194], suggesting an important role of glucose homeostasis in the progression of steatohepatitis and HCC.

Importantly, unlike the CD and CDAA diets, feeding mice or rats with MCD or CDE diets results in weight loss due to muscle wasting, reduced plasma TG and cholesterol levels and increased peripheral insulin sensitivity [9,106,163]. Therefore, these diets may not be an applicable animal model for studying the peripheral effects of the human metabolic syndrome. However, their ability to cause progressive and severe steatohepatitis suits them well to mechanistic studies of fat-related liver injury.

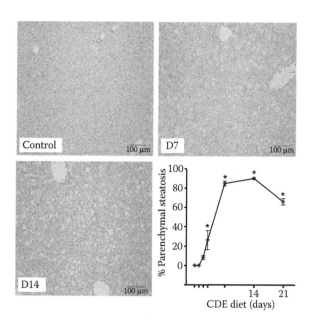

FIGURE 9.2 Development of steatosis in CDE- versus control-fed mice. C57BL/6J mice were fed with the CDE diet for up to 21 days. Liver morphology and fat accumulation were evaluated by H&E staining after the indicated time points (magnification ×200). The graph represents the percentage of parenchymal cells that contain fat vacuoles at each time point. $*p < 0.05$ compared with control. (Reprinted from Aharoni-Simon M. et al., *Lab Invest*, 91, 1018–28, 2011. With permission.)

SUMMARY AND CONCLUSIONS

This chapter discussed various nutritional aspects in the induction and development of NAFLD. Numerous works prove that nutritional factors impact the pathogenesis of NAFLD by many different signaling pathways, with complex cross-talk networks.

Overconsumption of total calories as well as increased fat and carbohydrates content appear to participate in the induction of obesity-related NAFLD. Epidemiological dietary studies performed in patients are of main importance for revealing the involvement of specific components of the Western diet in promotion of steatosis and in disease development. These investigations imply the roles played by characteristic components of the Western diet, such as high content of saturated fats, cholesterol, and simple carbohydrates. Further understanding of mechanistic explanations for these effects is achieved by numerous investigations of nutritional manipulations in animal models.

Unfortunately, existing models have not encompassed the full spectrum of human disease, and to date, the ideal model has not been developed. Still, these models provide crucial information by presenting many typical features of the human disease. Importantly, wide overview of accumulated experimental data indicates that the deleterious effect of Western diet components in combination can exceed their ability to harm separately. Therefore, diet composition is of high importance, beyond the simple impact of overnutrition. This issue requires further exploration.

Alternatively, fatty liver is also induced in conditions of undernutrition and by insufficient uptake of essential nutrients. This nutritional aspect is relevant in developing societies, but also in specific subpopulations of NAFLD patients with nutritional deficiencies. Mechanistic understanding of the involvement of nutrients deficiencies that have been implicated in steatosis development among malnourished people is important for correction of deficiencies and for providing proper treatment. Moreover, dietary deficiencies implemented in laboratory animals, such as choline deficiency, are commonly used as models for human disease.

Better understanding of nutrition-related factors involved in NAFLD induction and progression is of major importance, especially since, currently, there is still no widely accepted drug therapy for this pathology. Future research in this field may provide novel findings and enable to develop intervention strategies for the prevention and treatment of fatty liver disease and its complications.

REFERENCES

1. Hotamisligil GS, Arner P, Caro JF, Atkinson RL, Spiegelman BM: Increased adipose tissue expression of tumor necrosis factor-alpha in human obesity and insulin resistance. *J Clin Invest* 1995, 95:2409–2415.
2. Weisberg SP, McCann D, Desai M, Rosenbaum M, Leibel RL, Ferrante AW Jr: Obesity is associated with macrophage accumulation in adipose tissue. *J Clin Invest* 2003, 112:1796–1808.
3. Xu H, Barnes GT, Yang Q, Tan G, Yang D, Chou CJ, Sole J, Nichols A, Ross JS, Tartaglia LA, Chen H: Chronic inflammation in fat plays a crucial role in the development of obesity-related insulin resistance. *J Clin Invest* 2003, 112:1821–1830.

4. Coppack SW, Evans RD, Fisher RM, Frayn KN, Gibbons GF, Humphreys SM, Kirk ML, Potts JL, Hockaday TD: Adipose tissue metabolism in obesity: lipase action in vivo before and after a mixed meal. *Metabolism* 1992, 41:264–272.
5. Hickner RC, Racette SB, Binder EF, Fisher JS, Kohrt WM: Suppression of whole body and regional lipolysis by insulin: effects of obesity and exercise. *J Clin Endocrinol Metab* 1999, 84:3886–3895.
6. Jensen MD, Haymond MW, Rizza RA, Cryer PE, Miles JM: Influence of body fat distribution on free fatty acid metabolism in obesity. *J Clin Invest* 1989, 83:1168–1173.
7. Nellemann B, Gormsen LC, Sorensen LP, Christiansen JS, Nielsen S: Impaired insulin-mediated antilipolysis and lactate release in adipose tissue of upper-body obese women. *Obesity (Silver Spring)* 2012, 20:57–64.
8. Roust LR, Jensen MD: Postprandial free fatty acid kinetics are abnormal in upper body obesity. *Diabetes* 1993, 42:1567–1573.
9. Maher JJ: New insights from rodent models of fatty liver disease. *Antioxid Redox Signal* 2011, 15:535–550.
10. Stefan N, Kantartzis K, Haring HU: Causes and metabolic consequences of Fatty liver. *Endocr Rev* 2008, 29:939–960.
11. Cancello R, Tordjman J, Poitou C, Guilhem G, Bouillot JL, Hugol D, Coussieu C, Basdevant A, Bar Hen A, Bedossa P et al.: Increased infiltration of macrophages in omental adipose tissue is associated with marked hepatic lesions in morbid human obesity. *Diabetes* 2006, 55:1554–1561.
12. Kral JG, Schaffner F, Pierson RN Jr, Wang J: Body fat topography as an independent predictor of fatty liver. *Metabolism* 1993, 42:548–551.
13. Park SH, Kim BI, Kim SH, Kim HJ, Park DI, Cho YK, Sung IK, Sohn CI, Kim H, Keum DK et al.: Body fat distribution and insulin resistance: beyond obesity in nonalcoholic fatty liver disease among overweight men. *J Am Coll Nutr* 2007, 26:321–326.
14. Sabir N, Sermez Y, Kazil S, Zencir M: Correlation of abdominal fat accumulation and liver steatosis: importance of ultrasonographic and anthropometric measurements. *Eur J Ultrasound* 2001, 14:121–128.
15. Thomas EL, Hamilton G, Patel N, O'Dwyer R, Dore CJ, Goldin RD, Bell JD, Taylor-Robinson SD: Hepatic triglyceride content and its relation to body adiposity: a magnetic resonance imaging and proton magnetic resonance spectroscopy study. *Gut* 2005, 54:122–127.
16. Farrell GC, Larter CZ: Nonalcoholic fatty liver disease: from steatosis to cirrhosis. *Hepatology* 2006, 43:S99–S112.
17. Capristo E, Miele L, Forgione A, Vero V, Farnetti S, Mingrone G, Greco AV, Gasbarrini G, Grieco A: Nutritional aspects in patients with non-alcoholic steatohepatitis (NASH). *Eur Rev Med Pharmacol Sci* 2005, 9:265–268.
18. Gonzalez C, de Ledinghen V, Vergniol J, Foucher J, Le Bail B, Carlier S, Maury E, Gin H, Rigalleau V: Hepatic Steatosis, Carbohydrate Intake, and Food Quotient in Patients with NAFLD. *Int J Endocrinol* 2013, 2013:428542.
19. Drenick EJ, Simmons F, Murphy JF: Effect on hepatic morphology of treatment of obesity by fasting, reducing diets and small-bowel bypass. *N Engl J Med* 1970, 282:829–834.
20. Huang MA, Greenson JK, Chao C, Anderson L, Peterman D, Jacobson J, Emick D, Lok AS, Conjeevaram HS: One-year intense nutritional counseling results in histological improvement in patients with non-alcoholic steatohepatitis: a pilot study. *Am J Gastroenterol* 2005, 100:1072–1081.
21. Perfield JW 2nd, Ortinau LC, Pickering RT, Ruebel ML, Meers GM, Rector RS: Altered hepatic lipid metabolism contributes to nonalcoholic fatty liver disease in leptin-deficient Ob/Ob mice. *J Obes* 2013, 2013:296537.

22. Guo H, Xia M, Zou T, Ling W, Zhong R, Zhang W: Cyanidin 3-glucoside attenuates obesity-associated insulin resistance and hepatic steatosis in high-fat diet-fed and db/db mice via the transcription factor FoxO1. *J Nutr Biochem* 2012, 23:349–360.
23. Inui Y, Kawata S, Matsuzawa Y, Tokunaga K, Fujioka S, Tamura S, Kobatake T, Keno Y, Odaka H, Matsuo T et al.: Inhibitory effect of a new alpha-glucosidase inhibitor on fatty liver in Zucker fatty rats. *J Hepatol* 1990, 10:62–68.
24. Rector RS, Thyfault JP, Uptergrove GM, Morris EM, Naples SP, Borengasser SJ, Mikus CR, Laye MJ, Laughlin MH, Booth FW, Ibdah JA: Mitochondrial dysfunction precedes insulin resistance and hepatic steatosis and contributes to the natural history of non-alcoholic fatty liver disease in an obese rodent model. *J Hepatol* 2010, 52:727–736.
25. Kon K, Ikejima K, Okumura K, Arai K, Aoyama T, Watanabe S: Diabetic KK-A(y) mice are highly susceptible to oxidative hepatocellular damage induced by acetaminophen. *Am J Physiol Gastrointest Liver Physiol* 2010, 299:G329–337.
26. Arsov T, Larter CZ, Nolan CJ, Petrovsky N, Goodnow CC, Teoh NC, Yeh MM, Farrell GC: Adaptive failure to high-fat diet characterizes steatohepatitis in Alms1 mutant mice. *Biochem Biophys Res Commun* 2006, 342:1152–1159.
27. Anstee QM, Goldin RD: Mouse models in non-alcoholic fatty liver disease and steato-hepatitis research. *Int J Exp Pathol* 2006, 87:1–16.
28. Nanji AA: Animal models of nonalcoholic fatty liver disease and steatohepatitis. *Clin Liver Dis* 2004, 8:559–574, ix.
29. Kim JY, van de Wall E, Laplante M, Azzara A, Trujillo ME, Hofmann SM, Schraw T, Durand JL, Li H, Li G et al.: Obesity-associated improvements in metabolic profile through expansion of adipose tissue. *J Clin Invest* 2007, 117:2621–2637.
30. Rector RS, Thyfault JP, Morris RT, Laye MJ, Borengasser SJ, Booth FW, Ibdah JA: Daily exercise increases hepatic fatty acid oxidation and prevents steatosis in Otsuka Long-Evans Tokushima Fatty rats. *Am J Physiol Gastrointest Liver Physiol* 2008, 294:G619–626.
31. Bi S, Scott KA, Hyun J, Ladenheim EE, Moran TH: Running wheel activity prevents hyperphagia and obesity in Otsuka long-evans Tokushima Fatty rats: role of hypotha-lamic signaling. *Endocrinology* 2005, 146:1676–1685.
32. Johnson NA, Sachinwalla T, Walton DW, Smith K, Armstrong A, Thompson MW, George J: Aerobic exercise training reduces hepatic and visceral lipids in obese indi-viduals without weight loss. *Hepatology* 2009, 50:1105–1112.
33. Bedogni G, Bellentani S: Fatty liver: how frequent is it and why? *Ann Hepatol* 2004, 3:63–65.
34. Tiikkainen M, Bergholm R, Vehkavaara S, Rissanen A, Hakkinen AM, Tamminen M, Teramo K, Yki-Jarvinen H: Effects of identical weight loss on body composition and features of insulin resistance in obese women with high and low liver fat content. *Diabetes* 2003, 52:701–707.
35. Cortez-Pinto H, Jesus L, Barros H, Lopes C, Moura MC, Camilo ME: How differ-ent is the dietary pattern in non-alcoholic steatohepatitis patients? *Clin Nutr* 2006, 25:816–823.
36. Westerbacka J, Lammi K, Hakkinen AM, Rissanen A, Salminen I, Aro A, Yki-Jarvinen H: Dietary fat content modifies liver fat in overweight nondiabetic subjects. *J Clin Endocrinol Metab* 2005, 90:2804–2809.
37. Cai D, Yuan M, Frantz DF, Melendez PA, Hansen L, Lee J, Shoelson SE: Local and sys-temic insulin resistance resulting from hepatic activation of IKK-beta and NF-kappaB. *Nat Med* 2005, 11:183–190.
38. Park EJ, Lee JH, Yu GY, He G, Ali SR, Holzer RG, Osterreicher CH, Takahashi H, Karin M: Dietary and genetic obesity promote liver inflammation and tumorigenesis by enhancing IL-6 and TNF expression. *Cell* 2010, 140:197–208.

39. Wunderlich FT, Luedde T, Singer S, Schmidt-Supprian M, Baumgartl J, Schirmacher P, Pasparakis M, Bruning JC: Hepatic NF-kappa B essential modulator deficiency prevents obesity-induced insulin resistance but synergizes with high-fat feeding in tumorigenesis. *Proc Natl Acad Sci USA* 2008, 105:1297–1302.
40. Yoshimatsu M, Terasaki Y, Sakashita N, Kiyota E, Sato H, van der Laan LJ, Takeya M: Induction of macrophage scavenger receptor MARCO in nonalcoholic steatohepatitis indicates possible involvement of endotoxin in its pathogenic process. *Int J Exp Pathol* 2004, 85:335–343.
41. Solga SF, Diehl AM: Non-alcoholic fatty liver disease: lumen-liver interactions and possible role for probiotics. *J Hepatol* 2003, 38:681–687.
42. Ozcan U, Cao Q, Yilmaz E, Lee AH, Iwakoshi NN, Ozdelen E, Tuncman G, Gorgun C, Glimcher LH, Hotamisligil GS: Endoplasmic reticulum stress links obesity, insulin action, and type 2 diabetes. *Science* 2004, 306:457–461.
43. Kammoun HL, Hainault I, Ferre P, Foufelle F: Nutritional related liver disease: targeting the endoplasmic reticulum stress. *Curr Opin Clin Nutr Metab Care* 2009, 12: 575–582.
44. Alkhouri N, Gornicka A, Berk MP, Thapaliya S, Dixon LJ, Kashyap S, Schauer PR, Feldstein AE: Adipocyte apoptosis, a link between obesity, insulin resistance, and hepatic steatosis. *J Biol Chem* 2010, 285:3428–3438.
45. Wueest S, Rapold RA, Schumann DM, Rytka JM, Schildknecht A, Nov O, Chervonsky AV, Rudich A, Schoenle EJ, Donath MY, Konrad D: Deletion of Fas in adipocytes relieves adipose tissue inflammation and hepatic manifestations of obesity in mice. *J Clin Invest* 2010, 120:191–202.
46. Donnelly KL, Smith CI, Schwarzenberg SJ, Jessurun J, Boldt MD, Parks EJ: Sources of fatty acids stored in liver and secreted via lipoproteins in patients with nonalcoholic fatty liver disease. *J Clin Invest* 2005, 115:1343–1351.
47. Eaton S: Control of mitochondrial beta-oxidation flux. *Prog Lipid Res* 2002, 41:197–239.
48. Day CP, James OF: Hepatic steatosis: innocent bystander or guilty party? *Hepatology* 1998, 27:1463–1466.
49. Budick-Harmelin N, Dudas J, Demuth J, Madar Z, Ramadori G, Tirosh O: Triglycerides potentiate the inflammatory response in rat Kupffer cells. *Antioxid Redox Signal* 2008, 10:2009–2022.
50. Yamaguchi K, Yang L, McCall S, Huang J, Yu XX, Pandey SK, Bhanot S, Monia BP, Li YX, Diehl AM: Inhibiting triglyceride synthesis improves hepatic steatosis but exacerbates liver damage and fibrosis in obese mice with nonalcoholic steatohepatitis. *Hepatology* 2007, 45:1366–1374.
51. Alkhouri N, Dixon LJ, Feldstein AE: Lipotoxicity in nonalcoholic fatty liver disease: not all lipids are created equal. *Expert Rev Gastroenterol Hepatol* 2009, 3:445–451.
52. McClain CJ, Mokshagundam SP, Barve SS, Song Z, Hill DB, Chen T, Deaciuc I: Mechanisms of non-alcoholic steatohepatitis. *Alcohol* 2004, 34:67–79.
53. Joshi-Barve S, Barve SS, Amancherla K, Gobejishvili L, Hill D, Cave M, Hote P, McClain CJ: Palmitic acid induces production of proinflammatory cytokine interleukin-8 from hepatocytes. *Hepatology* 2007, 46:823–830.
54. Choi YJ, Choi SE, Ha ES, Kang Y, Han SJ, Kim DJ, Lee KW, Kim HJ: Involvement of visfatin in palmitate-induced upregulation of inflammatory cytokines in hepatocytes. *Metabolism* 2011, 60:1781–1789.
55. Feldstein AE, Werneburg NW, Canbay A, Guicciardi ME, Bronk SF, Rydzewski R, Burgart LJ, Gores GJ: Free fatty acids promote hepatic lipotoxicity by stimulating TNF-alpha expression via a lysosomal pathway. *Hepatology* 2004, 40:185–194.
56. Malhi H, Bronk SF, Werneburg NW, Gores GJ: Free fatty acids induce JNK-dependent hepatocyte lipoapoptosis. *J Biol Chem* 2006, 281:12093–12101.

57. Wei Y, Wang D, Topczewski F, Pagliassotti MJ: Saturated fatty acids induce endoplasmic reticulum stress and apoptosis independently of ceramide in liver cells. *Am J Physiol Endocrinol Metab* 2006, 291:E275–281.

58. Feldstein AE, Canbay A, Guicciardi ME, Higuchi H, Bronk SF, Gores GJ: Diet associated hepatic steatosis sensitizes to Fas mediated liver injury in mice. *J Hepatol* 2003, 39:978–983.

59. Gao D, Nong S, Huang X, Lu Y, Zhao H, Lin Y, Man Y, Wang S, Yang J, Li J: The effects of palmitate on hepatic insulin resistance are mediated by NADPH Oxidase 3-derived reactive oxygen species through JNK and p38MAPK pathways. *J Biol Chem* 2010, 285:29965–29973.

60. Ruddock MW, Stein A, Landaker E, Park J, Cooksey RC, McClain D, Patti ME: Saturated fatty acids inhibit hepatic insulin action by modulating insulin receptor expression and post-receptor signalling. *J Biochem* 2008, 144:599–607.

61. Wan XD, Yang WB, Xia YZ, Wang JF, Lu T, Wang XM: Disruption of glucose homeostasis and induction of insulin resistance by elevated free fatty acids in human L02 hepatocytes. *J Endocrinol Invest* 2009, 32:454–459.

62. Shi H, Kokoeva MV, Inouye K, Tzameli I, Yin H, Flier JS: TLR4 links innate immunity and fatty acid-induced insulin resistance. *J Clin Invest* 2006, 116:3015–3025.

63. de Lima TM, de Sa Lima L, Scavone C, Curi R: Fatty acid control of nitric oxide production by macrophages. *FEBS Lett* 2006, 580:3287–3295.

64. Chen J, Schenker S, Frosto TA, Henderson GI: Inhibition of cytochrome c oxidase activity by 4-hydroxynonenal (HNE). Role of HNE adduct formation with the enzyme subunits. *Biochim Biophys Acta* 1998, 1380:336–344.

65. Sanyal AJ, Campbell-Sargent C, Mirshahi F, Rizzo WB, Contos MJ, Sterling RK, Luketic VA, Shiffman ML, Clore JN: Nonalcoholic steatohepatitis: association of insulin resistance and mitochondrial abnormalities. *Gastroenterology* 2001, 120:1183–1192.

66. Pan M, Cederbaum AI, Zhang YL, Ginsberg HN, Williams KJ, Fisher EA: Lipid peroxidation and oxidant stress regulate hepatic apolipoprotein B degradation and VLDL production. *J Clin Invest* 2004, 113:1277–1287.

67. George J, Pera N, Phung N, Leclercq I, Yun Hou J, Farrell G: Lipid peroxidation, stellate cell activation and hepatic fibrogenesis in a rat model of chronic steatohepatitis. *J Hepatol* 2003, 39:756–764.

68. Gauthier MS, Couturier K, Latour JG, Lavoie JM: Concurrent exercise prevents high-fat-diet-induced macrovesicular hepatic steatosis. *J Appl Physiol* 2003, 94:2127–2134.

69. Pfluger PT, Herranz D, Velasco-Miguel S, Serrano M, Tschop MH: Sirt1 protects against high-fat diet-induced metabolic damage. *Proc Natl Acad Sci USA* 2008, 105:9793–9798.

70. Garbow JR, Doherty JM, Schugar RC, Travers S, Weber ML, Wentz AE, Ezenwajiaku N, Cotter DG, Brunt EM, Crawford PA: Hepatic steatosis, inflammation, and ER stress in mice maintained long term on a very low-carbohydrate ketogenic diet. *Am J Physiol Gastrointest Liver Physiol* 2011, 300:G956–967.

71. Kennedy AR, Pissios P, Otu H, Roberson R, Xue B, Asakura K, Furukawa N, Marino FE, Liu FF, Kahn BB et al.: A high-fat, ketogenic diet induces a unique metabolic state in mice. *Am J Physiol Endocrinol Metab* 2007, 292:E1724–1739.

72. Monetti M, Levin MC, Watt MJ, Sajan MP, Marmor S, Hubbard BK, Stevens RD, Bain JR, Newgard CB, Farese RV, Sr. et al.: Dissociation of hepatic steatosis and insulin resistance in mice overexpressing DGAT in the liver. *Cell Metab* 2007, 6:69–78.

73. Singh R, Wang Y, Xiang Y, Tanaka KE, Gaarde WA, Czaja MJ: Differential effects of JNK1 and JNK2 inhibition on murine steatohepatitis and insulin resistance. *Hepatology* 2009, 49:87–96.

74. Svegliati-Baroni G, Candelaresi C, Saccomanno S, Ferretti G, Bachetti T, Marzioni M, De Minicis S, Nobili L, Salzano R, Omenetti A et al.: A model of insulin resistance and nonalcoholic steatohepatitis in rats: role of peroxisome proliferator-activated

receptor-alpha and n-3 polyunsaturated fatty acid treatment on liver injury. *Am J Pathol* 2006, 169:846–860.

75. Ito M, Suzuki J, Tsujioka S, Sasaki M, Gomori A, Shirakura T, Hirose H, Ishihara A, Iwaasa H, Kanatani A: Longitudinal analysis of murine steatohepatitis model induced by chronic exposure to high-fat diet. *Hepatol Res* 2007, 37:50–57.
76. Baumgardner JN, Shankar K, Hennings L, Badger TM, Ronis MJ: A new model for nonalcoholic steatohepatitis in the rat utilizing total enteral nutrition to overfeed a high-polyunsaturated fat diet. *Am J Physiol Gastrointest Liver Physiol* 2008, 294:G27–38.
77. Lieber CS, Leo MA, Mak KM, Xu Y, Cao Q, Ren C, Ponomarenko A, DeCarli LM: Model of nonalcoholic steatohepatitis. *Am J Clin Nutr* 2004, 79:502–509.
78. Zou Y, Li J, Lu C, Wang J, Ge J, Huang Y, Zhang L, Wang Y: High-fat emulsion-induced rat model of nonalcoholic steatohepatitis. *Life Sci* 2006, 79:1100–1107.
79. Ogasawara M, Hirose A, Ono M, Aritake K, Nozaki Y, Takahashi M, Okamoto N, Sakamoto S, Iwasaki S, Asanuma T et al.: A novel and comprehensive mouse model of human non-alcoholic steatohepatitis with the full range of dysmetabolic and histological abnormalities induced by gold thioglucose and a high-fat diet. *Liver Int* 2011, 31: 542–551.
80. Schugar RC, Crawford PA: Low-carbohydrate ketogenic diets, glucose homeostasis, and nonalcoholic fatty liver disease. *Curr Opin Clin Nutr Metab Care* 2012, 15:374–380.
81. Borghjid S, Feinman RD: Response of C57Bl/6 mice to a carbohydrate-free diet. *Nutr Metab (Lond)* 2012, 9:69.
82. Musso G, Gambino R, De Michieli F, Cassader M, Rizzetto M, Durazzo M, Faga E, Silli B, Pagano G: Dietary habits and their relations to insulin resistance and postprandial lipemia in nonalcoholic steatohepatitis. *Hepatology* 2003, 37:909–916.
83. Tamura Y, Tanaka Y, Sato F, Choi JB, Watada H, Niwa M, Kinoshita J, Ooka A, Kumashiro N, Igarashi Y et al.: Effects of diet and exercise on muscle and liver intracellular lipid contents and insulin sensitivity in type 2 diabetic patients. *J Clin Endocrinol Metab* 2005, 90:3191–3196.
84. Lin J, Yang R, Tarr PT, Wu PH, Handschin C, Li S, Yang W, Pei L, Uldry M, Tontonoz P et al.: Hyperlipidemic effects of dietary saturated fats mediated through PGC-1beta coactivation of SREBP. *Cell* 2005, 120:261–273.
85. Sampath H, Miyazaki M, Dobrzyn A, Ntambi JM: Stearoyl-CoA desaturase-1 mediates the pro-lipogenic effects of dietary saturated fat. *J Biol Chem* 2007, 282:2483–2493.
86. Romestaing C, Piquet MA, Bedu E, Rouleau V, Dautresme M, Hourmand-Ollivier I, Filippi C, Duchamp C, Sibille B: Long term highly saturated fat diet does not induce NASH in Wistar rats. *Nutr Metab (Lond)* 2007, 4:4.
87. Ricchi M, Odoardi MR, Carulli L, Anzivino C, Ballestri S, Pinetti A, Fantoni LI, Marra F, Bertolotti M, Banni S et al.: Differential effect of oleic and palmitic acid on lipid accumulation and apoptosis in cultured hepatocytes. *J Gastroenterol Hepatol* 2009, 24:830–840.
88. Listenberger LL, Han X, Lewis SE, Cases S, Farese RV, Jr., Ory DS, Schaffer JE: Triglyceride accumulation protects against fatty acid-induced lipotoxicity. *Proc Natl Acad Sci USA* 2003, 100:3077–3082.
89. Deng QG, She H, Cheng JH, French SW, Koop DR, Xiong S, Tsukamoto H: Steatohepatitis induced by intragastric overfeeding in mice. *Hepatology* 2005, 42:905–914.
90. Tetri LH, Basaranoglu M, Brunt EM, Yerian LM, Neuschwander-Tetri BA: Severe NAFLD with hepatic necroinflammatory changes in mice fed *trans* fats and a high-fructose corn syrup equivalent. *Am J Physiol Gastrointest Liver Physiol* 2008, 295: G987–995.
91. Obara N, Fukushima K, Ueno Y, Wakui Y, Kimura O, Tamai K, Kakazu E, Inoue J, Kondo Y, Ogawa N et al.: Possible involvement and the mechanisms of excess *trans*-fatty acid consumption in severe NAFLD in mice. *J Hepatol* 2010, 53:326–334.

92. Koppe SW, Elias M, Moseley RH, Green RM: *trans* fat feeding results in higher serum alanine aminotransferase and increased insulin resistance compared with a standard murine high-fat diet. *Am J Physiol Gastrointest Liver Physiol* 2009, 297:G378–384.

93. Dhibi M, Brahmi F, Mnari A, Houas Z, Chargui I, Bchir L, Gazzah N, Alsaif MA, Hammami M: The intake of high fat diet with different *trans* fatty acid levels differentially induces oxidative stress and non alcoholic fatty liver disease (NAFLD) in rats. *Nutr Metab (Lond)* 2011, 8:65.

94. Bendsen NT, Chabanova E, Thomsen HS, Larsen TM, Newman JW, Stender S, Dyerberg J, Haugaard SB, Astrup A: Effect of *trans* fatty acid intake on abdominal and liver fat deposition and blood lipids: a randomized trial in overweight postmenopausal women. *Nutr Diabetes* 2011, 1:e4.

95. Ogawa T, Fujii H, Yoshizato K, Kawada N: A human-type nonalcoholic steatohepatitis model with advanced fibrosis in rabbits. *Am J Pathol* 2010, 177:153–165.

96. Larter CZ, Yeh MM: Animal models of NASH: getting both pathology and metabolic context right. *J Gastroenterol Hepatol* 2008, 23:1635–1648.

97. Biddinger SB, Almind K, Miyazaki M, Kokkotou E, Ntambi JM, Kahn CR: Effects of diet and genetic background on sterol regulatory element-binding protein-1c, stearoyl-CoA desaturase 1, and the development of the metabolic syndrome. *Diabetes* 2005, 54:1314–1323.

98. Nishikawa S, Yasoshima A, Doi K, Nakayama H, Uetsuka K: Involvement of sex, strain and age factors in high fat diet-induced obesity in C57BL/6J and BALB/cA mice. *Exp Anim* 2007, 56:263–272.

99. Matsuzawa N, Takamura T, Kurita S, Misu H, Ota T, Ando H, Yokoyama M, Honda M, Zen Y, Nakanuma Y et al.: Lipid-induced oxidative stress causes steatohepatitis in mice fed an atherogenic diet. *Hepatology* 2007, 46:1392–1403.

100. Sumiyoshi M, Sakanaka M, Kimura Y: Chronic intake of a high-cholesterol diet resulted in hepatic steatosis, focal nodular hyperplasia and fibrosis in non-obese mice. *Br J Nutr* 2010, 103:378–385.

101. Jeong WI, Jeong DH, Do SH, Kim YK, Park HY, Kwon OD, Kim TH, Jeong KS: Mild hepatic fibrosis in cholesterol and sodium cholate diet-fed rats. *J Vet Med Sci* 2005, 67:235–242.

102. Kainuma M, Fujimoto M, Sekiya N, Tsuneyama K, Cheng C, Takano Y, Terasawa K, Shimada Y: Cholesterol-fed rabbit as a unique model of nonalcoholic, nonobese, non-insulin-resistant fatty liver disease with characteristic fibrosis. *J Gastroenterol* 2006, 41:971–980.

103. Vergnes L, Phan J, Strauss M, Tafuri S, Reue K: Cholesterol and cholate components of an atherogenic diet induce distinct stages of hepatic inflammatory gene expression. *J Biol Chem* 2003, 278:42774–42784.

104. Nakamuta M, Fujino T, Yada R, Yada M, Yasutake K, Yoshimoto T, Harada N, Higuchi N, Kato M, Kohjima M et al.: Impact of cholesterol metabolism and the LXRalpha-SREBP-1c pathway on nonalcoholic fatty liver disease. *Int J Mol Med* 2009, 23:603–608.

105. Enjoji M, Nakamuta M: Is the control of dietary cholesterol intake sufficiently effective to ameliorate nonalcoholic fatty liver disease? *World J Gastroenterol* 2010, 16:800–803.

106. Hebbard L, George J: Animal models of nonalcoholic fatty liver disease. *Nat Rev Gastroenterol Hepatol* 2011, 8:35–44.

107. Mari M, Caballero F, Colell A, Morales A, Caballeria J, Fernandez A, Enrich C, Fernandez-Checa JC, Garcia-Ruiz C: Mitochondrial free cholesterol loading sensitizes to TNF- and Fas-mediated steatohepatitis. *Cell Metab* 2006, 4:185–198.

108. Wouters K, van Gorp PJ, Bieghs V, Gijbels MJ, Duimel H, Lutjohann D, Kerksiek A, van Kruchten R, Maeda N, Staels B et al.: Dietary cholesterol, rather than liver steatosis, leads to hepatic inflammation in hyperlipidemic mouse models of nonalcoholic steato-hepatitis. *Hepatology* 2008, 48:474–486.

109. Yasutake K, Nakamuta M, Shima Y, Ohyama A, Masuda K, Haruta N, Fujino T, Aoyagi Y, Fukuizumi K, Yoshimoto T et al.: Nutritional investigation of non-obese patients with non-alcoholic fatty liver disease: the significance of dietary cholesterol. *Scand J Gastroenterol* 2009, 44:471–477.

110. Enjoji M, Machida K, Kohjima M, Kato M, Kotoh K, Matsunaga K, Nakashima M, Nakamuta M: NPC1L1 inhibitor ezetimibe is a reliable therapeutic agent for non-obese patients with nonalcoholic fatty liver disease. *Lipids Health Dis* 2010, 9:29.

111. Solga S, Alkhuraishe AR, Clark JM, Torbenson M, Greenwald A, Diehl AM, Magnuson T: Dietary composition and nonalcoholic fatty liver disease. *Dig Dis Sci* 2004, 49:1578–1583.

112. Diraison F, Moulin P, Beylot M: Contribution of hepatic de novo lipogenesis and reesterification of plasma non esterified fatty acids to plasma triglyceride synthesis during non-alcoholic fatty liver disease. *Diabetes Metab* 2003, 29:478–485.

113. Sevastianova K, Santos A, Kotronen A, Hakkarainen A, Makkonen J, Silander K, Peltonen M, Romeo S, Lundbom J, Lundbom N et al.: Effect of short-term carbohydrate overfeeding and long-term weight loss on liver fat in overweight humans. *Am J Clin Nutr* 2012, 96:727–734.

114. Browning JD, Baker JA, Rogers T, Davis J, Satapati S, Burgess SC: Short-term weight loss and hepatic triglyceride reduction: evidence of a metabolic advantage with dietary carbohydrate restriction. *Am J Clin Nutr* 2011, 93:1048–1052.

115. Yamashita H, Takenoshita M, Sakurai M, Bruick RK, Henzel WJ, Shillinglaw W, Arnot D, Uyeda K: A glucose-responsive transcription factor that regulates carbohydrate metabolism in the liver. *Proc Natl Acad Sci USA* 2001, 98:9116–9121.

116. Iizuka K, Bruick RK, Liang G, Horton JD, Uyeda K: Deficiency of carbohydrate response element-binding protein (ChREBP) reduces lipogenesis as well as glycolysis. *Proc Natl Acad Sci USA* 2004, 101:7281–7286.

117. Dentin R, Girard J, Postic C: Carbohydrate responsive element binding protein (ChREBP) and sterol regulatory element binding protein-1c (SREBP-1c): two key regulators of glucose metabolism and lipid synthesis in liver. *Biochimie* 2005, 87:81–86.

118. Shimomura I, Shimano H, Korn BS, Bashmakov Y, Horton JD: Nuclear sterol regulatory element-binding proteins activate genes responsible for the entire program of unsaturated fatty acid biosynthesis in transgenic mouse liver. *J Biol Chem* 1998, 273:35299–35306.

119. Miyazaki M, Flowers MT, Sampath H, Chu K, Otzelberger C, Liu X, Ntambi JM: Hepatic stearoyl-CoA desaturase-1 deficiency protects mice from carbohydrate-induced adiposity and hepatic steatosis. *Cell Metab* 2007, 6:484–496.

120. Varela-Rey M, Embade N, Ariz U, Lu SC, Mato JM, Martinez-Chantar ML: Non-alcoholic steatohepatitis and animal models: understanding the human disease. *Int J Biochem Cell Biol* 2009, 41:969–976.

121. Kang H, Greenson JK, Omo JT, Chao C, Peterman D, Anderson L, Foess-Wood L, Sherbondy MA, Conjeevaram HS: Metabolic syndrome is associated with greater histologic severity, higher carbohydrate, and lower fat diet in patients with NAFLD. *Am J Gastroenterol* 2006, 101:2247–2253.

122. Bergheim I, Weber S, Vos M, Kramer S, Volynets V, Kaserouni S, McClain CJ, Bischoff SC: Antibiotics protect against fructose-induced hepatic lipid accumulation in mice: role of endotoxin. *J Hepatol* 2008, 48:983–992.

123. Li Z, Soloski MJ, Diehl AM: Dietary factors alter hepatic innate immune system in mice with nonalcoholic fatty liver disease. *Hepatology* 2005, 42:880–885.

124. Mayes PA: Intermediary metabolism of fructose. *Am J Clin Nutr* 1993, 58:754S–765S.

125. Kawasaki T, Igarashi K, Koeda T, Sugimoto K, Nakagawa K, Hayashi S, Yamaji R, Inui H, Fukusato T, Yamanouchi T: Rats fed fructose-enriched diets have characteristics of nonalcoholic hepatic steatosis. *J Nutr* 2009, 139:2067–2071.

126. Ackerman Z, Oron-Herman M, Grozovski M, Rosenthal T, Pappo O, Link G, Sela BA: Fructose-induced fatty liver disease: hepatic effects of blood pressure and plasma tri-glyceride reduction. *Hypertension* 2005, 45:1012–1018.
127. Jurgens H, Haass W, Castaneda TR, Schurmann A, Koebnick C, Dombrowski F, Otto B, Nawrocki AR, Scherer PE, Spranger J et al.: Consuming fructose-sweetened beverages increases body adiposity in mice. *Obes Res* 2005, 13:1146–1156.
128. Armutcu F, Coskun O, Gurel A, Kanter M, Can M, Ucar F, Unalacak M: Thymosin alpha 1 attenuates lipid peroxidation and improves fructose-induced steatohepatitis in rats. *Clin Biochem* 2005, 38:540–547.
129. Ouyang X, Cirillo P, Sautin Y, McCall S, Bruchette JL, Diehl AM, Johnson RJ, Abdelmalek MF: Fructose consumption as a risk factor for non-alcoholic fatty liver disease. *J Hepatol* 2008, 48:993–999.
130. Zelber-Sagi S, Nitzan-Kaluski D, Goldsmith R, Webb M, Blendis L, Halpern Z, Oren R: Long term nutritional intake and the risk for non-alcoholic fatty liver disease (NAFLD): a population based study. *J Hepatol* 2007, 47:711–717.
131. Abdelmalek MF, Suzuki A, Guy C, Unalp-Arida A, Colvin R, Johnson RJ, Diehl AM: Increased fructose consumption is associated with fibrosis severity in patients with non-alcoholic fatty liver disease. *Hepatology* 2010, 51:1961–1971.
132. Faeh D, Minehira K, Schwarz JM, Periasamy R, Park S, Tappy L: Effect of fructose overfeeding and fish oil administration on hepatic de novo lipogenesis and insulin sen-sitivity in healthy men. *Diabetes* 2005, 54:1907–1913.
133. Le KA, Faeh D, Stettler R, Ith M, Kreis R, Vermathen P, Boesch C, Ravussin E, Tappy L: A 4-wk high-fructose diet alters lipid metabolism without affecting insulin sensitivity or ectopic lipids in healthy humans. *Am J Clin Nutr* 2006, 84:1374–1379.
134. Nomura K, Yamanouchi T: The role of fructose-enriched diets in mechanisms of nonal-coholic fatty liver disease. *J Nutr Biochem* 2012, 23:203–208.
135. Takahashi Y, Soejima Y, Fukusato T: Animal models of nonalcoholic fatty liver disease/nonalcoholic steatohepatitis. *World J Gastroenterol* 2012, 18:2300–2308.
136. Spruss A, Kanuri G, Wagnerberger S, Haub S, Bischoff SC, Bergheim I: Toll-like receptor 4 is involved in the development of fructose-induced hepatic steatosis in mice. *Hepatology* 2009, 50:1094–1104.
137. Wada T, Kenmochi H, Miyashita Y, Sasaki M, Ojima M, Sasahara M, Koya D, Tsuneki H, Sasaoka T: Spironolactone improves glucose and lipid metabolism by ameliorating hepatic steatosis and inflammation and suppressing enhanced gluconeogenesis induced by high-fat and high-fructose diet. *Endocrinology* 2010, 151:2040–2049.
138. Kohli R, Kirby M, Xanthakos SA, Softic S, Feldstein AE, Saxena V, Tang PH, Miles L, Miles MV, Balistreri WF et al.: High-fructose, medium chain *trans* fat diet induces liver fibrosis and elevates plasma coenzyme Q9 in a novel murine model of obesity and nonalcoholic steatohepatitis. *Hepatology* 2010, 52:934–944.
139. Fong DG, Nehra V, Lindor KD, Buchman AL: Metabolic and nutritional considerations in nonalcoholic fatty liver. *Hepatology* 2000, 32:3–10.
140. Guglielmi FW, Boggio-Bertinet D, Federico A, Forte GB, Guglielmi A, Loguercio C, Mazzuoli S, Merli M, Palmo A, Panella C et al.: Total parenteral nutrition-related gas-troenterological complications. *Dig Liver Dis* 2006, 38:623–642.
141. Knapp AC, Todesco L, Torok M, Beier K, Krahenbuhl S: Effect of carnitine deprivation on carnitine homeostasis and energy metabolism in mice with systemic carnitine defi-ciency. *Ann Nutr Metab* 2008, 52:136–144.
142. Spaniol M, Kaufmann P, Beier K, Wuthrich J, Torok M, Scharnagl H, Marz W, Krahenbuhl S: Mechanisms of liver steatosis in rats with systemic carnitine defi-ciency due to treatment with trimethylhydraziniumpropionate. *J Lipid Res* 2003, 44: 144–153.

143. Alwayn IP, Javid PJ, Gura KM, Nose V, Ollero M, Puder M: Do polyunsaturated fatty acids ameliorate hepatic steatosis in obese mice by SREPB-1 suppression or by correcting essential fatty acid deficiency. *Hepatology* 2004, 39:1176–1177; author reply 1177–1178.

144. Ling PR, De Leon CE, Le H, Puder M, Bistrian BR: Early development of essential fatty acid deficiency in rats: fat-free vs. hydrogenated coconut oil diet. *Prostaglandins Leukot Essent Fatty Acids* 2010, 83:229–237.

145. Allard JP, Aghdassi E, Mohammed S, Raman M, Avand G, Arendt BM, Jalali P, Kandasamy T, Prayitno N, Sherman M et al.: Nutritional assessment and hepatic fatty acid composition in non-alcoholic fatty liver disease (NAFLD): a cross-sectional study. *J Hepatol* 2008, 48:300–307.

146. Clarke SD: Nonalcoholic steatosis and steatohepatitis. I. Molecular mechanism for polyunsaturated fatty acid regulation of gene transcription. *Am J Physiol Gastrointest Liver Physiol* 2001, 281:G865–869.

147. Neuschwander-Tetri BA: Betaine: an old therapy for a new scourge. *Am J Gastroenterol* 2001, 96:2534–2536.

148. Gulsen M, Yesilova Z, Bagci S, Uygun A, Ozcan A, Ercin CN, Erdil A, Sanisoglu SY, Cakir E, Ates Y et al.: Elevated plasma homocysteine concentrations as a predictor of steatohepatitis in patients with non-alcoholic fatty liver disease. *J Gastroenterol Hepatol* 2005, 20:1448–1455.

149. Polyzos SA, Kountouras J, Patsiaoura K, Katsiki E, Zafeiriadou E, Zavos C, Deretzi G, Tsiaousi E, Slavakis A: Serum vitamin B12 and folate levels in patients with nonalcoholic fatty liver disease. *Int J Food Sci Nutr* 2012, 63:659–666.

150. Compher CW, Kinosian BP, Stoner NE, Lentine DC, Buzby GP: Choline and vitamin B12 deficiencies are interrelated in folate-replete long-term total parenteral nutrition patients. *JPEN J Parenter Enteral Nutr* 2002, 26:57–62.

151. Buchman AL, Dubin M, Jenden D, Moukarzel A, Roch MH, Rice K, Gornbein J, Ament ME, Eckhert CD: Lecithin increases plasma free choline and decreases hepatic steatosis in long-term total parenteral nutrition patients. *Gastroenterology* 1992, 102:1363–1370.

152. Buchman AL, Dubin MD, Moukarzel AA, Jenden DJ, Roch M, Rice KM, Gornbein J, Ament ME: Choline deficiency: a cause of hepatic steatosis during parenteral nutrition that can be reversed with intravenous choline supplementation. *Hepatology* 1995, 22:1399–1403.

153. Fischer LM, daCosta KA, Kwock L, Stewart PW, Lu TS, Stabler SP, Allen RH, Zeisel SH: Sex and menopausal status influence human dietary requirements for the nutrient choline. *Am J Clin Nutr* 2007, 85:1275–1285.

154. Zeisel SH, Da Costa KA, Franklin PD, Alexander EA, Lamont JT, Sheard NF, Beiser A: Choline, an essential nutrient for humans. *FASEB J* 1991, 5:2093–2098.

155. Zeisel SH: Choline: critical role during fetal development and dietary requirements in adults. *Annu Rev Nutr* 2006, 26:229–250.

156. Zeisel SH, Mar MH, Howe JC, Holden JM: Concentrations of choline-containing compounds and betaine in common foods. *J Nutr* 2003, 133:1302–1307.

157. Fischer LM, da Costa KA, Kwock L, Galanko J, Zeisel SH: Dietary choline requirements of women: effects of estrogen and genetic variation. *Am J Clin Nutr* 2010, 92: 1113–1119.

158. Noga AA, Vance DE: A gender-specific role for phosphatidylethanolamine N-methyltransferase-derived phosphatidylcholine in the regulation of plasma high density and very low density lipoproteins in mice. *J Biol Chem* 2003, 278:21851–21859.

159. Resseguie M, Song J, Niculescu MD, da Costa KA, Randall TA, Zeisel SH: Phosphatidylethanolamine N-methyltransferase (PEMT) gene expression is induced by estrogen in human and mouse primary hepatocytes. *FASEB J* 2007, 21:2622–2632.

160. Resseguie ME, da Costa KA, Galanko JA, Patel M, Davis IJ, Zeisel SH: Aberrant estrogen regulation of PEMT results in choline deficiency-associated liver dysfunction. *J Biol Chem* 2011, 286:1649–1658.
161. Tessitore L, Sesca E, Greco M, Pani P, Dianzani MU: Sexually differentiated response to choline in choline deficiency and ethionine intoxication. *Int J Exp Pathol* 1995, 76:125–129.
162. Kulinski A, Vance DE, Vance JE: A choline-deficient diet in mice inhibits neither the CDP-choline pathway for phosphatidylcholine synthesis in hepatocytes nor apolipoprotein B secretion. *J Biol Chem* 2004, 279:23916–23924.
163. Vetelainen R, van Vliet A, van Gulik TM: Essential pathogenic and metabolic differences in steatosis induced by choline or methione-choline deficient diets in a rat model. *J Gastroenterol Hepatol* 2007, 22:1526–1533.
164. Yao ZM, Vance DE: Reduction in VLDL, but not HDL, in plasma of rats deficient in choline. *Biochem Cell Biol* 1990, 68:552–558.
165. Al-Humadi H, Zarros A, Kyriakaki A, Al-Saigh R, Liapi C: Choline deprivation: an overview of the major hepatic metabolic response pathways. *Scand J Gastroenterol* 2012, 47:874–886.
166. Nakae D, Mizumoto Y, Kobayashi E, Noguchi O, Konishi Y: Improved genomic/nuclear DNA extraction for 8-hydroxydeoxyguanosine analysis of small amounts of rat liver tissue. *Cancer Lett* 1995, 97:233–239.
167. Nakae D, Yoshiji H, Maruyama H, Kinugasa T, Denda A, Konishi Y: Production of both 8-hydroxydeoxyguanosine in liver DNA and gamma-glutamyltransferase-positive hepatocellular lesions in rats given a choline-deficient, L-amino acid–defined diet. *Jpn J Cancer Res Gann* 1990, 81:1081–1084.
168. Nakae D, Yoshiji H, Mizumoto Y, Horiguchi K, Shiraiwa K, Tamura K, Denda A, Konishi Y: High incidence of hepatocellular carcinomas induced by a choline deficient L-amino acid defined diet in rats. *Cancer Res* 1992, 52:5042–5045.
169. Nakae D, Mizumoto Y, Andoh N, Tamura K, Horiguchi K, Endoh T, Kobayashi E, Tsujiuchi T, Denda A, Lombardi B et al.: Comparative changes in the liver of female Fischer-344 rats after short-term feeding of a semipurified or a semisynthetic L-amino acid–defined choline-deficient diet. *Toxicol Pathol* 1995, 23:583–590.
170. Kodama Y, Kisseleva T, Iwaisako K, Miura K, Taura K, De Minicis S, Osterreicher CH, Schnabl B, Seki E, Brenner DA: c-Jun N-terminal kinase-1 from hematopoietic cells mediates progression from hepatic steatosis to steatohepatitis and fibrosis in mice. *Gastroenterology* 2009, 137:1467–1477 e1465.
171. Denda A, Kitayama W, Kishida H, Murata N, Tsutsumi M, Tsujiuchi T, Nakae D, Konishi Y: Development of hepatocellular adenomas and carcinomas associated with fibrosis in C57BL/6J male mice given a choline-deficient, L-amino acid–defined diet. *Jpn J Cancer Res Gann* 2002, 93:125–132.
172. Miura K, Yang L, van Rooijen N, Ohnishi H, Seki E: Hepatic recruitment of macrophages promotes nonalcoholic steatohepatitis through CCR2. *Am J Physiol Gastrointest Liver Physiol* 2012, 302:G1310–1321.
173. Miura K, Yang L, van Rooijen N, Brenner DA, Ohnishi H, Seki E: Toll-like receptor 2 and palmitic acid cooperatively contribute to the development of nonalcoholic steatohepatitis through inflammasome activation in mice. *Hepatology* 2013, 57:577–589.
174. Miura K, Kodama Y, Inokuchi S, Schnabl B, Aoyama T, Ohnishi H, Olefsky JM, Brenner DA, Seki E: Toll-like receptor 9 promotes steatohepatitis by induction of interleukin-1beta in mice. *Gastroenterology* 2010, 139:323–334 e327.
175. Endo H, Niioka M, Kobayashi N, Tanaka M, Watanabe T: Butyrate-producing probiotics reduce nonalcoholic Fatty liver disease progression in rats: new insight into the probiotics for the gut-liver axis. *PLoS One* 2013, 8:e63388.

176. Wang B, Hsu SH, Frankel W, Ghoshal K, Jacob ST: Stat3-mediated activation of microRNA-23a suppresses gluconeogenesis in hepatocellular carcinoma by down-regulating glucose-6-phosphatase and peroxisome proliferator-activated receptor gamma, coactivator 1 alpha. *Hepatology* 2012, 56:186–197.
177. Takeuchi-Yorimoto A, Noto T, Yamada A, Miyamae Y, Oishi Y, Matsumoto M: Persistent fibrosis in the liver of choline-deficient and iron-supplemented L-amino acid–defined diet-induced nonalcoholic steatohepatitis rat due to continuing oxidative stress after choline supplementation. *Toxicol Appl Pharmacol* 2013, 268:264–277.
178. Denda A, Kitayama W, Kishida H, Murata N, Tamura K, Kusuoka O, Tsutsumi M, Nishikawa F, Kita E, Nakae D et al.: Expression of inducible nitric oxide (NO) synthase but not prevention by its gene ablation of hepatocarcinogenesis with fibrosis caused by a choline-deficient, L-amino acid–defined diet in rats and mice. *Nitric Oxide Biol Chem* 2007, 16:164–176.
179. Fujita K, Nozaki Y, Yoneda M, Wada K, Takahashi H, Kirikoshi H, Inamori M, Saito S, Iwasaki T, Terauchi Y et al.: Nitric oxide plays a crucial role in the development/progression of nonalcoholic steatohepatitis in the choline-deficient, l-amino acid–defined diet-fed rat model. *Alcohol Clin Exp Res* 2010, 34 Suppl 1:S18–24.
180. Garcia-Trevijano ER, Martinez-Chantar ML, Latasa MU, Mato JM, Avila MA: NO sensitizes rat hepatocytes to proliferation by modifying S-adenosylmethionine levels. *Gastroenterology* 2002, 122:1355–1363.
181. Mato JM, Corrales FJ, Lu SC, Avila MA: S-Adenosylmethionine: a control switch that regulates liver function. *FASEB J* 2002, 16:15–26.
182. Mehedint MG, Zeisel SH: Choline's role in maintaining liver function: new evidence for epigenetic mechanisms. *Curr Opin Clin Nutr Metab Care* 2013, 16:339–345.
183. Rinella ME, Elias MS, Smolak RR, Fu T, Borensztajn J, Green RM: Mechanisms of hepatic steatosis in mice fed a lipogenic methionine choline-deficient diet. *J Lipid Res* 2008, 49:1068–1076.
184. Caballero F, Fernandez A, Matias N, Martinez L, Fucho R, Elena M, Caballeria J, Morales A, Fernandez-Checa JC, Garcia-Ruiz C: Specific contribution of methionine and choline in nutritional nonalcoholic steatohepatitis: impact on mitochondrial S-adenosyl-L-methionine and glutathione. *J Biol Chem* 2010, 285:18528–18536.
185. Schattenberg JM, Singh R, Wang Y, Lefkowitch JH, Rigoli RM, Scherer PE, Czaja MJ: JNK1 but not JNK2 promotes the development of steatohepatitis in mice. *Hepatology* 2006, 43:163–172.
186. Schattenberg JM, Wang Y, Singh R, Rigoli RM, Czaja MJ: Hepatocyte CYP2E1 overexpression and steatohepatitis lead to impaired hepatic insulin signaling. *J Biol Chem* 2005, 280:9887–9894.
187. Dixon LJ, Berk M, Thapaliya S, Papouchado BG, Feldstein AE: Caspase-1-mediated regulation of fibrogenesis in diet-induced steatohepatitis. *Lab Invest* 2012, 92:713–723.
188. Weltman MD, Farrell GC, Liddle C: Increased hepatocyte CYP2E1 expression in a rat nutritional model of hepatic steatosis with inflammation. *Gastroenterology* 1996, 111:1645–1653.
189. Aharoni-Simon M, Anavi S, Beifuss U, Madar Z, Tirosh O: Nitric oxide, can it be only good? Increasing the antioxidant properties of nitric oxide in hepatocytes by YC-1 compound. *Nitric Oxide Biol Chem* 2012, 27:248–256.
190. Avila MA, Mingorance J, Martinez-Chantar ML, Casado M, Martin-Sanz P, Bosca L, Mato JM: Regulation of rat liver S-adenosylmethionine synthetase during septic shock: role of nitric oxide. *Hepatology* 1997, 25:391–396.
191. Aharoni-Simon M, Hann-Obercyger M, Pen S, Madar Z, Tirosh O: Fatty liver is associated with impaired activity of PPARgamma-coactivator 1alpha (PGC1alpha) and mitochondrial biogenesis in mice. *Lab Invest* 2011, 91:1018–1028.

192. Akhurst B, Croager EJ, Farley-Roche CA, Ong JK, Dumble ML, Knight B, Yeoh GC: A modified choline-deficient, ethionine-supplemented diet protocol effectively induces oval cells in mouse liver. *Hepatology* 2001, 34:519–522.

193. Knight B, Matthews VB, Akhurst B, Croager EJ, Klinken E, Abraham LJ, Olynyk JK, Yeoh G: Liver inflammation and cytokine production, but not acute phase protein synthesis, accompany the adult liver progenitor (oval) cell response to chronic liver injury. *Immunol Cell Biol* 2005, 83:364–374.

194. Tirosh O, Artan A, Aharoni-Simon M, Ramadori G, Madar Z: Impaired liver glucose production in a murine model of steatosis and endotoxemia: protection by inducible nitric oxide synthase. *Antioxid Redox Signal* 2010, 13:13–26.

10 The Double-Edged Sword of Hepatic Iron Metabolism in Health and Diseases

Guiliano Ramadori and Ihtzaz Ahmed Malik

CONTENTS

INTRODUCTION

THE BODY'S NEED FOR IRON

Iron is a fundamental element of almost every organism. It contributes in a wide variety of metabolic processes including oxygen transport, heme and nonheme iron proteins, electron transfer, neurotransmitter synthesis, myelin production, energy metabolism, and mitochondrial function in the organs (Camaschella, 2005; Hentze et al., 2004; Napier et al., 2005; Stankiewicz et al., 2007). Ribonucleotide reductase (the rate-limiting enzyme of DNA synthesis) and succinate dehydrogenase and aconitase of the TCA cycle are also iron-dependent enzymes (Crowe and Morgan, 1992). However, the excess of iron can lead to the production of oxygen free radicals, which can damage various cellular components. In contrast to many other nutrients, the body has no defined excretory mechanism for iron; for this reason, organisms must regulate the body iron at intestinal absorption levels to provide the body with sufficient iron for cellular needs without developing the toxicity due to iron excess (Frazer and Anderson, 2005).

The Iron Metabolism Proteins and Normal Iron Homeostasis

Iron homeostasis is controlled by a large group of iron regulatory proteins. Heme iron is transported across the apical membrane of enterocytes and is converted into ferrous iron by heme-oxygenase 1 (HO-1) (Camaschella, 2005; Hentze et al., 2004; Napier et al., 2005; Stankiewicz et al., 2007).

Absorption of dietary iron begins by its transport across the duodenal brush border membrane mediated by duodenal metal transporter 1 (DMT-1) and a ferroreductase known as duodenum cytochrome B (Dcytb) that is thought to reduce ferric (Fe^{3+}) to ferrous (Fe^{2+}) iron (McKie et al., 2001) for transport by DMT-1. DMT-1 is also essential for iron acquisition necessary for erythropoiesis (Gunshin et al., 1997). DMT-1 has been detected in the endosomal compartment of different cell types, suggesting that it may also participate in transport of transferrin-bound iron across the membrane of acidified endosomes and into the cytoplasm (Gruenheid et al., 1999; Tabuchi et al., 2000). Transferrin (Tf) carries iron to the reticuloendothelial system, liver parenchymal cells, and all proliferating cells in the body. Interaction of diferric Tf with the transferrin receptor 1 (TfR1) and internalization of the complex by receptor-mediated endocytosis leads to iron uptake in the cells (Conner and Schmid, 2003; Frazer and Anderson, 2005; Jandl et al., 1959; Morgan and Appleton, 1969) (Figure 10.1). The synthesis of the TfR1 is generally known to be regulated at the mRNA level through iron-responsive elements (IRE) present in the untranslated region of the mRNA. If the cellular iron level is low, these IREs interact with iron regulatory proteins to protect

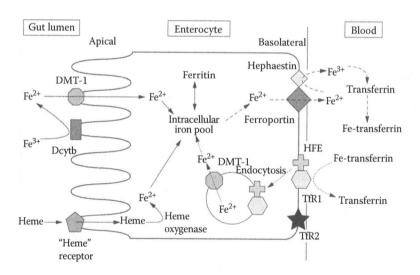

FIGURE 10.1 A model of iron absorption pathways by duodenal enterocyte. This shows the uptake of ionic iron and heme iron from the gut lumen and transfer of iron to blood. DMT-1, divalent metal transporter 1; HFE, hemochromatosis protein; TfR1, transferrin receptor 1; TfR2, transferrin receptor 2. (From Trinder, D. et al., *Gut*, 51, 290–295, 2002.)

mRNA from cleavage and degradation and thereby increase protein synthesis (Casey et al., 1989; Rouault, 2006).

A second transferrin-mediated route of iron uptake is via TfR2. Although the role of TfR1 is well defined for transporting iron across the plasma membrane, the role of TfR2 is not yet clearly understood. TfR2 knockout mice results in embryonic lethality due to severe anemia (Levy et al., 1999). Because TfR2 mutation or knockout results in hepatic iron overload, TfR2 appears to function, not principally in cellular iron uptake and delivery, but rather in systemic iron homeostasis (Roetto et al., 2010).

Several other genes involved in iron homeostasis have been characterized including ferroportin 1 (Fpn-1) (McKie et al., 2000), ferritin (FTL) (Ganz and Nemeth, 2012), hepcidin (Pigeon et al., 2001), and hemojuvelin (HJV) (Lanzara et al., 2004).

Within the cell, iron is mainly stored as ferritin (Ganz and Nemeth, 2012). In human, ferritin is composed of two subunits: ferritin L 125 amino acid (19 kDa) and ferritin H 183 amino acid (21 kDa). Both subunits are highly conserved (Arosio et al., 2009), but are genetically separated (Caskey et al., 1983; Worwood et al., 1985) and maintain distinct functions (Sammarco et al., 2008). The L and H subunits spontaneously assemble in a 24-subunit protein "cage" with a flexible H/L ratio. The H/L ratio can vary between different cell types (Arosio et al., 2009; Sammarco et al., 2008). The FTL gene has very little tissue-specific regulations, whereas multiple conditions activate FTH gene transcription (Briat et al., 2010; Ponka et al., 1998) including cell differentiation, changes in the cell proliferation status (Cozzi et al., 2004), cytokines, and heme. However, iron does not change the transcription rate of the FTH gene, whereas it stimulates transcription of the FTL gene, at least in the liver (Hentze et al., 2010; Meyron-Holtz et al., 2011).

Hepcidin previously reported as liver-expressed antimicrobial peptide (Krause et al., 2000) is a recently discovered circulating antimicrobial peptide mainly synthesized by hepatocytes in the liver. It regulates intestinal iron absorption as well as maternal fetal iron transport across the placenta (Ganz, 2006). It affects the release of iron from hepatic stores and from macrophages involved in the recycling of iron from hemoglobin (Ganz, 2013). Hepcidin (30) is 25–amino acid, 2- to 3-kDa, cationic peptide (Park et al., 2001) and is an acute-phase protein (Sheikh et al., 2007). Its production is increased during inflammation and in iron-overload conditions (Krause et al., 2000). It is a major regulator of iron balance in the intestinal mucosa, which seems to have a significant role during inflammation, and it is a major contributor to the hypoferremia associated with inflammation (Ganz, 2011; Krause et al., 2000). Hepcidin is also found to control iron levels by directly interacting with Fpn-1, leading to internalization and degradation of Fpn-1 when iron levels are high, consequently blocking release of iron from storage sites, hepatocytes, and macrophages (Nemeth et al., 2004b).

Fpn-1 (also known as MTP1, IREG-1, or SLC11A3) is the main iron-export protein. It was first characterized as an iron exporter in zebrafish where embryos carrying mutations in the Fpn-1 orthologue showed a lack of iron transfer ability from the yolk sac to embryo (Donovan et al., 2000). It is highly expressed in numerous cells, including duodenal enterocytes, reticuloendothelial macrophages, and Kupffer cells

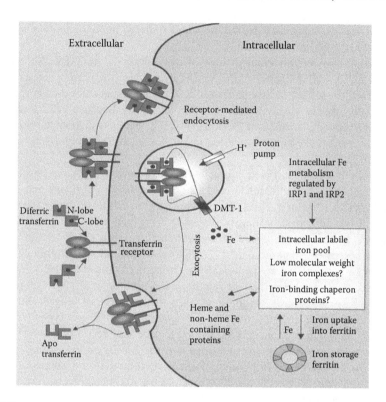

FIGURE 10.2 Schematic diagram illustrating the mechanisms involved in iron uptake. Diferric Tf undergoes endocytosis after binding to TfR1. Iron is released from Tf mediated by a decrease in pH and is exported out of the endosome by DMT-1, where it enters the labile iron pool (LIP). Iron in the LIP can subsequently be incorporated into ferritin for iron storage or into iron-containing proteins. (From Kalinowski, D.S., Richardson, D.R., *Pharmacol Rev*, 57, 547–583, 2005.)

(Donovan et al., 2000; Ganz, 2005). After entering the enterocytes, iron is used for metabolic purposes, stored in ferritin subunits (heavy and light chain), or translocated to the plasma by Fpn-1 (Figure 10.2). It is also suggested that Fpn-1 mediates iron export in hepatocytes (Abboud and Haile, 2000). In the presence of an iron exporter (Fpn-1) and a ferroxidase, hephastin, the newly released ferrous iron could be oxidized to its ferric form, allowing binding to transferrin (Song et al., 2010). Hephastin is proposed to have a multi–copper oxidase activity due to its homology with ceruloplasmin and to be located on the basolateral membrane in intestinal enterocytes because it has a single predicted transmembrane domain (Anderson et al., 2002; Vulpe et al., 1999). The previous study showed that hephastin protein was located on the basolateral membrane of small intestine in mice (Han and Kim, 2007; Kuo et al., 2004; Yeh et al., 2009). The colocalization of Fpn-1 and hephastin suggested a collaborative role of both proteins in transport of iron out of enterocytes, but it is not known whether these two proteins interact during iron absorption.

IRON-RELATED DISORDERS

Hereditary hemochromatosis (HH) is an autosomal recessive disorder of iron metabolism due to mutations in the HFE-gene (Allen et al., 2008; Pietrangelo, 2006). HH is an inherited condition of dysregulated iron absorption that can lead to total-body iron overload with secondary tissue damage in a wide range of organs. This condition can lead to diseases such as hepatic cirrhosis and hepatocellular carcinoma (Allen et al., 2008; Pietrangelo, 2006).

Most cases of adult HH are the result of a single faulty gene on chromosome 6 that codes for a protein called HFE (Feder et al., 1996; Simon et al., 1976). Two common mutations are described which are designated as C282Y and H63D. The C282Y mutation, a single point mutation with substitution of tyrosine for cysteine at position 282, is found 85%–90% cases of HH (Bacon et al., 1999; Feder et al., 1996).

As the liver is the primary organ of iron storage in the body, it is usually the first organ affected in this disorder. Ferritin and haemosiderin deposits are mainly found in hepatocytes, rather than in the reticuloendothelial cells such as Kupffer cells (Allen et al., 2008; Dubois and Kowdley, 2004). However, the precise physiological mechanism of increased iron absorption of HH is still not described.

In normal adults, iron loss and iron absorption are in balance, each amounting to approximately 1 mg/day in men, and 1.5–2 mg/day in women. The total body iron content in adult men is approximately 35–45 mg/kg of body weight, with lower levels in premenopausal women secondary to menstrual loss (Alexander and Kowdley, 2009; Bacon et al., 1999; Olynyk et al., 2008). Erythrocyte hemoglobin comprises more than two thirds of the iron pool, with storage iron in the liver accounting for most of the rest (Alexander and Kowdley, 2009; Olynyk et al., 2008). Increased metabolic demand for iron results in increased intestinal iron absorption and mobilization of iron from tissue stores; the reverse happens in conditions of decreased iron demand. Sloughing of intestinal mucosal cells and menstrual blood loss are the main physiological processes responsible for loss of iron from the body (Alexander and Kowdley, 2009; Olynyk et al., 2008). Because there are no regulatory mechanisms to control these processes according to body iron status, regulation of the amount of iron in the body takes place mainly at the level of absorption (Anderson and Frazer, 2005).

Defective hepcidin synthesis in the liver is postulated to be the central pathogenic factor in HH-HFE. However, the link between HFE gene mutations and defective hepcidin synthesis has not yet been elucidated (Alexander and Kowdley, 2009; Gehrke et al., 2003).

Elevation of serum transferrin-iron saturation, in association with increased nontransferrin-bound iron is the first biochemical abnormality in HH. This is followed by elevation of serum ferritin, which reflects iron overload in parenchymal cells. Because serum iron is high, and as the iron transport to bone marrow and incorporation into hemoglobin are unaffected, erythropoiesis is characteristically unimpaired in HH (Alexander and Kowdley, 2009; Gehrke et al., 2003; Pietrangelo, 2006).

LIVER AND IRON METABOLISM

Liver is a major organ in iron homeostasis. Hepatocytes (major; 70%, cell population of liver) are key cells to regulate absorption of dietary iron and reutilization of iron after senescent red cells are phagocytosed and digested by macrophages by secreting the regulatory peptide hormone, hepcidin. Hepcidin, a liver derived hormone (Krause et al., 2000), is a 25-amino acid, 2- to 3-kDa, cationic peptide (McGrath and Rigby, 2004). Hepatocytes judge the total-body iron stores and secrete hepcidin in direct proportion to hepatocytic iron stores.

Kupffer cells regulate the return of iron to the circulation by regulating expression of ferroportin, which appears to be the major mammalian iron exporter (Ganz, 2005). The expression of Fpn-1 is supposed to be regulated by liver-derived hormone, hepcidin. Hepcidin is reported to cause internalization and degradation of Fpn-1; as a result, the cells lack the iron exporter (Figure 10.3). Decreased expression of intestinal Fpn-1 reduces intestinal iron absorption, and decreased expression of Fpn-1 in macrophages simultaneously reduces the return of iron to the circulation. By decreasing iron absorption from the intestine and increasing macrophage iron sequestration, hepcidin causes a decrease in serum iron levels (Cairo et al., 2011; Ganz and Nemeth, 2006).

In hepcidin knockout mice, hepcidin deficiency induces periportal Fpn-1 stabilization and, thus, iron is exported along the pericentral axis and progressively accumulated in the centrolobular region where it is trapped due to the absence of Fpn-1 in this area (Ramey et al., 2010). However, several studies also demonstrated direct iron regulatory effects on Fpn-1 gene expression (Aydemir et al., 2009; Yeh et al., 2009). In addition, a recent study identifies and characterized two isoforms of Fpn-1 (Fpn-1a and Fpn-1b), which differs from each other by existence/absence of iron

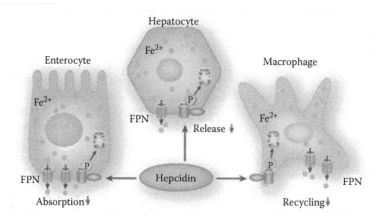

FIGURE 10.3 Hepcidin downregulates ferroportin expression. Ferroportin (FPN) is expressed in enterocytes, hepatocytes, and tissue macrophages. The binding of hepcidin to Fpn-1 leads to its phosphorylation, internalization, and degradation. Low levels of Fpn-1 expression reduce iron absorption in the gut, lower iron release from the liver, and prevent iron recycling by tissue macrophages. (From Cui, Y. et al., *Kidney Int*, 76, 1137–1141, 2009.)

regulatory elements proposing that the isoform that could escape repression through the IRE/IRP system in iron deficiency might be expressed in the duodenum to allow active export of iron into the blood stream to meet systemic iron demands (Zhang et al., 2009).

THE MODEL OF ACUTE-PHASE STUDY AND IRON METABOLISM

There are two well-established animal models to study the APR- and acute phase-mediated changes in acute-phase proteins. Induction of APR by bacterial endotoxin lipopolysaccharide (LPS) administration induces systemic APR together with liver damage (Boelen et al., 2005; Ramadori et al., 1985). The other model of APR is turpentine oil (TO)-induced sterile muscle abscess without a detectable injury to liver and other tissues (Boelen et al., 2005; Ramadori et al., 1990; Tron et al., 2005; Wusteman et al., 1990). Thus, the TO-induced acute-phase response (APR) model allows studying the effect of cytokines produced at distant sites on the liver. It reproduces changes observed in human disease states (Boelen et al., 2005; Gabay and Kushner, 1999).

Under inflammatory conditions induced by microbial attack or during liver injury, a diversion of iron traffic from the circulation to storage sites of reticuloendothelial system occurs to minimize the availability of this essential element for the microbial proliferation and growth (Weiss, 2005). However, during APR induced by sterile muscle abscess by TO-intramuscular administration, the acute-phase cytokines mediates the expressional changes of iron metabolism proteins, which in turn leads to serum iron turnover and deposition of iron in metabolically active tissue (Cairo et al., 2011; Sheikh et al., 2007) (Figure 10.4).

In fact, recently, an increase in liver cytoplasmic and an even stronger increase in liver nuclear iron concentration during APR have also been shown. However, in the spleen, the iron concentration decreased during APR (Naz et al., 2012). As a bacteriostatic response, decrease in serum iron concentration is a characteristic response of infection and endotoxin-induced APR (Chlosta et al., 2006; Nairz et al., 2007; Wessling-Resnick, 2010). The increased concentration of iron in rat liver tissue during acute-phase reaction in a model of sterile inflammation could suggest an increased need of iron supply to satisfy the increased metabolic work under acute-phase conditions as it is known for liver (Ramadori and Christ, 1999). The previous studies show that in iron loading in HFE knockout mice with hemochromatosis was associated with limited iron deposition into the spleen (Ahmad et al., 2002; Zhou et al., 1998). In rat liver, apart from the difference of magnitude, the gene expression of iron export proteins (Fpn-1, Fpn-1a, Fpn-1b, and hephastin) was downregulated during APR. Moreover, an upregulation of gene expression of iron import proteins (Tf, TfR1, TfR2, and DMT-1) and iron storage proteins (ferritin H and L) was observed in rat liver (Malik et al., 2011; Naz et al., 2012; Sheikh et al., 2007).

It indicates that iron is temporarily sequestered in the liver as Fpn-1, and hephastin (the iron exporters) gene expression in this tissue is dramatically downregulated during APR. This also suggests that extra iron may be needed to satisfy the increased metabolic work under acute-phase conditions, as is known for the liver (Ramadori and Christ, 1999). The increased gene expression of the transport molecules may be

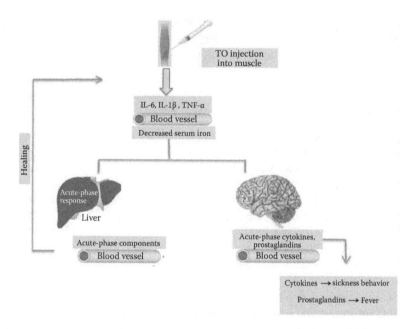

FIGURE 10.4 The acute-phase model of study. Turpentine injection into the limb muscle results in cytokine production at the site of injury. These cytokines are released into the blood, and when they reach the liver, liver becomes metabolically active and releases acute-phase mediators to start the healing process at the site of injury. The decreased iron concentration in the serum is the hallmark of APR. The fever and illness behavior during acute-phase response is induced by local production of cytokines and prostaglandins by brain.

due to the action of the major acute-phase cytokine (IL-6), as shown in vitro (Sheikh et al., 2006), and the increased iron concentration, maybe on its own, further induces an upregulation of gene expression of some proteins such as DMT-1, TfR1, and TfR2 (Tacchini et al., 2002; Trinder et al., 2000).

THE DIFFERENTIAL CELLULAR LOCALIZATION OF IRON TRANSPORT PROTEINS IN RAT LIVER

Recently, by means of immunohistochemical analysis, a membranous and cytoplasmic expression of TfR1 was observed in the liver and liver cells (Kupffer cells and hepatocytes) and human hepatoma cell (HepG2) (Malik et al., 2011). In contrast, TfR2 and DMT-1 were exclusively located in the nuclei of the rat liver and liver cells. Similarly, Fpn-1 was also localized to the nuclei of the liver. Furthermore, these iron transport proteins were expressed in hepatocytes and Kupffer cells, but not in myofibroblasts (Naz et al., 2012).

The nuclear expression of ferritin-H has been described in hepatocytes only under supra-physiological conditions (Smith et al., 1990). However, the nuclear expression of MT-1, TfR2, and Fpn-1 in rat liver is a very recent advancement. This may suggest iron sequestration not only in the cytoplasm but also in the nucleus of liver cells, as observed by the increased cytoplasmic and nuclear iron concentrations in liver, and an important role of iron for hepatocyte metabolism under stress conditions. Moreover, an increase in the mRNA expression of iron-dependent cytoplasmic enzyme ribonucleotide reductase (RNR) in the present model of study supports the increased iron needs during APR. Increased nuclear iron uptake indicates the increased activity of nuclear enzymes for DNA synthesis and repair (Roth et al., 2000), as demonstrated by increased mRNA and protein concentrations of cyclin E, and/or to regulate the initiation of transcription (Roth et al., 2000). As transcription function is strongly upregulated under stress conditions, nuclear uptake of iron may indicate an important role of this metal. A previous study reported the evidence of stainable iron in the nuclei of hepatocytes and Kupffer cells in mice liver under iron overload conditions. This finding may support not only the presence of iron transport proteins in the nuclei of liver cells under nonphysiological conditions as a defense mechanism (Magens et al., 2005), but also the need of iron for nuclear metabolism.

MT-1 and TfR2 nuclear expression has been demonstrated in rat PC12 cells (Roth et al., 2000) and in mice glioblastomas cancer cell lines, respectively (Calzolari et al., 2010). Nuclear localization of Fpn-1 in liver and brain tissue is quite surprising and mystifies its function as a membrane iron export protein. There are conflicting reports that demonstrate the localization of Fpn-1 protein in different organs of human, rat, and mice by means of immunohistochemical analysis. Membrane positivity of Fpn-1 protein was shown in extra-embryonic visceral endoderm and duodenal enterocytes of mice (Donovan et al., 2005). In one study on human lung tissues, the membrane localization of Fpn-1 in airway epithelial cells was described where it was also visible in the nucleoli of these cells. Anyhow, in alveolar macrophages, Fpn-1 was detected only in the membrane, cytoplasm, and intracellular vesicles. Moreover, a study by Yang et al. (2005) demonstrates the tissue-specific subcellular localization of Fpn-1 in the lung and duodenum of rat. However, D'Anna et al. (2009) report supranuclear expression of Fpn-1 protein in mice liver macrophages. The differential subcellular localization of Fpn-1 in different organs suggests that hepcidin might not be the only one that regulates Fpn-1, but different regulatory mechanisms may exist in different organs depending on cellular iron needs. A recent study reports hepcidin-independent regulation of Fpn-1 in human embryonic kidney (De Domenico et al., 2010). Similarly, a study reports on both inflammation-mediated transcriptional and IRE-dependent post-transcriptional mechanisms for inhibiting ferroportin expression in mononuclear phagocyte cells (Liu et al., 2002).

Fpn-1, a Negative Acute-Phase Protein

Under iron overload conditions, Fpn-1 is bounded by hepcidin and degraded, leading to cellular iron retention (Canonne-Hergaux et al., 2006). Furthermore, the downregulation of Fpn-1 could probably be controlled by acute-phase cytokines (mainly IL-6) released at the site of injury during APR, as these cytokines are able to modulate the expression of iron transport proteins (Liu et al., 2005; Nemeth et al. 2004a).

Moreover, the Fpn-1 protein expression in the liver that almost diminished during APR with a slight upregulation of IL-6 gene expression in liver can, at the same time, possibly justify the intense decrease in Fpn-1 protein expression in the liver at this time point; this indicates a direct or combination effect (with hepcidin) of acute-phase cytokine (IL-6 in this case) on regulating Fpn-1 gene expression (Naz et al., 2012). In fact, a downregulation of *Fpn-1* gene expression in parallel to an increase in acute-phase cytokines (IL-1β, IL-6, and TNF-α) was also reported in different rat models (Christiansen et al., 2007; Moriconi et al., 2009; Sheikh et al., 2006, 2007). The cytokine-induced Fpn-1 downregulation is most probably a mechanism occurring independently of hepcidin, as downregulation of Fpn-1 gene expression starts before hepcidin gene expression is upregulated.

A recent study showed the expression pattern of Fpn-1–, Fpn-1a–, Fpn-1b–, and hepcidin–mRNA in wild-type and IL-6 knockout mice, under the similar acute-phase conditions as for rats. It was reported that Fpn-1, Fpn-1a, and Fpn-1b gene expression was downregulated in wild-type and IL-6 knockout mice under acute-phase conditions. However, in wild-type mice, the decrease in the mRNA amount of *Fpn-1* and its isoforms was higher and significant compared to their IL-6 knockout counterparts (Naz et al., 2012). The upregulation of hepcidin and a slight downregulation of *Fpn-1* and its isoforms in IL-6 knockout mice under acute-phase conditions might be due to the existence of other acute-phase cytokines, IL-1β and TNF-α, produced at the site of injury (Ramadori et al., 2010). This study was further confirmed in isolated hepatocytes. As was observed in vivo, IL-6-treated hepatocytes, with a difference of magnitude, and the stimulation of hepatocytes with IL-1β and TNF-α led to a downregulation of Fpn-1 and its isoforms, with a slight upregulation of hepcidin gene expression (Naz et al., 2012), which indicates that these cytokines, to some extent, also regulate the gene expression of Fpn-1 and its isoforms (Naz et al., 2012; Sheikh et al., 2006). Similarly, a study on rat C6 glioma cells reports the modulation of Fpn-1 synthesis by IL-1β cytokine (di Patti et al., 2004). In fact, a similar finding was confirmed in cultured hepatocytes, where a dose-dependent downregulation of Fpn-1 gene expression was detected after acute-phase cytokines treatment (Sheikh et al., 2006), indicating a direct regulative effect. A similar study also reported a direct effect of acute inflammation mediators on downregulation of *Fpn-1* in the reticuloendothelial system (Yang et al., 2002). Taken together, these data may suggest that Fpn-1 can be considered as a negative intracellular (nuclear) acute-phase protein (APP).

CONCLUSION

In conclusion, we propose that under normal conditions, transferrin-bound iron of the portal blood is taken up by liver cells through TfR1-mediated iron uptake. Once in the cell, it is in part delivered not only to cytoplasmic organelles such as the mitochondria (Richardson et al., 2010) but also to the nucleus to meet the cellular functional requirements including DNA synthesis. Under acute-phase conditions, the liver behaves like a "sponge" for iron, as the reduction in serum iron concentration is most probably achieved by increased hepatic uptake of transferrin bound iron by TfR1-mediated iron transport into the hepatocytes. Increased DMT-1 also serves to transport iron inside the cell nuclei. On the same side, a reduction in Fpn-1 (mediated mainly by IL-6 cytokine) and hephastin leads to transient iron retention inside the cell and/or cell nucleus. All these events lead to iron retention inside the cell most probably to fulfil functional requirements of acute-phase situations. These findings have significant implications for further understanding of the importance of iron metabolism in the liver (Figures 10.5 and 10.6).

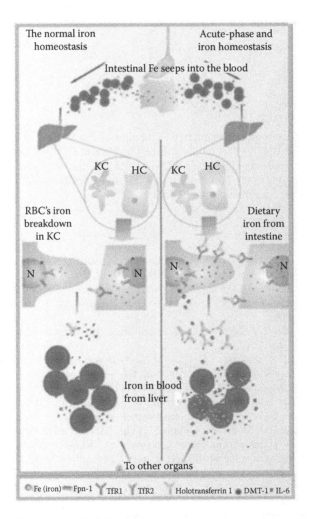

FIGURE 10.5 The proposed mechanism of iron metabolism in liver cells (HC, hepatocytes; KC, Kupffer cells) under physiological and acute-phase conditions. The iron absorbed at intestinal level seeps into blood and is taken up by Tf, which translocates iron inside the cell by TfR1 mediated endocytosis. TfR2 and DMT-1 help serve the iron transportation into the cell nuclei (N). During APR, the increased level of serum cytokine (IL-6) induces a downregulation of nuclear iron exporter (Fpn-1) and aids the cells to retain iron inside the cell and cell nuclei to meet the higher metabolic requirements under APR.

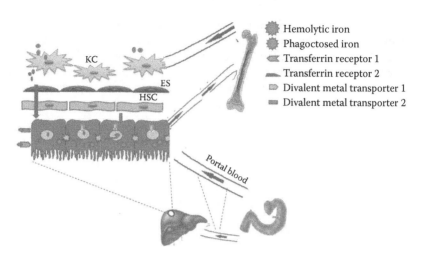

Hemolytic iron
Phagoctosed iron
Transferrin receptor 1
Transferrin receptor 2
Divalent metal transporter 1
Divalent metal transporter 2

FIGURE 10.6 Dietary iron is transferred to the liver via portal blood. Liver cells uptake iron via TfR 1 and DMT-1. This iron is utilized for different cellular functions and a part of it is also transferred within the liver via DMT-1 and TfR 2. Kupffer cells obtain iron via phagocytosis of the sunset erythrocytes and pass this iron to hepatocytes. Hepatocytes store and ultimately is use it for different bodily functions.

REFERENCES

Abboud S, Haile DJ (2000) A novel mammalian iron-regulated protein involved in intracellular iron metabolism. *J Biol Chem* 275:19906–19912.

Ahmad KA, Ahmann JR, Migas MC, Waheed A, Britton RS, Bacon BR, Sly WS, Fleming RE (2002) Decreased liver hepcidin expression in the Hfe knockout mouse. *Blood Cells Mol Dis* 29:361–366.

Alexander J, Kowdley KV (2009) HFE-associated hereditary hemochromatosis. *Genet Med* 11:307–313.

Allen KJ, Gurrin LC, Constantine CC, Osborne NJ, Delatycki MB, Nicoll AJ, McLaren CE, Bahlo M, Nisselle AE, Vulpe CD, Anderson GJ, Southey MC, Giles GG, English DR, Hopper JL, Olynyk JK, Powell LW, Gertig DM (2008) Iron-overload-related disease in HFE hereditary hemochromatosis. *N Engl J Med* 358:221–230.

Anderson GJ, Frazer DM (2005) Hepatic iron metabolism. *Semin Liver Dis* 25:420–432.

Anderson GJ, Frazer DM, McKie AT, Wilkins SJ, Vulpe CD (2002) The expression and regulation of the iron transport molecules hephaestin and IREG1: implications for the control of iron export from the small intestine. *Cell Biochem Biophys* 36:137–146.

Arosio P, Ingrassia R, Cavadini P (2009) Ferritins: a family of molecules for iron storage, antioxidation and more. *Biochim Biophys Acta* 1790:589–599.

Aydemir F, Jenkitkasemwong S, Gulec S, Knutson MD (2009) Iron loading increases ferroportin heterogeneous nuclear RNA and mRNA levels in murine J774 macrophages. *J Nutr* 139:434–438.

Bacon BR, Powell LW, Adams PC, Kresina TF, Hoofnagle JH (1999) Molecular medicine and hemochromatosis: at the crossroads. *Gastroenterology* 116:193–207.

Boelen A, Kwakkel J, Alkemade A, Renckens R, Kaptein E, Kuiper G, Wiersinga WM, Visser TJ (2005) Induction of type 3 deiodinase activity in inflammatory cells of mice with chronic local inflammation. *Endocrinology* 146:5128–5134.

Briat JF, Ravet K, Arnaud N, Duc C, Boucherez J, Touraine B, Cellier F, Gaymard F (2010) New insights into ferritin synthesis and function highlight a link between iron homeostasis and oxidative stress in plants. *Ann Bot* 105:811–822.

Cairo G, Recalcati S, Mantovani A, Locati M (2011) Iron trafficking and metabolism in macrophages: contribution to the polarized phenotype. *Trends Immunol* 32:241–247.

Calzolari A, Larocca LM, Deaglio S, Finisguerra V, Boe A, Raggi C, Ricci-Vitani L, Pierconti F, Malavasi F, De Maria R, Testa U, Pallini R (2010) Transferrin receptor 2 is frequently and highly expressed in glioblastomas. *Transl Oncol* 3:123–134.

Camaschella C (2005) Understanding iron homeostasis through genetic analysis of hemochromatosis and related disorders. *Blood* 106:3710–3717.

Canonne-Hergaux F, Donovan A, Delaby C, Wang HJ, Gros P (2006) Comparative studies of duodenal and macrophage ferroportin proteins. *Am J Physiol Gastrointest Liver Physiol* 290:G156–G163.

Casey JL, Koeller DM, Ramin VC, Klausner RD, Harford JB (1989) Iron regulation of transferrin receptor mRNA levels requires iron-responsive elements and a rapid turnover determinant in the 3′ untranslated region of the mRNA. *EMBO J* 8:3693–3699.

Caskey JH, Jones C, Miller YE, Seligman PA (1983) Human ferritin gene is assigned to chromosome 19. *Proc Natl Acad Sci U S A* 80:482–486.

Chlosta S, Fishman DS, Harrington L, Johnson EE, Knutson MD, Wessling-Resnick M, Cherayil BJ (2006) The iron efflux protein ferroportin regulates the intracellular growth of Salmonella enterica. *Infect Immun* 74:3065–3067.

Christiansen H, Sheikh N, Saile B, Reuter F, Rave-Frank M, Hermann RM, Dudas J, Hille A, Hess CF, Ramadori G (2007) x-Irradiation in rat liver: consequent upregulation of hepcidin and downregulation of hemojuvelin and ferroportin-1 gene expression. *Radiology* 242:189–197.

Conner SD, Schmid SL (2003) Differential requirements for AP-2 in clathrin-mediated endocytosis. *J Cell Biol* 162:773–779.

Cozzi A, Corsi B, Levi S, Santambrogio P, Biasiotto G, Arosio P (2004) Analysis of the biologic functions of H- and L-ferritins in HeLa cells by transfection with siRNAs and cDNAs: evidence for a proliferative role of L-ferritin. *Blood* 103:2377–2383.

Crowe A, Morgan EH (1992) Iron and transferrin uptake by brain and cerebrospinal fluid in the rat. *Brain Res* 592:8–16.

Cui Y, Wu Q, Zhou Y (2009) Iron-refractory iron deficiency anemia: new molecular mechanisms. *Kidney Int* 76:1137–1141.

D'Anna MC, Veuthey TV, Roque ME (2009) Immunolocalization of ferroportin in healthy and anemic mice. *J Histochem Cytochem* 57:9–16.

De Domenico I, Lo E, Ward DM, Kaplan J (2010) Human mutation D157G in ferroportin leads to hepcidin-independent binding of Jak2 and ferroportin down-regulation. *Blood* 115:2956–2959.

di Patti MC, Persichini T, Mazzone V, Polticelli F, Colasanti M, Musci G (2004) Interleukin-1beta up-regulates iron efflux in rat C6 glioma cells through modulation of ceruloplasmin and ferroportin-1 synthesis. *Neurosci Lett* 363:182–186.

Donovan A, Brownlie A, Zhou Y, Shepard J, Pratt SJ, Moynihan J, Paw BH, Drejer A, Barut B, Zapata A, Law TC, Brugnara C, Lux SE, Pinkus GS, Pinkus JL, Kingsley PD, Palis J, Fleming MD, Andrews NC, Zon LI (2000) Positional cloning of zebrafish ferroportin1 identifies a conserved vertebrate iron exporter. *Nature* 403:776–781.

Donovan A, Lima CA, Pinkus JL, Pinkus GS, Zon LI, Robine S, Andrews NC (2005) The iron exporter ferroportin/Slc40a1 is essential for iron homeostasis. *Cell Metab* 1:191–200.

Dubois S, Kowdley KV (2004) Review article: targeted screening for hereditary haemochromatosis in high-risk groups. *Aliment Pharmacol Ther* 20:1–14.

Feder JN, Gnirke A, Thomas W, Tsuchihashi Z, Ruddy DA, Basava A, Dormishian F, Domingo R, Jr., Ellis MC, Fullan A, Hinton LM, Jones NL, Kimmel BE, Kronmal GS, Lauer P, Lee VK, Loeb DB, Mapa FA, McClelland E, Meyer NC, Mintier GA, Moeller N, Moore T, Morikang E, Prass CE, Quintana L, Starnes SM, Schatzman RC, Brunke KJ, Drayna DT, Risch NJ, Bacon BR, Wolff RK (1996) A novel MHC class I-like gene is mutated in patients with hereditary haemochromatosis. *Nat Genet* 13:399–408.

Frazer DM, Anderson GJ (2005) Iron imports. I. Intestinal iron absorption and its regulation. *Am J Physiol Gastrointest Liver Physiol* 289:G631–G635.

Gabay C, Kushner I (1999) Acute-phase proteins and other systemic responses to inflammation. *N Engl J Med* 340:448–54.

Ganz T (2005) Cellular iron: ferroportin is the only way out. *Cell Metab* 1:155–157.

Ganz T (2006) Hepcidin and its role in regulating systemic iron metabolism. *Hematology Am Soc Hematol Educ Program* 29–35, 507.

Ganz T (2011) Hepcidin and iron regulation, 10 years later. *Blood* 117:4425–4433.

Ganz T (2013) Systemic iron homeostasis. *Physiol Rev* 93:1721–1741.

Ganz T, Nemeth E (2006) Iron imports. IV. Hepcidin and regulation of body iron metabolism. *Am J Physiol Gastrointest Liver Physiol* 290:G199–G203.

Ganz T, Nemeth E (2012) Iron metabolism: interactions with normal and disordered erythropoiesis. *Cold Spring Harb Perspect Med* 2:a011668.

Gehrke SG, Kulaksiz H, Herrmann T, Riedel HD, Bents K, Veltkamp C, Stremmel W (2003) Expression of hepcidin in hereditary hemochromatosis: evidence for a regulation in response to the serum transferrin saturation and to non-transferrin-bound iron. *Blood* 102:371–376.

Gruenheid S, Canonne-Hergaux F, Gauthier S, Hackam DJ, Grinstein S, Gros P (1999) The iron transport protein NRAMP2 is an integral membrane glycoprotein that colocalizes with transferrin in recycling endosomes. *J Exp Med* 189:831–841.

Gunshin H, Mackenzie B, Berger UV, Gunshin Y, Romero MF, Boron WF, Nussberger S, Gollan JL, Hediger MA (1997) Cloning and characterization of a mammalian proton–coupled metal-ion transporter. *Nature* 388:482–488.

Han O, Kim EY (2007) Colocalization of ferroportin-1 with hephaestin on the basolateral membrane of human intestinal absorptive cells. *J Cell Biochem* 101:1000–1010.

Hentze MW, Muckenthaler MU, Andrews NC (2004) Balancing acts: molecular control of mammalian iron metabolism. *Cell* 117:285–297.

Hentze MW, Muckenthaler MU, Galy B, Camaschella C (2010) Two to tango: regulation of Mammalian iron metabolism. *Cell* 142:24–38.

Jandl JH, Inman JK, Simmons RL, Allen DW (1959) Transfer of iron from serum iron-binding protein to human reticulocytes. *J Clin Invest* 38:161–185.

Kalinowski DS, Richardson DR (2005) The evolution of iron chelators for the treatment of iron overload disease and cancer. *Pharmacol Rev* 57:547–583.

Krause A, Neitz S, Magert HJ, Schulz A, Forssmann WG, Schulz-Knappe P, Adermann K (2000) LEAP-1, a novel highly disulfide-bonded human peptide, exhibits antimicrobial activity. *FEBS Lett* 480:147–150.

Kuo YM, Su T, Chen H, Attieh Z, Syed BA, McKie AT, Anderson GJ, Gitschier J, Vulpe CD (2004) Mislocalisation of hephaestin, a multicopper ferroxidase involved in basolateral intestinal iron transport, in the sex linked anaemia mouse. *Gut* 53:201–206.

Lanzara C, Roetto A, Daraio F, Rivard S, Ficarella R, Simard H, Cox TM, Cazzola M, Piperno A, Gimenez-Roqueplo AP, Grammatico P, Volinia S, Gasparini P, Camaschella C (2004) Spectrum of hemojuvelin gene mutations in 1q-linked juvenile hemochromatosis. *Blood* 103:4317–4321.

Levy JE, Jin O, Fujiwara Y, Kuo F, Andrews NC (1999) Transferrin receptor is necessary for development of erythrocytes and the nervous system. *Nat Genet* 21:396–399.

Liu XB, Hill P, Haile DJ (2002) Role of the ferroportin iron-responsive element in iron and nitric oxide dependent gene regulation. *Blood Cells Mol Dis* 29:315–326.

Liu XB, Nguyen NB, Marquess KD, Yang F, Haile DJ (2005) Regulation of hepcidin and ferroportin expression by lipopolysaccharide in splenic macrophages. *Blood Cells Mol Dis* 35:47–56.

Magens B, Dullmann J, Schumann K, Wulfhekel U, Nielsen P (2005) Nuclear iron deposits in hepatocytes of iron-loaded HFE-knock-out mice: a morphometric and immunocyto-chemical analysis. *Acta Histochem* 107:57–65.

Malik IA, Naz N, Sheikh N, Khan S, Moriconi F, Blaschke M, Ramadori G (2011) Comparison of changes in gene expression of transferrin receptor-1 and other iron-regulatory proteins in rat liver and brain during acute-phase response. *Cell Tissue Res.*

McGrath H, Rigby PG (2004) Hepcidin: inflammation's iron curtain. *Rheumatology* 43:1323–1325.

McKie AT, Marciani P, Rolfs A, Brennan K, Wehr K, Barrow D, Miret S, Bomford A, Peters TJ, Farzaneh F, Hediger MA, Hentze MW, Simpson RJ (2000) A novel duodenal iron-regulated transporter, IREG1, implicated in the basolateral transfer of iron to the circulation. *Mol Cell* 5:299–309.

McKie AT, Barrow D, Latunde-Dada GO, Rolfs A, Sager G, Mudaly E, Mudaly M, Richardson C, Barlow D, Bomford A, Peters TJ, Raja KB, Shirali S, Hediger MA, Farzaneh F, Simpson RJ (2001) An iron-regulated ferric reductase associated with the absorption of dietary iron. *Science* 291:1755–1759.

Meyron-Holtz EG, Moshe-Belizowski S, Cohen LA (2011) A possible role for secreted ferritin in tissue iron distribution. *J Neural Transm* 118:337–347.

Morgan EH, Appleton TC (1969) Autoradiographic localization of 125-I–labelled transferrin in rabbit reticulocytes. *Nature* 223:1371–1372.

Moriconi F, Ahmad G, Ramadori P, Malik I, Sheikh N, Merli M, Riggio O, Dudas J, Ramadori G (2009) Phagocytosis of gadolinium chloride or zymosan induces simultaneous upregulation of hepcidin- and downregulation of hemojuvelin- and Fpn-1–gene expression in murine liver. *Lab Invest* 89:1252–1260.

Nairz M, Theurl I, Ludwiczek S, Theurl M, Mair SM, Fritsche G, Weiss G (2007) The co-ordinated regulation of iron homeostasis in murine macrophages limits the availability of iron for intracellular Salmonella typhimurium. *Cell Microbiol* 9:2126–2140.

Napier I, Ponka P, Richardson DR (2005) Iron trafficking in the mitochondrion: novel pathways revealed by disease. *Blood* 105:1867–1874.

Naz N, Malik IA, Sheikh N, Ahmad S, Khan S, Blaschke M, Schultze F, Ramadori G (2012) Ferroportin-1 is a 'nuclear'-negative acute-phase protein in rat liver: a comparison with other iron-transport proteins. *Lab Invest* 92:842–856.

Nemeth E, Rivera S, Gabayan V, Keller C, Taudorf S, Pedersen BK, Ganz T (2004a) IL-6 mediates hypoferremia of inflammation by inducing the synthesis of the iron regulatory hormone hepcidin. *J Clin Invest* 113:1271–1276.

Nemeth E, Tuttle MS, Powelson J, Vaughn MB, Donovan A, Ward DM, Ganz T, Kaplan J (2004b) Hepcidin regulates cellular iron efflux by binding to ferroportin and inducing its internalization. *Science* 306:2090–2093.

Olynyk JK, Trinder D, Ramm GA, Britton RS, Bacon BR (2008) Hereditary hemochromatosis in the post-HFE era. *Hepatology* 48:991–1001.

Park CH, Valore EV, Waring AJ, Ganz T (2001) Hepcidin, a urinary antimicrobial peptide synthesized in the liver. *J Biol Chem* 276:7806–7810.

Pietrangelo A (2006) Hereditary hemochromatosis. *Biochim Biophys Acta* 1763:700–710.

Pigeon C, Ilyin G, Courselaud B, Leroyer P, Turlin B, Brissot P, Loreal O (2001) A new mouse liver-specific gene, encoding a protein homologous to human antimicrobial peptide hepcidin, is overexpressed during iron overload. *J Biol Chem* 276:7811–7819.

Ponka P, Beaumont C, Richardson DR (1998) Function and regulation of transferrin and ferritin. *Semin Hematol* 35:35–54.

Ramadori G, Christ B (1999) Cytokines and the hepatic acute-phase response. *Semin Liver Dis* 19:141–155.

Ramadori G, Meyer Zum Buschenfelde KH, Tobias PS, Mathison JC, Ulevitch RJ (1990) Biosynthesis of lipopolysaccharide-binding protein in rabbit hepatocytes. *Pathobiology* 58:89–94.

Ramadori G, Sipe JD, Colten HR (1985) Expression and regulation of the murine serum amyloid A (SAA) gene in extrahepatic sites. *J Immunol* 135:3645–3647.

Ramadori P, Ahmad G, Ramadori G (2010) Cellular and molecular mechanisms regulating the hepatic erythropoietin expression during acute-phase response: a role for IL-6. *Lab Invest* 90:1306–1324.

Ramey G, Deschemin JC, Durel B, Canonne-Hergaux F, Nicolas G, Vaulont S (2010) Hepcidin targets ferroportin for degradation in hepatocytes. *Haematologica* 95:501–504.

Richardson DR, Lane DJ, Becker EM, Huang ML, Whitnall M, Suryo RY, Sheftel AD, Ponka P (2010) Mitochondrial iron trafficking and the integration of iron metabolism between the mitochondrion and cytosol. *Proc Natl Acad Sci U S A* 107:10775–10782.

Roetto A, Di CF, Pellegrino RM, Hirsch E, Azzolino O, Bondi A, Defilippi I, Carturan S, Miniscalco B, Riondato F, Cilloni D, Silengo L, Altruda F, Camaschella C, Saglio G (2010) Comparison of 3 Tfr2-deficient murine models suggests distinct functions for Tfr2-alpha and Tfr2-beta isoforms in different tissues. *Blood* 115:3382–3389.

Roth JA, Horbinski C, Feng L, Dolan KG, Higgins D, Garrick MD (2000) Differential localization of divalent metal transporter 1 with and without iron response element in rat PC12 and sympathetic neuronal cells. *J Neurosci* 20:7595–7601.

Rouault TA (2006) The role of iron regulatory proteins in mammalian iron homeostasis and disease. *Nat Chem Biol* 2:406–414.

Sammarco MC, Ditch S, Banerjee A, Grabczyk E (2008) Ferritin L and H subunits are differentially regulated on a post-transcriptional level. *J Biol Chem* 283:4578–4587.

Sheikh N, Batusic DS, Dudas J, Tron K, Neubauer K, Saile B, Ramadori G (2006) Hepcidin and hemojuvelin gene expression in rat liver damage: in vivo and in vitro studies. *Am J Physiol Gastrointest Liver Physiol* 291:G482–G490.

Sheikh N, Dudas J, Ramadori G (2007) Changes of gene expression of iron regulatory proteins during turpentine oil-induced acute-phase response in the rat. *Lab Invest* 87:713–725.

Simon M, Bourel M, Fauchet R, Genetet B (1976) Association of HLA-A3 and HLA-B14 antigens with idiopathic haemochromatosis. *Gut* 17:332–334.

Smith AG, Carthew P, Francis JE, Edwards RE, Dinsdale D (1990) Characterization and accumulation of ferritin in hepatocyte nuclei of mice with iron overload. *Hepatology* 12:1399–1405.

Song N, Wang J, Jiang H, Xie J (2010) Ferroportin 1 but not hephaestin contributes to iron accumulation in a cell model of Parkinson's disease. *Free Radic Biol Med* 48:332–341.

Stankiewicz J, Panter SS, Neema M, Arora A, Batt CE, Bakshi R (2007) Iron in chronic brain disorders: imaging and neurotherapeutic implications. *Neurotherapeutics* 4:371–386.

Tabuchi M, Yoshimori T, Yamaguchi K, Yoshida T, Kishi F (2000) Human NRAMP2/DMT1, which mediates iron transport across endosomal membranes, is localized to late endosomes and lysosomes in HEp-2 cells. *J Biol Chem* 275:22220–22228.

Tacchini L, Fusar PD, Bernelli-Zazzera A, Cairo G (2002) Transferrin receptor gene expression and transferrin-bound iron uptake are increased during postischemic rat liver reperfusion. *Hepatology* 36:103–111.

Trinder D, Fox C, Vautier G, Olynyk JK (2002) Molecular pathogenesis of iron overload. *Gut* 51:290–295.

Trinder D, Oates PS, Thomas C, Sadleir J, Morgan EH (2000) Localisation of divalent metal transporter 1 (DMT1) to the microvillus membrane of rat duodenal enterocytes in iron deficiency, but to hepatocytes in iron overload. *Gut* 46:270–276.

Tron K, Novosyadlyy R, Dudas J, Samoylenko A, Kietzmann T, Ramadori G (2005) Upregulation of heme oxygenase-1 gene by turpentine oil-induced localized inflammation: involvement of interleukin-6. *Lab Invest* 85:376–387.

Vulpe CD, Kuo YM, Murphy TL, Cowley L, Askwith C, Libina N, Gitschier J, Anderson GJ (1999) Hephaestin, a ceruloplasmin homologue implicated in intestinal iron transport, is defective in the sla mouse. *Nat Genet* 21:195–199.

Weiss G (2005) Modification of iron regulation by the inflammatory response. *Best Pract Res Clin Haematol* 18:183–201.

Wessling-Resnick M (2010) Iron homeostasis and the inflammatory response. *Annu Rev Nutr* 30:105–122.

Worwood M, Brook JD, Cragg SJ, Hellkuhl B, Jones BM, Perera P, Roberts SH, Shaw DJ (1985) Assignment of human ferritin genes to chromosomes 11 and 19q13.3–19qter. *Hum Genet* 69:371–374.

Wusteman M, Wight DG, Elia M (1990) Protein metabolism after injury with turpentine: a rat model for clinical trauma. *Am J Physiol* 259:E763–E769.

Yang F, Haile DJ, Wang X, Dailey LA, Stonehuerner JG, Ghio AJ (2005) Apical location of ferroportin 1 in airway epithelia and its role in iron detoxification in the lung. *Am J Physiol Lung Cell Mol Physiol* 289:L14–L23.

Yang F, Liu XB, Quinones M, Melby PC, Ghio A, Haile DJ (2002) Regulation of reticuloendothelial iron transporter MTP1 (Slc11a3) by inflammation. *J Biol Chem* 277:39786–39791.

Yeh KY, Yeh M, Mims L, Glass J (2009) Iron feeding induces ferroportin 1 and hephaestin migration and interaction in rat duodenal epithelium. *Am J Physiol Gastrointest Liver Physiol* 296:G55–G65.

Zhang DL, Hughes RM, Ollivierre-Wilson H, Ghosh MC, Rouault TA (2009) A ferroportin transcript that lacks an iron-responsive element enables duodenal and erythroid precursor cells to evade translational repression. *Cell Metab* 9:461–473.

Zhou XY, Tomatsu S, Fleming RE, Parkkila S, Waheed A, Jiang J, Fei Y, Brunt EM, Ruddy DA, Prass CE, Schatzman RC, OGÇÖNeill R, Britton RS, Bacon BR, Sly WS (1998) HFE gene knockout produces mouse model of hereditary hemochromatosis. *Proc Natl Acad Sci U S A* 95:2492–2497.

11 Diet and Lifestyle Changes as Treatment for Nonalcoholic Fatty Liver Disease

Shira Zelber-Sagi

CONTENTS

OBESITY AND WEIGHT GAIN

Nonalcoholic fatty liver disease (NAFLD) has been recognized as a major health burden. Estimates suggest that about 20% to 30% of adults in developed countries have excess fat accumulation in the liver (Zelber-Sagi et al., 2006; Bedogni and Bellentani, 2004; Bellentani et al., 2000; Falck-Ytter et al., 2001; Propst et al.,

1995), 50% among people with diabetes, and about 80% in obese and morbidly obese (Bellentani et al., 2000; Gupte et al., 2004; Del Gaudio et al., 2002). The U.S. National Health and Nutrition Examination Surveys data, collected from 1988 to 2008, show a 2-fold increased prevalence of NAFLD, along with the increasing prevalence of metabolic conditions as obesity and insulin resistance (Younossi et al., 2011). A 7-year prospective follow-up data emphasize the importance of even a modest weight change of 3–5 kg as an independent predictor for the development and remission of NAFLD (Zelber-Sagi et al., 2012). The importance of modest weight gain, as low as 2 kg, in the development of NAFLD is also demonstrated in two large Korean cohorts (Kim et al., 2009; Chang et al., 2009). Indeed, it has been demonstrated that insulin resistance already develops during weight gain within the normal range of body weight (Erdmann et al., 2008) and even modest weight gain results in increases in abdominal fat (Orr et al., 2008), which causes free fatty acid (FFA) levels to increase in the portal and peripheral circulations (Ruderman et al., 1998).

Because the efficacy and safety profile of pharmacotherapy in the treatment of NAFLD remains uncertain (Cheung and Sanyal, 2010) and obesity is strongly associated with hepatic steatosis (Koteish and Diehl, 2001), the first line of treatment remains lifestyle modification.

This chapter will discuss the existing epidemiological evidence for the association between human NAFLD and dietary composition, weight reduction, and physical activity (PA).

NUTRITIONAL COMPOSITION IN THE PREVENTION AND TREATMENT OF NAFLD

In light of the difficulty in reducing weight and maintaining the weight reduction in the long term (Katan, 2009), changing dietary composition without necessarily reducing caloric intake, may offer a more realistic and feasible alternative to treat NAFLD patients. Furthermore, an increasing number of patients have been described with normal body mass index, although these individuals may have central adiposity and occult insulin resistance (Chitturi et al., 2002; Pagano et al., 2002; Lee et al., 1998; Banerji et al., 1999). In fact, the prevalence of "lean NAFLD" is as high as 7% as indicated in data from National Health and Nutrition Examination Survey III in the United States (Younossi et al., 2012).

Moreover, epidemiological studies (Assy et al., 2008; Musso et al., 2003; Yasutake et al., 2009) indicate that this unique group of normal weight patients is characterized in particular with unhealthy dietary composition as will be discussed later.

DIETARY MACRONUTRIENTS

Multiple studies in animals have documented that a HFD rapidly induces hepatic steatosis (McCuskey et al., 2004; Samuel et al., 2004; Kim et al., 2003), but data in humans are scarce.

The association between total dietary fat and hepatic fat content has been directly tested in humans by placing 10 obese women on two successive 2-week isocaloric diets, which contained either 16% or 56% of energy from fat in randomized order using crossover design and assessing the liver fat by proton spectroscopy. Liver fat decreased by 20% during the low-fat diet and increased by 35% during the HFD. The changes in liver fat were paralleled by changes in fasting serum insulin concentrations. Importantly, these changes were independent of body weight that did not change during the study (Westerbacka et al., 2005). Similar effect was observed in men (Sobrecases et al., 2010).

In morbidly obese patients, dietary evaluation indicated that carbohydrate intake (above 54% of calories) was associated with significantly higher odds of inflammation, whereas higher fat intake was associated with significantly lower odds of inflammation on liver biopsy. However, this study was unable to discern any differences in specific dietary fat composition and did not differentiate between simple versus complex carbohydrates (Solga et al., 2004). The association with carbohydrates is supported and sharpened by a study from Japan comparing dietary habits between 28 patients with NASH and 18 with simple steatosis indicating an excess intake of carbohydrates, especially of sweets and not cereals, in the NASH group (Toshimitsu et al., 2007). In 63 morbid obese patients, high fatty liver disease fibrosis score (NFS) or elevated ALT were positively associated with excessive dietary intake of protein (>116 g/day), animal protein (>70 g/day), fat (>150 g/day), and carbohydrate (>394 g/day) (Ricci et al., 2011). Thus, it seems that overconsumption of fat, carbohydrates, and protein may be related to NAFLD pathogenesis and that all macronutrients should be consumed according to the accepted recommendations as part of a balanced diet. As demonstrated later in this chapter, the specific subtypes of fat (saturated versus unsaturated and its subgroups) and carbohydrates (complex versus simple and its subgroups) may be more important than their total amount.

Type of Dietary Fat

Contrary to cardiovascular disease, there is little epidemiological evidence that the type of dietary fat is associated with fatty liver (Bedogni and Bellentani, 2004). The diet of normal-weight NASH patients as compared with age-, gender-, and BMI-matched controls seems to be richer in saturated fat and cholesterol and poorer in polyunsaturated fat (Musso et al., 2003). These results are supported by another study in which the ratio polyunsaturated/saturated fatty acid intake in both the NASH and simple steatosis patients was lower than the ratio in randomly selected controls (Toshimitsu et al., 2007).

n-3 Polyunsaturated Fatty Acids

Different types of fats can have a protective effect in NAFLD. The most established one is the n-3 polyunsaturated fatty acid (n-3 PUFA).

Experimental studies have shown that diets enriched with n-3 PUFA increase insulin sensitivity in rats (Storlien et al., 1987), reduce intrahepatic triglyceride content, and ameliorate steatohepatitis (Sekiya et al., 2003; Levy et al., 2004).

Two observational studies provide evidence of a lower consumption of ω-3 PUFA among NAFLD patients. NASH patients, compared with a large sample of controls and matched for sex and age, had a significantly higher intake of n-6 fatty acids and n-6/n-3 ratio. An excessive amount of n-6 fatty acids could be implicated in promoting necro-inflammation (Cortez-Pinto et al., 2006). In a cross-sectional study of volunteers from the general population, those diagnosed with NAFLD had a significantly higher meat intake (p < 0.001) and a tendency (p = 0.056) to a lower intake of fish rich in n-3 PUFA. Since n-6 fatty acids are abundant in meat, these data suggest a higher intake of n-6/n-3 ratio in NAFLD patients (Zelber-Sagi et al., 2007).

Pilot clinical trials support the protective role of n-3 PUFA in NAFLD. A nonrandomized open-label controlled trial that assessed the effect of a one year n-3 PUFA supplementation (containing both eicosapentaenoic acid [EPA] and docosahexaenoic acid [DHA]) at a dose of 1000 mg/day in 42 NAFLD patients versus 14 patients who refused the treatment and were analyzed as controls. PUFA supplementation significantly decreased serum liver enzymes (ALT, AST, GGT) and reduced liver fat (as measured by ultrasonography) as compared with controls (Capanni et al., 2006). In a noncontrolled trial in 23 NASH patients who were supplemented with 2700 mg/day of EPA for 1 year, ALT levels were significantly improved. Seven of the 23 patients underwent posttreatment liver biopsy, which showed improvement of hepatic steatosis and fibrosis, hepatocyte ballooning, and lobular inflammation in six patients (Tanaka et al., 2008). In both trials, body weight remained unchanged.

A recent meta-analysis for studies pertaining to the effect of n-3 PUFA supplementation on NAFLD in humans included nine eligible studies that were heterogenic in study design (some uncontrolled and some controlled with or without placebo or alternative medication), population (mostly NAFLD, few with proven NASH and some dyslipidemic) duration (2–12 months), and dose (0.83–13.7 g). The data show that despite the significant heterogeneity, marine ω-3 fatty acid supplementation in humans is associated with a positive effect on liver fat, and this effect was also observed when only RCTs were included in analysis. However, when only RCT data were analyzed, there was no significant efficacy of PUFA therapy on ALT. The optimal dose of n-3 PUFA supplementation in NAFLD is currently unknown (Parker et al., 2012).

Trans-Fatty Acids

Little is known about the role of TFA in promoting liver injury in NAFLD. The association between *trans*-fatty acids (TFA) and increased risk of developing insulin resistance (Ibrahim et al., 2005) and coronary heart disease by raising LDL cholesterol levels, lowering HDL cholesterol levels, raising triglyceride levels, and increasing CRP (Hu et al., 1997) suggest that it may be involved in NAFLD pathogenesis.

Compared with PUFA- and saturated fatty acid-fed mice, TFA-fed mice had impaired glucose tolerance and NASH-like lesions (Machado et al., 2010). In another experiment in mice, isocaloric replacement of TFA with lard indicated that TFA played a major role in promoting hepatic steatosis and injury (Tetri et al., 2008). Therefore, the role of TFA in human NAFLD needs to be evaluated, facing a challenge to nutritional epidemiologists since information on TFA content in food is unknown in many cases.

Monounsaturated Fat

n-9 Oleic acid is the most prevalent monounsaturated fat (MUFA) in the diet, and olive oil is one of its major sources (other sources are nuts and avocado). Importantly for NAFLD patients, MUFA has been demonstrated to have favorable effect on lipid profile (Mensink et al., 2003). High-MUFA diets reduce fasting plasma triacylglycerol and VLDL-cholesterol concentrations by 19% and 22%, respectively, and cause a modest increase in HDL-cholesterol concentrations without adversely affecting LDL-cholesterol concentrations (Garg, 1998). In rats, olive oil was demonstrated to decrease the accumulation of triglycerides in the liver by 30% (Hussein et al., 2007), contributed to the recovery of the liver from hepatic steatosis (Hernandez et al., 2005) and protected against the development of fibrosis (Szende et al., 1994).

In a recent randomized parallel-group design trial, 37 men and 8 women with type 2 diabetes were assigned to two isocaloric diets: either high-carbohydrate, high-fiber diet or high-MUFA diet for an 8-week period. Liver fat content decreased more in the MUFA group (−29%) than in the CHO/fiber group (−4%), despite stable weight in both groups. The different dietary composition was carbohydrate, 52% versus 40%; fat, 30% versus 42%; and MUFA (mostly olive oil), 16% versus 28% for high-carbohydrate/high-fiber diet and MUFA diet, respectively. The other components, including the saturated fat (7%), protein (18%), and PUFA (4%), were similar in the two diets (Bozzetto et al., 2012). These results are in agreement with the benefits of a Mediterranean (MD) dietary pattern that were recently demonstrated among 12 non-diabetic NAFLD patients in a randomized, crossover 6-week dietary intervention. All subjects undertook both the MD and a control diet, a low-fat/high-carbohydrate diet (LF/HCD). There was a significant relative reduction in hepatic steatosis after the MD compared with the LF/HCD: 39% versus 7%, despite a very modest weight loss that was not different between the two diets. The MD diet was based on the traditional Cretan MD: olives, dried fruit, nuts, Greek yoghurt, fish, and olive oil. The approximate macronutrient composition of the diet was 40% energy from fat (MUFA and ω-3 PUFA) and 40% from carbohydrates. The LF/HCD was low in saturated and unsaturated fat and higher in carbohydrate than the MD. The approximate macronutrient composition was 30% of the energy from fat and 50% from carbohydrates (Ryan et al., 2013).

Cholesterol

In mice, excess cholesterol intake leads to the development of NAFLD, even in the absence of obesity (Wouters et al., 2008; Matsuzawa et al., 2007), and a diet containing 1% cholesterol induces steatohepatitis more than a simple high-fat diet (Savard et al., 2013).

However, results from observational studies have been conflicting. Some studies did not demonstrate different dietary intakes of cholesterol between NAFLD patients and controls (Cortez-Pinto et al., 2006; Zelber-Sagi et al., 2007), but Musso et al. (2003) did demonstrate a higher cholesterol consumption among normal weight NASH patients versus BMI-matched controls. A study that supports the role of dietary cholesterol in NAFLD compared 12 normal weight NAFLD patients with 44 obese NAFLD patients, demonstrating that dietary cholesterol intake was significantly higher, whereas the intake of PUFAs was significantly lower in the nonobese group. Therefore, this altered cholesterol and PUFA intake may be associated with the development of NAFLD in nonobese patients (Yasutake et al., 2009). In a large, nationally representative epidemiological study, dietary cholesterol consumption was independently associated with the development of cirrhosis (Ioannou et al., 2009). These findings may indicate that impairment of cholesterol regulation may have a causal relationship with liver steatogenesis. Indeed, excess intracellular cholesterol activates liver X receptor (LXRs), which regulates cholesterol homeostasis (Repa and Mangelsdorf, 2002) but induces hepatic steatosis (Fon Tacer and Rozman, 2011) by activating SREBP-1c, a master transcriptional regulator of fatty acid synthesis in the liver (Schultz et al., 2000; Chen et al., 2004).

Added Sugar, Fructose, and Soft Drinks

Simple carbohydrate refers to monosaccharides and disaccharides. The most common disaccharide is sucrose (glucose and fructose) found in sugar cane, sugar beets, honey, and corn syrup. The most common naturally occurring monosaccharide is fructose (found in fruits and vegetables). Naturally occurring sugar refers to the sugar that is an integral constituent of whole fruit, vegetable, and milk products, whereas added sugar refers to sucrose or other refined sugars in soft drinks and incorporated into food, fruit drinks, and other beverages (Howard and Wylie-Rosett, 2002).

Soft drinks are the leading source of added sugar in the world (Gaby, 2005). In recent decades, intake of sugar-sweetened beverages has increased around the globe (Brownell et al., 2009). Data from the years 2005 to 2006 show that children and adults in the United States consume 175 kcal/day from sugar-sweetened beverages (Duffey and Popkin, 2007), which is a little more than one can (330 cc) of sweetened soda or fruit juice a day (130–160 kcal) and contributes 9 teaspoons of sugar and/or fructose. The increasing quantity of fructose in the diet comes from sugar additives (most commonly sucrose and high-fructose corn syrup [HFCS]) in beverages and processed foods (Vos and Lavine, 2013).

The consumption of sugar-sweetened beverages, either soda or fruit juice, has been linked to risks for obesity, diabetes, metabolic syndrome, fatty liver, and heart disease, possibly by providing excess calories and large amounts of rapidly absorbable sugars (Schulze et al., 2004; Poulsom, 1986; Malik et al., 2006, 2010; Vartanian et al., 2007; Fung et al., 2009; Zelber-Sagi et al., 2007).

A sucrose-rich diet increases the hepatic synthesis of triglycerides. Rats and humans that are fed either sucrose- or fructose-enriched diets develop fatty livers (Poulsom, 1986; Herman et al., 1970; Sobrecases et al., 2010; Le et al., 2009). Therefore, it is reasonable to suggest that NAFLD patients should limit their fructose consumption (Cave et al., 2007). In addition, cola soft drinks contain caramel coloring, which is rich in advanced glycation end (AGEs) products that may increase insulin resistance and inflammation (Gaby, 2005). Fructose also seems to be associated with alteration in intestinal microflora, and a growing body of evidence supports a role for increased gut permeability and endotoxin in human NAFLD (Vos and Lavine, 2013). In animal studies, a high-fructose diet induces changes similar to those seen in models of chronic alcohol intake and high-fat diets, including increased gut permeability, endotoxemia, increased hepatic tumor necrosis factor (TNF) production, and hepatic steatosis (Vos and McClain, 2009). In mice, hepatic lipid accumulation, endotoxin levels in portal blood, lipid peroxidation, and TNF-α expression were significantly higher in mice consuming fructose compared with glucose, sucrose, or controls. Concomitant treatment of fructose fed mice with antibiotics markedly reduced hepatic lipid accumulation (Bergheim et al., 2008).

In recent years, several studies have been published on the association between soft drink consumption and NAFLD, demonstrating a positive association (Zelber-Sagi et al., 2007; Ouyang et al., 2008; Assy et al., 2008; Abid et al., 2009). In a subsample (n = 375) of the Israeli National Health and Nutrition Survey, NAFLD patients had a higher intake of soft drinks that was associated with an increased risk of NAFLD, independently of age, gender, BMI, and total calories (Zelber-Sagi et al., 2007). Similarly, the consumption of fructose containing beverages was 2-fold higher in NAFLD patients compared with controls matched for gender, age, and BMI (Ouyang et al., 2008). Furthermore, normal-weight NAFLD patients without classic risk factors compared with healthy controls consumed higher amounts of added sugar, most of it (43%) from soft drinks and juices as compared with only 8% in the controls (Assy et al., 2008).

A large-scale study of 427 NAFLD patients expanded the understanding of the hepatic damage that may be related to overconsumption of fructose-containing beverages. After controlling for age, sex, BMI, and total calorie intake, daily fructose-containing beverages consumption was significantly associated with higher fibrosis stage (OR = 3.2, 1.4–7.4, 95% CI for ≥7 servings versus <7 per week) (Abdelmalek et al., 2010). Recently, overweight subjects (n = 47) were randomly assigned to four different test drinks (1 L/day for 6 months): regular cola, isocaloric semi-skimmed milk, aspartame-sweetened diet cola, and water. The relative change in liver fat between baseline and the end of 6-month intervention was significantly higher in the regular cola group than in the three other groups (132%–143%) (Maersk et al., 2012).

Questions that remain controversial are whether in a regular human diet fructose alone has more deleterious hepatic implications as compared with fructose combined with glucose (in the form of sucrose)? Experimental short-term overfeeding with fructose or glucose in healthy young males led to a similar intrahepatic fat deposition (Ngo Sock et al., 2010). However, in a nonexperimental diet, pure fructose is rarely consumed because processed and natural foods mostly containing a mixture of fructose and glucose. Because of this, studies that use the typically consumed substances (sucrose or HFCS) are more relevant to "real life" (Vos and Lavine, 2013). Another question is if it matters whether fructose is delivered as free fructose (e.g., HFCS) or as a disaccharide (sucrose). Observational "real-life" studies (Zelber-Sagi et al., 2007; Abid et al., 2009; Abdelmalek et al., 2010) reporting an association between soft drinks and NAFLD could not differentiate among consumption of sucrose, glucose, fructose, or HFCS that are all found, alone, or in combination in common soft drinks.

In summary, studies performed so far identified soft drinks as an important modifiable risk factor. Physicians and dietitians should routinely include questions regarding soft drink consumption as part of the patient's history and advise patients to avoid it.

WESTERN DIETARY PATTERN AND FAST FOOD

Examination of overall dietary patterns would more closely parallel the real world, where people eat meals consisting of a variety of foods with complex combinations of nutrients that may be interactive or synergistic (Hu et al., 2000). The studies presented above regarding dietary composition usually indicate on several nutrients or foods that characterize the dietary intake of NAFLD patients and may be looked at as a pattern of unhealthy or Western dietary pattern. This pattern includes overconsumption of fructose and soft drinks (Zelber-Sagi et al., 2007; Assy et al., 2008; Ouyang et al., 2008) along with lower consumption of fiber (Cortez-Pinto et al., 2006) plus overconsumption of meat (Zelber-Sagi et al., 2007) or saturated fat and cholesterol (Musso et al., 2003; Yasutake et al., 2009) along with lower consumption of fish or ω-3 fatty acids (Zelber-Sagi et al., 2007; Cortez-Pinto et al., 2006) or PUFA (Yasutake et al., 2009) and lower consumption of some vitamins (Musso et al., 2003) that may indicate below recommended consumption of vegetables and an unbalanced diet in general.

Fast-food consumption has strong positive associations with weight gain and insulin resistance in humans (Pereira et al., 2005). In men, 7 days of excess fat, fructose, and fat-plus-fructose intakes increased hepatic steatosis, but the combination increased hepatic steatosis more than either alone and also prevented the increase in hepatic VLDL secretion seen with isolated fructose overfeeding (Sobrecases et al., 2010). Healthy young students that were put on a fast-food diet (at least two fast-food meals/day) during 4 weeks increased their hepatic triglyceride content, and within only 1 week, 11 out of 15 with normal ALT levels at baseline had elevated ALT levels. Thus, in clinical evaluations of subjects with elevated ALT levels, medical history should include not only questions about alcohol and soft drink intake but also explore whether recent excessive intake of fast food has occurred (Kechagias et al., 2008).

Potential mechanisms of fast-food hepatoxicity are high energy density and portion size, high fat and saturated fat, high refined carbohydrate, low fiber, high fructose corn syrup, caramel coloring, red meat, industrially produced *trans*-fatty acids, all together promoting free fatty acid overflow to the liver and local inflammation (Marchesini et al., 2008).

DIFFERENT WEIGHT REDUCTION REGIMENS IN THE TREATMENT OF NAFLD

The usual management of NAFLD includes gradual weight reduction and increased PA leading to an improvement in serum liver enzymes, reduced hepatic fatty infiltration, and in some cases, a reduced degree of hepatic inflammation and fibrosis (Andersen et al., 1991; Dixon et al., 2004; Eriksson et al., 1986; Luyckx et al., 1998; Palmer and Schaffner, 1990; Ueno et al., 1997; Shah et al., 2009). However, most studies did not include repeated liver biopsy and, thus, histological improvement could not be determined.

Are Very Low Calorie Diets Effective?

Small sample trials from the 1960s (Rozental et al., 1967) and 1970s (Drenick et al., 1970) included fasting or very low calorie diet (about 500 kcal), leading to drastic weight reduction. Steatosis was reduced in all patients, but liver damage, as indicated by fibrosis and focal necrosis, was observed in some patients during the acute weight loss. In a later study from 1991, Andersen et al. provided 41 morbidly obese patients with a 400-kcal formula-based diet, leading again to improved steatosis. However, 24% developed slight portal inflammation (p = 0.04) or slight portal fibrosis (p = 0.06). This study helps in setting the upper limit for the rate of weight reduction in NAFLD patients because none of the patients who lost less than 1.6 kg/week developed fibrosis. Interestingly, liver biochemistry improved regardless of the histological changes (Andersen et al., 1991). In another study with very-low-calorie diet, a weight reduction of greater than or equal to 10% normalized abnormal hepatic test results in most patients; however, liver biopsies were not obtained (Palmer and Schaffner, 1990). Because very-low-calorie diets did not show advantage over moderately low-calorie diets in the long term (Tsai and Wadden, 2006), are very difficult to maintain, and might lead to hepatic damage in some patients, they usually cannot be recommended to NAFLD patients.

Balanced Diets and Gradual Weight Reduction

Pilot uncontrolled or nonrandomized small sample size studies that had histological outcome demonstrated a beneficial effect of a balanced diet. A 3-month gradual weight reduction resulted in reduced hepatic steatosis, inflammation, and a tendency for fibrosis, although not significant (Ueno et al., 1997). In a longer 1-year trial, 9 out of 15 patients who lost an average of 7% of their body weight had an improved NASH score (Huang et al., 2005).

In a randomized controlled trial, 32 NASH patients were randomized to receive intensive 48 weeks of lifestyle intervention or basic education about healthy lifestyle (controls). The moderate, balanced diet was combined with moderate-intensity activities, with particular emphasis on walking with pedometers. NASH histological activity score (NAS) improved significantly in the treatment arm. Participants who achieved weight loss of >7% compared with those who lost less than 7% had significant improvements in steatosis, lobular inflammation, ballooning injury, and NAS (Promrat et al., 2010). In the orlistat trial by Harrison et al. (2009), a somewhat bigger weight reduction of at least 9% was necessary to achieve significant improvement in NAS, although 5% reduction was sufficient for improving steatosis. Recently, another RCT tested the effect of a 12-month intensive lifestyle intervention on hepatic steatosis in a specific subgroup of patients with type 2 diabetes. The intervention included a moderate caloric restriction plus increased PA and weekly meetings, whereas the control group received only general information on nutrition and PA. After 12 months, participants assigned to the intensive intervention as compared with controls lost more weight (−8.5% versus −0.05%; p < 0.01) and had a greater decline in steatosis (−50.8% versus −22.8%, p = 0.04). Furthermore, a dose–response relationship was observed with weight loss, with the greatest reduction, of 80% steatosis, observed in those with the greatest weight loss (10% or more). The intervention was also beneficial in prevention of NAFLD as 26% of controls versus 3% of intervention participants, without NAFLD at baseline, developed NAFLD at 12 months (Lazo et al., 2010).

Three recent, relatively large sample size studies, addressed the effect of diet, provided in different settings, on ALT levels (St George et al., 2009a; Suzuki et al.,

2005; Oza et al., 2009). In the trial by Suzuki et al. (2005), 348 male subjects with elevated ALT were recruited from annual health checkups and were given health-care instructions using customized brochures and then followed at health checkups three times a year. At 1-year follow-up, all subjects achieving ≥5% weight reduc-tion showed improvement in serum ALT and 136 subjects had ALT normalization (Suzuki et al., 2005). In the second trial, 152 patients with elevated liver enzymes were randomized to either a moderate (6 sessions/10 weeks) or low-intensity (3 sessions/4 weeks) lifestyle counseling intervention or control group. Reduction in liver enzymes was greatest in the moderate-intensity intervention group and the least in the control group, in parallel to the proportion of subjects achieving weight loss (St George et al., 2009a). In the third trial, with a smaller sample size, 67 patients with NAFLD were enrolled into a 6-month home-based lifestyle modification inter-vention that included monthly visits with a physician and nutritional counseling every 3 months. At 6 months, there were significant improvements in terms of body weight, liver/spleen ratio, and liver enzymes. This study's flaw was a large attrition rate with only 22 patients (33%) completing the 6-month intervention (Oza et al., 2009), perhaps indicating that patients require a more intensive follow-up.

In summary, a recent meta-analysis of 23 trials (6 randomized, 5 with repeated liver biopsy) concludes that lifestyle modifications leading to weight reduction and/ or increased PA consistently reduced liver fat, and limited data also suggest benefits for liver histopathology (Thoma et al., 2012).

ARE LOW-CARBOHYDRATE DIETS BETTER THAN LOW-FAT DIETS?

In general, low-carbohydrate diets have been shown to be at least as effective as low-fat diets in inducing long-term weight loss and to confer favorable changes in tri-glyceride and high-density lipoprotein cholesterol and unfavorable changes in low-density lipoprotein cholesterol (Nordmann et al., 2006).

On the short term, low carbohydrates may seem more effective in reducing liver fat. Obese insulin-resistant individuals randomized to 16 weeks' hypocaloric diets containing either 60% carbohydrate/25% fat or 40% carbohydrate/45% fat had a greater decrease in ALT levels with the low carbohydrate diet that correlated with a greater decline in daylong insulin concentrations, despite equal weight loss (Ryan et al., 2007). In a shorter-term study, during 2 weeks of diet, liver triglycerides decreased significantly more in carbohydrate-restricted diet than in calorie-restricted diet (Browning et al., 2011). At 48 h, intrahepatic lipid content has been shown to decrease more with low-carbohydrate diet versus a low-fat diet, but reduction was similar in both diets after 7% weight loss (Kirk et al., 2009).

In a large long-term RCT, a total of 102 overweight and obese subjects were ran-domized to 6 months' reduced carbohydrate (<90 g carbohydrates and a minimum of 30% fat of total energy intake) or reduced fat (<20% fat of total energy intake), both energy-restricted diets (70% of regular-energy intake). Significant reductions were observed in both diets in intrahepatic lipid content and alanine aminotransfer-ase without any difference between the two diet regimens. Thus, it seems that a pro-longed hypocaloric diet low in carbohydrates and high in fat has the same beneficial effects on intrahepatic lipid accumulation as the traditional low-fat hypocaloric diet

(Haufe et al., 2011). It should be mentioned that in both diets, there was a reduction in saturated fat intake and patients received information on healthy food choices. In summary, there is presently no convincing evidence that over the long-term low carbohydrates diets are better than low-fat diets, and the diet of choice should be the one that individuals are able to adhere for years rather than weeks (Boden, 2009).

HOW MUCH PA IS ENOUGH AND WHICH TYPE IS MOST EFFECTIVE?

PA has been shown to reduce the risk of type 2 diabetes mellitus, insulin resistance, hypertension, dyslipidemia, impaired fasting glucose (IFG), and the metabolic syndrome (Bassuk and Manson, 2005; LaMonte et al., 2005; Bauman, 2004; Pan et al., 1997), all strongly associated with NAFLD. PA benefits NAFLD beyond encouraging weight reduction. Exercise alone, in the absence of any change in body weight or composition, may enhance insulin sensitivity and glucose homeostasis (Boule et al., 2001). Exercise also has a beneficial effect on free fatty acid (FFA) metabolism by enhancing whole-body lipid oxidation (Hannukainen et al., 2007) and reducing hepatic FFA uptake (Iozzo et al., 2004).

OBSERVATIONAL STUDIES

Several observational studies indicated an inverse association between reported leisure time PA or cardiorespiratory fitness and the prevalence of NAFLD or hepatic fat content independently of body mass index) (Magkos, 2010).

In a large-scale study with 191 participants, a higher reported level of habitual PA was associated with a lower intrahepatic fat content regardless of BMI, insulin resistance, and circulating adiponectin levels (Perseghin et al., 2007). Similar results were demonstrated in another study (n = 349) of the general population in which the NAFLD group engaged in less reported leisure time PA including total, aerobic, and resistance training (RT). The association between NAFLD and engaging in any kind of PA remained significant after adjusting for insulin resistance and circulating adiponectin plus nutritional factors but not BMI. Only the association with resistance PA remained significant with further adjustment for BMI (Zelber-Sagi et al., 2008). Another study (n = 218 men) demonstrated an inverse association between fitness categories and the prevalence of NAFLD regardless of BMI (Church et al., 2006).

Few studies tested the association with liver histology. In a small study on 37 NAFLD patients with liver biopsy, there was a lower cardiorespiratory fitness among patients with higher NAFLD activity score and NASH versus no NASH (Krasnoff et al., 2008). Exercise intensity and histological severity of NAFLD was tested in a large cohort of adults with biopsy-proven NAFLD. Self-reported PA was classified according to the accepted recommendations for either moderate or vigorous intensity exercise. Moderate-intensity exercise was not associated with NASH or stage of fibrosis. However, meeting vigorous recommendations was associated with a decreased BMI-adjusted risk of having NASH in both minimum (≥75 min/week) and extensive time (≥150 min/week) of PA (in 35% and 44%, respectively). However, only extensive time spent in vigorous exercise was sufficient for a reduced risk of advanced fibrosis in almost 50% (Kistler et al., 2011).

CLINICAL TRIALS WITH AEROBIC TRAINING

The beneficial effect of exercise is supported by clinical trials and by a recent meta-analysis concluding that "there is a clear evidence for a benefit of exercise therapy on liver fat with minimal or no weight loss and at exercise levels below current exercise recommendations for obesity management" (Keating et al., 2012). However, the ability of exercise alone to improve other aspects of liver histology remains unknown (Chalasani et al., 2012).

One of the first trials included 141 patients with suspected NAFLD based on abnormal liver enzymes in which those who increased their PA by ≥60 min per week (n = 85) significantly reduced weight (−2.4 kg on average), HOMA, and all liver enzymes. Importantly, these improvements were independent of the change in weight (St George et al., 2009b). Thus, it seems that among NAFLD patients, even small increments in regular PA can improve liver enzymes. Another RCT assessed the effect of a short-term 4-week aerobic exercise training (3 cycle sessions per week of 30–45 min each versus stretching) in 19 sedentary obese men and women resulting in s reduction of 21% in hepatic triglyceride concentration along with reduction in visceral adipose tissue volume by 12% and 14% reduction in plasma free fatty acids. Importantly, no change in weight or dietary intake was noted, thus isolating the net effect of aerobic exercise (Johnson et al., 2009). Two other clinical trials one in obese adolescents (van der Heijden et al., 2009) and the other in healthy elderly (Finucane et al., 2010) support the beneficial effect of aerobic exercise. A 12-week aerobic exercise led to about 35% reduction in hepatic fat without diet or weight loss.

CLINICAL TRIALS WITH RT

In recent years, increasing attention has been paid to RT as a useful adjunctive tool of exercise (Albright et al., 2000; Pollock et al., 2000). RT, without a concomitant weight loss diet, improves insulin sensitivity and fasting glycemia and decreases abdominal fat (Ibanez et al., 2005). Tsuzuku et al. (2007) demonstrated that non-instrumental RT, using body weight as a load, appears to be effective in decreasing visceral fat and improving metabolic profiles, without weight loss. The results of a randomized trial comparing the effect of aerobic versus RT on coronary risk factors, demonstrated that only the RT group showed a reduction in total body fat with an associated increase in lean body mass (Banz et al., 2003). A meta-analysis comparing aerobic training with weight training concluded that weight training resulted in greater increases in fat-free mass (Ballor and Keesey, 1991). An increase in muscle mass may improve insulin sensitivity by increasing the available glucose storage area, thereby reducing the amount of insulin required to maintain a normal glucose tolerance (Miller et al., 1984).

Two small trials found beneficial effects for RT as a single treatment in NAFLD patients, but results regarding reduction in steatosis were conflicting (van der Heijden et al., 2010; Hallsworth et al., 2011). In RCT including 19 sedentary adult NAFLD patients, 8 weeks of RT consisting of 45 min sessions trice weekly led to a reduction in liver fat without weight loss, but this was only significant within group (Hallsworth et al., 2011). In an uncontrolled clinical trial including 12 obese adolescents, a 3-month RT program consisting of 1-h sessions twice weekly did not change hepatic fat content but improved hepatic insulin sensitivity (van der Heijden et al., 2010).

In a large RCT that compared the effect of 8 months of aerobic training versus RT and versus the combination of both in overweight sedentary subjects, aerobic training led to significant reductions in liver fat and alanine aminotransferase, whereas RT did not. The effect of the combined training was statistically indistinguishable from the effect of aerobic training alone (Slentz et al., 2011). However, the aerobic training and the combined training groups lost small but significant body weight (2 kg), whereas the RT group did not, a difference that may partially explain the difference in outcomes.

Although aerobic exercise seems to have more extensive effects, a longer duration and/or a more intensive resistance exercise program may be required for reduction of hepatic fat content. For those who have physical limitations or low motivation that prevents them from performance of aerobic PA, resistance exercise can serve as an alternative option.

PREVENTION IS BETTER THAN CURE

NAFLD is not only a cause of chronic liver disease but might also predict the tendency to develop diabetes mellitus (Vozarova et al., 2002; Hanley et al., 2004; Wannamethee et al., 2005) and recently was suggested to be associated with coronary artery disease as well (Marchesini and Forlani, 2002; Fracanzani et al., 2006; Ekstedt et al., 2006; Villanova et al., 2005; Targher et al., 2005; Jepsen et al., 2003; Kessler et al., 2005). In a recent randomized trial, participants who were at high cardiovascular risk, somewhat similar to most NAFLD patients, received either a Mediterranean diet supplemented with extra-virgin olive oil, a Mediterranean diet supplemented with mixed nuts, or a control diet (advice to reduce dietary fat) with a median follow-up of 4.8 years. The Mediterranean diet supplemented with extra-virgin olive oil or nuts reduced the incidence of major cardiovascular events in about 30% as compared with the standard low-fat diet (Estruch et al., 2013). Future studies should focus on testing the potential for prevention of cardiovascular disease among NAFLD patients by lifestyle changes.

SUMMARY AND IMPLICATIONS

Nutrition has been demonstrated to be associated with NAFLD and NASH in both animals (Poulsom, 1986; Bogin et al., 1986), and humans (Zelber-Sagi et al., 2011) and thus serves as a major route of prevention and treatment. Based on available data patients should optimally achieve a 5%–10% weight reduction. A position statement by the EASL on NAFLD/NASH (Ratziu et al., 2010) recommended on a weight loss of 7%, as proposed by international societies on the basis of an extensive body of literature. An American Association for the Study of Liver Diseases (AASLD) Practice

Guideline indicate that loss of at least 3%–5% of body weight appears necessary to improve steatosis, but a greater weight loss (up to 10%) may be needed to improve necro-inflammation (Chalasani et al., 2012).

Setting realistic goals is essential for long-term successful lifestyle modification (Fabricatore, 2007; Anderson, 2000) because obese patients tend to have unrealistic weight loss expectations (about 25%–35%) that, if unmet, lead to adverse effects such as lower satisfaction with treatment and a lower self-esteem (Wadden et al., 2001). More effort must be devoted to informing NAFLD patients of the health benefits of even a modest weight reduction, and feedback should be provided not only on weight loss but also on individual changes in behavior and risk factors (Anderson, 2000).

Furthermore, all NAFLD patients, whether obese or of normal weight, should be informed that a healthy diet has benefits beyond weight reduction. They should be advised to reduce saturated/*trans*-fat and increase polyunsaturated ω-3 fatty acids. They should reduce added sugar to its minimum, try to avoid soft drinks containing sugar/fructose including fruit juices that contain a lot of fructose, and increase fiber intake. For the heavy meat eaters, especially those of red and processed meats, less meat and increased fish intake should be recommended. Minimizing fast-food intake will also help maintain a healthy diet. PA should be integrated into behavioral therapy in NAFLD as even small gains in PA and fitness may have significant health benefits.

A combination of educational, behavioral, and motivational strategies is required to help patients achieve lifestyle change (Anderson, 2000), preferably by multidisciplinary teams including dietitians, psychologists, and PA supervisors (Marchesini et al., 2008; Bellentani et al., 2008).

REFERENCES

Abdelmalek, M. F., A. Suzuki, C. Guy et al. 2010. Increased fructose consumption is associated with fibrosis severity in patients with nonalcoholic fatty liver disease. *Hepatology* 51:1961–71.

Abid, A., O. Taha, W. Nseir, R. Farah, M. Grosovski, and N. Assy. 2009. Soft drink consumption is associated with fatty liver disease independent of metabolic syndrome. *J Hepatol* 51:918–24.

Albright, A., M. Franz, G. Hornsby et al. 2000. American College of Sports Medicine position stand. Exercise and type 2 diabetes. *Med Sci Sports Exerc* 32:1345–60.

Andersen, T., C. Gluud, M. B. Franzmann, and P. Christoffersen. 1991. Hepatic effects of dietary weight loss in morbidly obese subjects. *J Hepatol* 12:224–9.

Anderson, A. S. 2000. How to implement dietary changes to prevent the development of metabolic syndrome. *Br J Nutr* 83:S165–8.

Assy, N., G. Nasser, I. Kamayse et al. 2008. Soft drink consumption linked with fatty liver in the absence of traditional risk factors. *Can J Gastroenterol* 22:811–6.

Ballor, D. L., and R. E. Keesey. 1991. A meta-analysis of the factors affecting exercise-induced changes in body mass, fat mass and fat-free mass in males and females. *International Journal of Obesity* 15:717–26.

Banerji, M. A., N. Faridi, R. Atluri, R. L. Chaiken, and H. E. Lebovitz. 1999. Body composition, visceral fat, leptin, and insulin resistance in Asian Indian men. *J Clin Endocrinol Metab* 84:137–44.

Banz, W. J., M. A. Maher, W. G. Thompson et al. 2003. Effects of resistance versus aerobic training on coronary artery disease risk factors. *Exp Biol Med (Maywood)* 228:434–40.

Bassuk, S. S., and J. E. Manson. 2005. Epidemiological evidence for the role of physical activity in reducing risk of type 2 diabetes and cardiovascular disease. *J Appl Physiol* 99:1193–204.

Bauman, A. E. 2004. Updating the evidence that physical activity is good for health: an epidemiological review 2000–2003. *J Sci Med Sport* 7:6–19.

Bedogni, G., and S. Bellentani. 2004. Fatty liver: how frequent is it and why? *Ann Hepatol* 3:63–65.

Bellentani, S., R. Dalle Grave, A. Suppini, and G. Marchesini. 2008. Behavior therapy for nonalcoholic fatty liver disease: the need for a multidisciplinary approach. *Hepatology* 47:746–54.

Bellentani, S., G. Saccoccio, F. Masutti et al. 2000. Prevalence of and risk factors for hepatic steatosis in Northern Italy. *Ann Intern Med* 132:112–7.

Bergheim, I., S. Weber, M. Vos et al. 2008. Antibiotics protect against fructose-induced hepatic lipid accumulation in mice: role of endotoxin. *J Hepatol* 48:983–92.

Boden, G. 2009. High- or low-carbohydrate diets: which is better for weight loss, insulin resistance, and fatty livers? *Gastroenterology* 136:1490–2.

Bogin, E., Y. Avidar, and M. Merom. 1986. Biochemical changes in liver and blood during liver fattening in rats. *J Clin Chem Clin Biochem* 24:621–6.

Boule, N. G., E. Haddad, G. P. Kenny, G. A. Wells, and R. J. Sigal. 2001. Effects of exercise on glycemic control and body mass in type 2 diabetes mellitus: a meta-analysis of controlled clinical trials. *JAMA* 286:1218–27.

Bozzetto, L., A. Prinster, G. Annuzzi et al. 2012. Liver fat is reduced by an isoenergetic MUFA diet in a controlled randomized study in type 2 diabetic patients. *Diabetes Care* 35:1429–35.

Brownell, K. D., T. Farley, W. C. Willett et al. 2009. The public health and economic benefits of taxing sugar-sweetened beverages. *N Engl J Med* 361:1599–605.

Browning, J. D., J. A. Baker, T. Rogers, J. Davis, S. Satapati, and S. C. Burgess. 2011. Short-term weight loss and hepatic triglyceride reduction: evidence of a metabolic advantage with dietary carbohydrate restriction. *Am J Clin Nutr* 93:1048–52.

Capanni, M., F. Calella, M. R. Biagini et al. 2006. Prolonged n-3 polyunsaturated fatty acid supplementation ameliorates hepatic steatosis in patients with non-alcoholic fatty liver disease: a pilot study. *Aliment Pharmacol Ther* 23:1143–51.

Cave, M., I. Deaciuc, C. Mendez et al. 2007. Nonalcoholic fatty liver disease: predisposing factors and the role of nutrition. *J Nutr Biochem* 18:184–95.

Chalasani, N., Z. Younossi, J. E. Lavine et al. 2012. The diagnosis and management of non-alcoholic fatty liver disease: practice Guideline by the American Association for the Study of Liver Diseases, American College of Gastroenterology, and the American Gastroenterological Association. *Hepatology* 55:2005–23.

Chang, Y., S. Ryu, E. Sung et al. 2009. Weight gain within the normal weight range predicts ultrasonographically detected fatty liver in healthy Korean men. *Gut* 58:1419–25.

Chen, G., G. Liang, J. Ou, J. L. Goldstein, and M. S. Brown. 2004. Central role for liver X receptor in insulin-mediated activation of Srebp-1c transcription and stimulation of fatty acid synthesis in liver. *Proc Natl Acad Sci USA* 101:11245–50.

Cheung, O., and A. J. Sanyal. 2010. Recent advances in nonalcoholic fatty liver disease. *Curr Opin Gastroenterol* 26:202–8.

Chitturi, S., S. Abeygunasekera, G. C. Farrell et al. 2002. NASH and insulin resistance: insulin hypersecretion and specific association with the insulin resistance syndrome. *Hepatology* 35:373–9.

Church, T. S., J. L. Kuk, R. Ross, E. L. Priest, E. Biltoft, and S. N. Blair. 2006. Association of cardiorespiratory fitness, body mass index, and waist circumference to nonalcoholic fatty liver disease. *Gastroenterology* 130:2023–30.

Cortez-Pinto, H., L. Jesus, H. Barros, C. Lopes, M. C. Moura, and M. E. Camilo. 2006. How different is the dietary pattern in non-alcoholic steatohepatitis patients? *Clin Nutr* 25:816–23.

Del Gaudio, A., L. Boschi, G. A. Del Gaudio, L. Mastrangelo, and D. Munari. 2002. Liver damage in obese patients. *Obes Surg* 12:802–4.

Dixon, J. B., P. S. Bhathal, N. R. Hughes, and P. E. O'Brien. 2004. Nonalcoholic fatty liver disease: Improvement in liver histological analysis with weight loss. *Hepatology* 39:1647–54.

Drenick, E. J., F. Simmons, and J. F. Murphy. 1970. Effect on hepatic morphology of treatment of obesity by fasting, reducing diets and small-bowel bypass. *N Engl J Med* 282:829–34.

Duffey, K. J., and B. M. Popkin. 2007. Shifts in patterns and consumption of beverages between 1965 and 2002. *Obesity (Silver Spring)* 15:2739–47.

Ekstedt, M., L. E. Franzén, U. L. Mathiesen, M. Holmqvist, G. Bodemar, and S. Kechagias. 2006. Survival and causes of death in patients with elevated liver enzymes associated with NAFLD. *J Hepatol* 44:S40.

Erdmann, J., B. Kallabis, U. Oppel, O. Sypchenko, S. Wagenpfeil, and V. Schusdziarra. 2008. Development of hyperinsulinemia and insulin resistance during the early stage of weight gain. *Am J Physiol Endocrinol Metab* 294:E568–75.

Eriksson, S., K. F. Eriksson, and L. Bondesson. 1986. Nonalcoholic steatohepatitis in obesity: a reversible condition. *Acta Med Scand* 220:83–88.

Estruch, R., E. Ros, J. Salas-Salvado et al. 2013. Primary prevention of cardiovascular disease with a Mediterranean diet. *N Engl J Med* 368:1279–90.

Fabricatore, A. N. 2007. Behavior therapy and cognitive-behavioral therapy of obesity: is there a difference? *J Am Diet Assoc* 107:92–9.

Falck-Ytter, Y., Z. M. Younossi, G. Marchesini, and A. J. McCullough. 2001. Clinical features and natural history of nonalcoholic steatosis syndromes. *Semin Liver Dis* 21:17–26.

Finucane, F. M., S. J. Sharp, L. R. Purslow et al. 2010. The effects of aerobic exercise on metabolic risk, insulin sensitivity and intrahepatic lipid in healthy older people from the Hertfordshire Cohort Study: a randomised controlled trial. *Diabetologia* 53:624–31.

Fon Tacer, K., and D. Rozman. 2011. Nonalcoholic Fatty liver disease: focus on lipoprotein and lipid deregulation. *J Lipids* 2011:783976.

Fracanzani, A. L., L. Burdick, S. Rasselli et al. 2006. Risk of early atherosclerosis evaluated by carotid artery intima-media thickness in patients with NAFLD: a case control study. *J Hepatol* 44:S39.

Fung, T. T., V. Malik, K. M. Rexrode, J. E. Manson, W. C. Willett, and F. B. Hu. 2009. Sweetened beverage consumption and risk of coronary heart disease in women. *Am J Clin Nutr* 89:1037–42.

Gaby, A. R. 2005. Adverse effects of dietary fructose. *Altern Med Rev* 10:294–306.

Garg, A. 1998. High-monounsaturated-fat diets for patients with diabetes mellitus: a meta-analysis. *Am J Clin Nutr* 67:577S–582S.

Gupte, P., D. Amarapurkar, S. Agal et al. 2004. Non-alcoholic steatohepatitis in type 2 diabetes mellitus. *J Gastroenterol Hepatol* 19:854–8.

Hallsworth, K., G. Fattakhova, K. G. Hollingsworth et al. 2011. Resistance exercise reduces liver fat and its mediators in non-alcoholic fatty liver disease independent of weight loss. *Gut* 60:1278–83.

Hanley, A. J., K. Williams, A. Festa et al. 2004. Elevations in markers of liver injury and risk of type 2 diabetes: the insulin resistance atherosclerosis study. *Diabetes* 53:2623–32.

Hannukainen, J. C., P. Nuutila, R. Borra et al. 2007. Increased physical activity decreases hepatic free fatty acid uptake: a study in human monozygotic twins. *J Physiol* 578:347–58.

Harrison, S. A., W. Fecht, E. M. Brunt, and B. A. Neuschwander-Tetri. 2009. Orlistat for overweight subjects with nonalcoholic steatohepatitis: A randomized, prospective trial. *Hepatology* 49:80–6.

Haufe, S., S. Engeli, P. Kast et al. 2011. Randomized comparison of reduced fat and reduced carbohydrate hypocaloric diets on intrahepatic fat in overweight and obese human subjects. *Hepatology* 53:1504–14.

Herman, R. H., D. Zakim, and F. B. Stifel. 1970. Effect of diet on lipid metabolism in experimental animals and man. *Fed Proc* 29:1302–7.

Hernandez, R., E. Martinez-Lara, A. Canuelo et al. 2005. Steatosis recovery after treatment with a balanced sunflower or olive oil-based diet: involvement of perisinusoidal stellate cells. *World J Gastroenterol* 11:7480–5.

Howard, B. V., and J. Wylie-Rosett. 2002. Sugar and cardiovascular disease: a statement for healthcare professionals from the Committee on Nutrition of the Council on Nutrition, Physical Activity, and Metabolism of the American Heart Association. *Circulation* 106:523–7.

Hu, F. B., E. B. Rimm, M. J. Stampfer, A. Ascherio, D. Spiegelman, and W. C. Willett. 2000. Prospective study of major dietary patterns and risk of coronary heart disease in men. *Am J Clin Nutr* 72:912–21.

Hu, F. B., M. J. Stampfer, J. E. Manson et al. 1997. Dietary fat intake and the risk of coronary heart disease in women. *N Engl J Med* 337:1491–9.

Huang, M. A., J. K. Greenson, C. Chao et al. 2005. One-year intense nutritional counseling results in histological improvement in patients with non-alcoholic steatohepatitis: a pilot study. *Am J Gastroenterol* 100:1072–81.

Hussein, O., M. Grosovski, E. Lasri, S. Svalb, U. Ravid, and N. Assy. 2007. Monounsaturated fat decreases hepatic lipid content in non-alcoholic fatty liver disease in rats. *World J Gastroenterol* 13:361–8.

Ibanez, J., M. Izquierdo, I. Arguelles et al. 2005. Twice-weekly progressive resistance training decreases abdominal fat and improves insulin sensitivity in older men with type 2 diabetes. *Diabetes Care* 28:662–7.

Ibrahim, A., S. Natrajan, and R. Ghafoorunissa. 2005. Dietary *trans*-fatty acids alter adipocyte plasma membrane fatty acid composition and insulin sensitivity in rats. *Metabolism* 54:240–6.

Ioannou, G. N., O. B. Morrow, M. L. Connole, and S. P. Lee. 2009. Association between dietary nutrient composition and the incidence of cirrhosis or liver cancer in the united states population. *Hepatology* 50:175–84.

Iozzo, P., T. Takala, V. Oikonen et al. 2004. Effect of training status on regional disposal of circulating free fatty acids in the liver and skeletal muscle during physiological hyperinsulinemia. *Diabetes Care* 27:2172–7.

Jepsen, P., H. Vilstrup, L. Mellemkjaer et al. 2003. Prognosis of patients with a diagnosis of fatty liver—a registry-based cohort study. *Hepatogastroenterology* 50:2101–4.

Johnson, N. A., T. Sachinwalla, D. W. Walton et al. 2009. Aerobic exercise training reduces hepatic and visceral lipids in obese individuals without weight loss. *Hepatology* 50:1105–12.

Katan, M. B. 2009. Weight-loss diets for the prevention and treatment of obesity. *N Engl J Med* 360:923–5.

Keating, S. E., D. A. Hackett, J. George, and N. A. Johnson. 2012. Exercise and non-alcoholic fatty liver disease: a systematic review and meta-analysis. *J Hepatol* 57:157–66.

Kechagias, S., A. Ernersson, O. Dahlqvist, P. Lundberg, T. Lindstrom, and F. H. Nystrom. 2008. Fast-food-based hyper-alimentation can induce rapid and profound elevation of serum alanine aminotransferase in healthy subjects. *Gut* 57:649–54.

Kessler, A., Y. Levy, A. Roth et al. 2005. Increased prevalence of NAFLD in patients with acute myocardial infarction independent of BMI. *Hepatology* 42:A623.

Kim, H. K., J. Y. Park, K. U. Lee et al. 2009. Effect of body weight and lifestyle changes on long-term course of nonalcoholic fatty liver disease in Koreans. *Am J Med Sci* 337:98–102.

Kim, S. P., M. Ellmerer, G. W. Van Citters, and R. N. Bergman. 2003. Primacy of hepatic insulin resistance in the development of the metabolic syndrome induced by an isocaloric moderate-fat diet in the dog. *Diabetes* 52:2453–60.

Kirk, E., D. N. Reeds, B. N. Finck, S. M. Mayurranjan, B. W. Patterson, and S. Klein. 2009. Dietary fat and carbohydrates differentially alter insulin sensitivity during caloric restriction. *Gastroenterology* 136:1552–60.

Kistler, K. D., E. M. Brunt, J. M. Clark, A. M. Diehl, J. F. Sallis, and J. B. Schwimmer. 2011. Physical activity recommendations, exercise intensity, and histological severity of nonalcoholic fatty liver disease. *Am J Gastroenterol* 106:460–8; quiz 469.

Koteish, A., and A. M. Diehl. 2001. Animal models of steatosis. *Semin Liver Dis* 21:89–104.

Krasnoff, J. B., P. L. Painter, J. P. Wallace, N. M. Bass, and R. B. Merriman. 2008. Health-related fitness and physical activity in patients with nonalcoholic fatty liver disease. *Hepatology* 47:1158–66.

LaMonte, M. J., S. N. Blair, and T. S. Church. 2005. Physical activity and diabetes prevention. *J Appl Physiol* 99:1205–13.

Lazo, M., S. F. Solga, A. Horska et al. 2010. The effect of a 12-month intensive lifestyle intervention on hepatic steatosis in adults with type 2 diabetes. *Diabetes Care* 33:2156–63.

Le, K. A., M. Ith, R. Kreis et al. 2009. Fructose overconsumption causes dyslipidemia and ectopic lipid deposition in healthy subjects with and without a family history of type 2 diabetes. *Am J Clin Nutr* 89:1760–5.

Lee, J. H., P. L. Rhee, J. K. Lee et al. 1998. Role of hyperinsulinemia and glucose intolerance in the pathogenesis of nonalcoholic fatty liver in patients with normal body weight. *Korean J Intern Med* 13:12–4.

Levy, J. R., J. N. Clore, and W. Stevens. 2004. Dietary n-3 polyunsaturated fatty acids decrease hepatic triglycerides in Fischer 344 rats. *Hepatology* 39:608–16.

Luyckx, F. H., C. Desaive, A. Thiry et al. 1998. Liver abnormalities in severely obese subjects: effect of drastic weight loss after gastroplasty. *Int J Obes Relat Metab Disord* 22:222–6.

Machado, R. M., J. T. Stefano, C. P. Oliveira et al. 2010. Intake of *trans* fatty acids causes nonalcoholic steatohepatitis and reduces adipose tissue fat content. *J Nutr* 140:1127–32.

Maersk, M., A. Belza, H. Stodkilde-Jorgensen et al. 2012. Sucrose-sweetened beverages increase fat storage in the liver, muscle, and visceral fat depot: a 6-mo randomized intervention study. *Am J Clin Nutr* 95:283–9.

Magkos, F. 2010. Exercise and fat accumulation in the human liver. *Curr Opin Lipidol* 21:507–17.

Malik, V. S., B. M. Popkin, G. A. Bray, J. P. Despres, W. C. Willett, and F. B. Hu. 2010. Sugar sweetened beverages and risk of metabolic syndrome and type 2 diabetes: a meta-analysis. *Diabetes Care* 33:2477–83.

Malik, V. S., M. B. Schulze, and F. B. Hu. 2006. Intake of sugar-sweetened beverages and weight gain: a systematic review. *Am J Clin Nutr* 84:274–88.

Marchesini, G., and G. Forlani. 2002. NASH: from liver diseases to metabolic disorders and back to clinical hepatology. *Hepatology* 35:497–9.

Marchesini, G., S. Moscatiello, S. Di Domizio, and G. Forlani. 2008. Obesity-associated liver disease. *J Clin Endocrinol Metab* 93:S74–80.

Marchesini, G., V. Ridolfi, and V. Nepoti. 2008. Hepatotoxicity of fast food? *Gut* 57:568–70.

Matsuzawa, N., T. Takamura, S. Kurita et al. 2007. Lipid-induced oxidative stress causes steatohepatitis in mice fed an atherogenic diet. *Hepatology* 46:1392–403.

McCuskey, R. S., Y. Ito, G. R. Robertson, M. K. McCuskey, M. Perry, and G. C. Farrell. 2004. Hepatic microvascular dysfunction during evolution of dietary steatohepatitis in mice. *Hepatology* 40:386–93.

Mensink, R. P., P. L. Zock, A. D. Kester, and M. B. Katan. 2003. Effects of dietary fatty acids and carbohydrates on the ratio of serum total to HDL cholesterol and on serum lipids and apolipoproteins: a meta-analysis of 60 controlled trials. *Am J Clin Nutr* 77:1146–55.

Miller, W. J., W. M. Sherman, and J. L. Ivy. 1984. Effect of strength training on glucose tolerance and post-glucose insulin response. *Med Sci Sports Exerc* 16:539–43.

Musso, G., R. Gambino, F. De Michieli et al. 2003. Dietary habits and their relations to insulin resistance and postprandial lipemia in nonalcoholic steatohepatitis. *Hepatology* 37:909–16.

Ngo Sock, E. T., K. A. Le, M. Ith, R. Kreis, C. Boesch, and L. Tappy. 2010. Effects of a short-term overfeeding with fructose or glucose in healthy young males. *Br J Nutr* 103:939–43.

Nordmann, A. J., A. Nordmann, M. Briel et al. 2006. Effects of low-carbohydrate vs low-fat diets on weight loss and cardiovascular risk factors: a meta-analysis of randomized controlled trials. *Arch Intern Med* 166:285–93.

Orr, J. S., C. L. Gentile, B. M. Davy, and K. P. Davy. 2008. Large artery stiffening with weight gain in humans: role of visceral fat accumulation. *Hypertension* 51:1519–24.

Ouyang, X., P. Cirillo, Y. Sautin et al. 2008. Fructose consumption as a risk factor for nonalcoholic fatty liver disease. *J Hepatol* 48:993–9.

Oza, N., Y. Eguchi, T. Mizuta et al. 2009. A pilot trial of body weight reduction for nonalcoholic fatty liver disease with a home-based lifestyle modification intervention delivered in collaboration with interdisciplinary medical staff. *J Gastroenterol* 44:1203–8.

Pagano, G., G. Pacini, G. Musso et al. 2002. Nonalcoholic steatohepatitis, insulin resistance, and metabolic syndrome: further evidence for an etiologic association. *Hepatology* 35:367–72.

Palmer, M., and F. Schaffner. 1990. Effect of weight reduction on hepatic abnormalities in overweight patients. *Gastroenterology* 99:1408–13.

Pan, X. R., G. W. Li, Y. H. Hu et al. 1997. Effects of diet and exercise in preventing NIDDM in people with impaired glucose tolerance. The Da Qing IGT and Diabetes Study. *Diabetes Care* 20:537–44.

Parker, H. M., N. A. Johnson, C. A. Burdon, J. S. Cohn, H. T. O'Connor, and J. George. 2012. Omega-3 supplementation and non-alcoholic fatty liver disease: a systematic review and meta-analysis. *J Hepatol* 56:944–51.

Pereira, M. A., A. I. Kartashov, C. B. Ebbeling et al. 2005. Fast-food habits, weight gain, and insulin resistance (the CARDIA study): 15-year prospective analysis. *Lancet* 365:36–42.

Perseghin, G., G. Lattuada, F. De Cobelli et al. 2007. Habitual physical activity is associated with intrahepatic fat content in humans. *Diabetes Care* 30:683–8.

Pollock, M. L., B. A. Franklin, G. J. Balady et al. 2000. AHA Science Advisory. Resistance exercise in individuals with and without cardiovascular disease: benefits, rationale, safety, and prescription: an advisory from the Committee on Exercise, Rehabilitation, and Prevention, Council on Clinical Cardiology, American Heart Association; position paper endorsed by the American College of Sports Medicine. *Circulation* 101:828–33.

Poulsom, R. 1986. Morphological changes of organs after sucrose or fructose feeding. *Prog Biochem Pharmacol* 21:104–34.

Promrat, K., D. E. Kleiner, H. M. Niemeier et al. 2010. Randomized controlled trial testing the effects of weight loss on nonalcoholic steatohepatitis. *Hepatology* 51:121–9.

Propst, A., T. Propst, G. Judmaier, and W. Vogel. 1995. Prognosis in nonalcoholic steatohepatitis. *Gastroenterology* 108:1607.

Ratziu, V., S. Bellentani, H. Cortez-Pinto, C. Day, and G. Marchesini. 2010. A position statement on NAFLD/NASH based on the EASL 2009 special conference. *J Hepatol* 53:372–84.

Repa, J. J., and D. J. Mangelsdorf. 2002. The liver X receptor gene team: potential new players in atherosclerosis. *Nat Med* 8:1243–8.

Ricci, G., E. Canducci, V. Pasini et al. 2011. Nutrient intake in Italian obese patients: relationships with insulin resistance and markers of non-alcoholic fatty liver disease. *Nutrition* 27:672–6.

Rozental, P., C. Biava, H. Spencer, and H. J. Zimmerman. 1967. Liver morphology and function tests in obesity and during total starvation. *Am J Dig Dis* 12:198–208.

Ruderman, N., D. Chisholm, X. Pi-Sunyer, and S. Schneider. 1998. The metabolically obese, normal-weight individual revisited. *Diabetes* 47:699–713.

Ryan, M. C., F. Abbasi, C. Lamendola, S. Carter, and T. L. McLaughlin. 2007. Serum alanine aminotransferase levels decrease further with carbohydrate than fat restriction in insulin-resistant adults. *Diabetes Care* 30:1075–80.

Ryan, M. C., C. Itsiopoulos, T. Thodis et al. 2013. The Mediterranean diet improves hepatic steatosis and insulin sensitivity in individuals with nonalcoholic fatty liver disease. *J Hepatol* 59:138–43.

Samuel, V. T., Z. X. Liu, X. Qu et al. 2004. Mechanism of hepatic insulin resistance in non-alcoholic fatty liver disease. *J Biol Chem* 279:32345–53.

Savard, C., E. V. Tartaglione, R. Kuver et al. 2013. Synergistic interaction of dietary cholesterol and dietary fat in inducing experimental steatohepatitis. *Hepatology* 57:81–92.

Schultz, J. R., H. Tu, A. Luk et al. 2000. Role of LXRs in control of lipogenesis. *Genes Dev* 14:2831–8.

Schulze, M. B., J. E. Manson, D. S. Ludwig et al. 2004. Sugar-sweetened beverages, weight gain, and incidence of type 2 diabetes in young and middle-aged women. *JAMA* 292:927–34.

Sekiya, M., N. Yahagi, T. Matsuzaka et al. 2003. Polyunsaturated fatty acids ameliorate hepatic steatosis in obese mice by SREBP-1 suppression. *Hepatology* 38:1529–39.

Shah, K., A. Stufflebam, T. N. Hilton, D. R. Sinacore, S. Klein, and D. T. Villareal. 2009. Diet and exercise interventions reduce intrahepatic fat content and improve insulin sensitivity in obese older adults. *Obesity (Silver Spring)* 17:2162–8.

Slentz, C. A., L. A. Bateman, L. H. Willis et al. 2011. Effects of aerobic vs. resistance training on visceral and liver fat stores, liver enzymes, and insulin resistance by HOMA in overweight adults from STRRIDE AT/RT. *Am J Physiol Endocrinol Metab* 301: E1033–9.

Sobrecases, H., K. A. Le, M. Bortolotti et al. 2010. Effects of short-term overfeeding with fructose, fat and fructose plus fat on plasma and hepatic lipids in healthy men. *Diabetes Metab* 36:244–6.

Solga, S., A. R. Alkhuraishe, J. M. Clark et al. 2004. Dietary composition and nonalcoholic fatty liver disease. *Dig Dis Sci* 49:1578–83.

St George, A., A. Bauman, A. Johnston, G. Farrell, T. Chey, and J. George. 2009a. Effect of a lifestyle intervention in patients with abnormal liver enzymes and metabolic risk factors. *J Gastroenterol Hepatol* 24:399–407.

St George, A., A. Bauman, A. Johnston, G. Farrell, T. Chey, and J. George. 2009b. Independent effects of physical activity in patients with nonalcoholic fatty liver disease. *Hepatology* 50:68–76.

Storlien, L. H., E. W. Kraegen, D. J. Chisholm, G. L. Ford, D. G. Bruce, and W. S. Pascoe. 1987. Fish oil prevents insulin resistance induced by high-fat feeding in rats. *Science* 237:885–8.

Suzuki, A., K. Lindor, J. St Saver et al. 2005. Effect of changes on body weight and lifestyle in nonalcoholic fatty liver disease. *J Hepatol* 43:1060–6.

Szende, B., F. Timar, and B. Hargitai. 1994. Olive oil decreases liver damage in rats caused by carbon tetrachloride (CCl4). *Exp Toxicol Pathol* 46:355–9.

Tanaka, N., K. Sano, A. Horiuchi, E. Tanaka, K. Kiyosawa, and T. Aoyama. 2008. Highly purified eicosapentaenoic acid treatment improves nonalcoholic steatohepatitis. *J Clin Gastroenterol* 42:413–8.

Targher, G., L. Bertolini, F. Poli et al. 2005. Nonalcoholic fatty liver disease and risk of future cardiovascular events among type 2 diabetic patients. *Diabetes* 54:3541–6.

Tetri, L. H., M. Basaranoglu, E. M. Brunt, L. M. Yerian, and B. A. Neuschwander-Tetri. 2008. Severe NAFLD with hepatic necroinflammatory changes in mice fed *trans* fats and a high-fructose corn syrup equivalent. *Am J Physiol Gastrointest Liver Physiol* 295:G987–95.

Thoma, C., C. P. Day, and M. I. Trenell. 2012. Lifestyle interventions for the treatment of nonalcoholic fatty liver disease in adults: a systematic review. *J Hepatol* 56:255–66.

Toshimitsu, K., B. Matsuura, I. Ohkubo et al. 2007. Dietary habits and nutrient intake in nonalcoholic steatohepatitis. *Nutrition* 23:46–52.

Tsai, A. G., and T. A. Wadden. 2006. The evolution of very-low-calorie diets: an update and meta-analysis. *Obesity (Silver Spring)* 14:1283–93.

Tsuzuku, S., T. Kajioka, H. Endo, R. D. Abbott, J. D. Curb, and K. Yano. 2007. Favorable effects of non-instrumental resistance training on fat distribution and metabolic profiles in healthy elderly people. *Eur J Appl Physiol Occup Physiol* 99:549–55.

Ueno, T., H. Sugawara, K. Sujaku et al. 1997. Therapeutic effects of restricted diet and exercise in obese patients with fatty liver. *J Hepatol* 27:103–7.

van der Heijden, G. J., Z. J. Wang, Z. D. Chu et al. 2009. A 12-week aerobic exercise program reduces hepatic fat accumulation and insulin resistance in obese, Hispanic adolescents. *Obesity (Silver Spring)* 18:384–90.

van der Heijden, G. J., Z. J. Wang, Z. Chu et al. 2010. Strength exercise improves muscle mass and hepatic insulin sensitivity in obese youth. *Med Sci Sports Exerc* 42:1973–80.

Vartanian, L. R., M. B. Schwartz, and K. D. Brownell. 2007. Effects of soft drink consumption on nutrition and health: a systematic review and meta-analysis. *Am J Public Health* 97:667–75.

Villanova, N., S. Moscatiello, S. Ramilli et al. 2005. Endothelial dysfunction and cardiovascular risk profile in nonalcoholic fatty liver disease. *Hepatology* 42:473–80.

Vos, M. B., and J. E. Lavine. 2013. Dietary fructose in nonalcoholic fatty liver disease. *Hepatology* 57:2525–31.

Vos, M. B., and C. J. McClain. 2009. Fructose takes a toll. *Hepatology* 50:1004–6.

Vozarova, B., N. Stefan, R. S. Lindsay et al. 2002. High alanine aminotransferase is associated with decreased hepatic insulin sensitivity and predicts the development of type 2 diabetes. *Diabetes* 51:1889–95.

Wadden, T. A., R. I. Berkowitz, D. B. Sarwer, R. Prus-Wisniewski, and C. Steinberg. 2001. Benefits of lifestyle modification in the pharmacologic treatment of obesity: a randomized trial. *Arch Intern Med* 161:218–27.

Wannamethee, S. G., A. G. Shaper, L. Lennon, and P. H. Whincup. 2005. Hepatic enzymes, the metabolic syndrome, and the risk of type 2 diabetes in older men. *Diabetes Care* 28:2913–8.

Westerbacka, J., K. Lammi, A. M. Hakkinen et al. 2005. Dietary fat content modifies liver fat in overweight nondiabetic subjects. *J Clin Endocrinol Metab* 90:2804–9.

Wouters, K., P. J. van Gorp, V. Bieghs et al. 2008. Dietary cholesterol, rather than liver steatosis, leads to hepatic inflammation in hyperlipidemic mouse models of nonalcoholic steatohepatitis. *Hepatology* 48:474–86.

Yasutake, K., M. Nakamuta, Y. Shima et al. 2009. Nutritional investigation of non-obese patients with non-alcoholic fatty liver disease: the significance of dietary cholesterol. *Scand J Gastroenterol* 44:471–7.

Younossi, Z. M., M. Stepanova, M. Afendy et al. 2011. Changes in the prevalence of the most common causes of chronic liver diseases in the United States from 1988 to 2008. *Clin Gastroenterol Hepatol* 9:524–30.

Younossi, Z. M., M. Stepanova, F. Negro et al. 2012. Nonalcoholic fatty liver disease in lean individuals in the United States. *Medicine (Baltimore)* 91:319–27.

Zelber-Sagi, S., R. Lotan, A. Shlomai et al. 2012. Predictors for incidence and remission of NAFLD in the general population during a seven-year prospective follow-up. *J Hepatol* 56:1145–51.

Zelber-Sagi, S., D. Nitzan-Kaluski, R. Goldsmith et al. 2007. Long term nutritional intake and the risk for non-alcoholic fatty liver disease (NAFLD): a population based study. *J Hepatol* 47:711–7.

Zelber-Sagi, S., D. Nitzan-Kaluski, R. Goldsmith et al. 2008. Role of leisure-time physical activity in nonalcoholic fatty liver disease: a population-based study. *Hepatology* 48:1791–8.

Zelber-Sagi, S., D. Nitzan-Kaluski, Z. Halpern, and R. Oren. 2006. Prevalence of primary non-alcoholic fatty liver disease in a population-based study and its association with biochemical and anthropometric measures. *Liver Int* 26:856–63.

Zelber-Sagi, S., V. Ratziu, and R. Oren. 2011. Nutrition and physical activity in NAFLD: an overview of the epidemiological evidence. *World J Gastroenterol* 17:3377–89.

12 Role of Antioxidants in the Nonalcoholic Fatty Liver Disease Spectrum

Tommy Pacana and Arun J. Sanyal

CONTENTS

INTRODUCTION

Nonalcoholic fatty liver disease (NAFLD), the leading cause of chronic liver disease in the United States and other Western countries, encompasses a histological spectrum of liver diseases ranging from simple steatosis to nonalcoholic steatohepatitis (NASH), which can progress to cirrhosis and liver cancer [1,2]. NAFLD is associated with increased mortality; cardiovascular-, liver-, and cancer-related deaths account for much of this excess mortality [3–5]. The disease is closely associated with obesity and diabetes, and due to their ongoing epidemics, the prevalence of NAFLD is likely to increase over time and continue to become a serious public health burden.

The mechanisms underlying the progression of NAFLD are poorly understood. It is believed that hepatic lipid accumulation sensitizes the liver to additional necro-inflammatory insults promoting injury, inflammation, and fibrosis [6]. Oxidative stress has been regarded as a major player in this process, triggering the progression of simple steatosis to NASH [7]. Animal and human studies of NAFLD have demonstrated evidence of increased reactive oxygen species (ROS) production and lipid peroxidation [8–10]. Thus, an effective therapeutic strategy is to target reduction in oxidative stress to prevent the progression of NAFLD to a more advance liver disease.

A meta-analysis evaluating the effects of several antioxidants on the progression of NAFLD has reported insufficient evidence to support or refute a role of antioxidants in NAFLD [11]. However, the American Association for the Study of Liver Diseases (AASLD) has recommended using vitamin E in nondiabetic adult patients with NASH based on the PIVENS (Pioglitazone, Vitamin E or Placebo for Treatment of Non-diabetic Patients with Nonalcoholic Steatohepatitis) trial that was published more recently [12]. Substantial evidence on the therapeutic efficacy of other antioxidants in NAFLD is lacking, and available literature mostly comes from observational studies with small sample sizes and no histological end points. The aim of this article is to discuss briefly the role of oxidative stress in NAFLD, biological activities of vitamin E, and present available evidence of the therapeutic efficacy of vitamin E and other antioxidants in NAFLD.

ROLE OF OXIDATIVE STRESS IN NAFLD

Oxidative stress results from an imbalance between excessive production of ROS and decreased antioxidant defenses (Figure 12.1). Experimental and human studies suggest a strong association between the degree of oxidative stress and severity of NAFLD [13–16]. The mitochondria are the major sites of fatty acid oxidation and ROS formation. In NAFLD, the increased hepatic uptake and synthesis of free fatty acids (FFA) is compensated by increased ability of the mitochondria to oxidize fatty acids, consequently impairing its oxidative capacity [17]. In the process, the increased delivery of electrons to the electron transport chain creates a state of overreduction of respiratory chain components reacting abnormally with oxygen to form the superoxide anion radical [7].

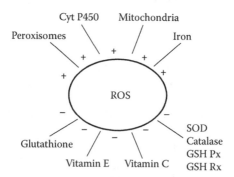

FIGURE 12.1 Imbalance between excessive production of reactive oxygen species and decreased antioxidant defenses leads to oxidative stress. Abbreviations: glutathione peroxidase (GSH Px), glutathione reductase (GSH Rx), superoxide dismutase (SOD).

The radical is dismutated by manganese superoxide dismutase to hydrogen peroxide, which is sequentially detoxified into water by glutathione peroxidase under physiological conditions [18]. However, without adequate amount of mitochondrial reduced glutathione as observed in NAFLD, the glutathione peroxidase loses its ability to detoxify hydrogen peroxide favoring mitochondrial dysfunction and cell death [19–21]. The superoxide anion radical may also react with nitric oxide leading to the formation of another pro-oxidant peroxynitrate [22]. Increased mitochondrial ROS formation has been demonstrated in animal models of NAFLD [8,14]. Mitochondrial dysfunction is evident particularly in NASH as shown by decreased mitochondrial respiratory chain complex activity, hepatic ATP depletion, and decreased mitochondrial DNA and their encoded polypeptides [21,23–27]. Furthermore, structural abnormalities in the mitochondria have been observed, consisting of enlargement (megamitochondria), loss of cristae, and paracrystalline inclusions [25,28].

Endogenous sources of ROS can also originate from defective microsomal P450 and peroxisomal oxidation activities. Lipooxygenation of long-chain fatty acids by cytochrome P450 system, particularly CYP2E1 and CYP4A, results in concomitant ROS overproduction [29]. In NASH patients, hepatic CYP2E1 expression and activity is increased and distributed in the perivenular (acinar zone 3) region, which relates to maximal hepatocellular injury [30–32]. Following fatty acid metabolism by microsomal CYP4A, dicarboxylic acids are generated serving as substrates for peroxisomal β-oxidation [33]. Peroxisomes are involved in the metabolism of very-long-chain fatty acids and branched-chain fatty acids that cannot readily undergo mitochondrial β-oxidation [34]. Proliferation and enlargement of hepatic peroxisomes are observed in hepatic steatosis [35]. Microsomal and peroxisomal oxidations are relatively minor pathways of fatty acid disposal, but become significant when CYP2E1 levels are low- and long-chain fatty acids accumulate. In CYP2E1 knockout mice, CYP4A enzymes are upregulated, thus playing an important role as alternative initiators of oxidative stress in the liver [36].

Insufficient antioxidant defenses are also a major factor promoting oxidative stress in NAFLD. Glutathione, a major hepatic antioxidant, is decreased in patients with NAFLD [37]. The conversion of methionine to cysteine via the *trans*-sulfuration pathway for glutathione synthesis is illustrated in Figure 12.2. Studies have also shown evidence of decreased vitamin E and antioxidant enzymes (e.g., superoxide dismutase, glutathione peroxidase, glutathione reductase, and catalase), thus allowing the accumulation of more ROS [37–39]. Single nucleotide polymorphism of superoxide dismutase is found to be present in NASH [40]. The antioxidant capacity of the liver is further diminished with progression from steatosis to steatohepatitis [37]. This is in agreement with reduced hepatic glutathione (GSH) as well as decreased reduced/oxidized GSH observed during NAFLD progression in another study [10]. In addition, the activity of glutathione transferase activity is decreased as NAFLD progresses [10].

As a result of the imbalance between pro-oxidants and antioxidants, ROS overproduction enhances lipid peroxidation, leading to the formation of aldehyde by-products (4-hydroxynonenal and malondialdehyde). Excess ROS also increases the expression of several cytokines such as tumor necrosis factor (TNF) α, TGF-β, Fas ligand, and interleukin 8 [41]. Both lipid peroxidation products and cytokines, in turn, further damage the mitochondrial DNA and respiratory chain polypeptides

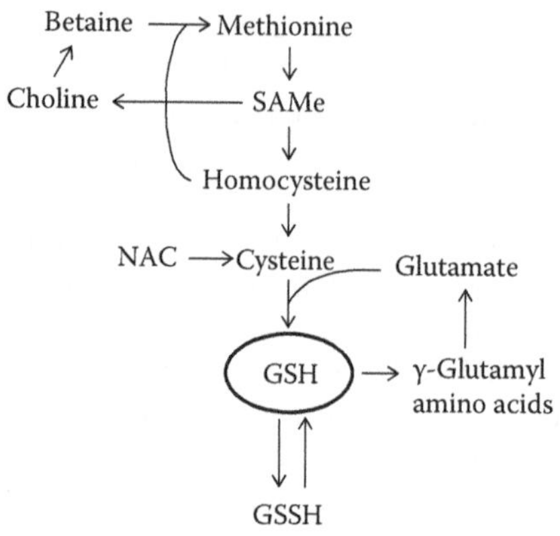

FIGURE 12.2 Glutathione (GSH) synthesis via methionine metabolism. Abbreviations: N-acetylcysteine (NAC), oxidized glutathione (GSSH), s-adenosyl methionine (SAMe).

triggering a vicious cycle by generating more ROS [17,42]. These events have the potential to induce apoptosis, inflammation, and liver fibrosis by impairing nucleotide and protein synthesis, promoting inflammatory cytokine production, and activating hepatic stellate cells.

ANTIOXIDANT THERAPY IN NAFLD

Majority of the studies that utilize antioxidant therapy in NAFLD do not have pretreatment and posttreatment histological data to support therapeutic efficacy. Only few randomized controlled trials are available in the literature that assesses both the biochemical and the histological changes following antioxidant treatment in biopsy-proven NAFLD or NASH. They are summarized in Table 12.1.

VITAMIN E

PHARMACOKINETICS AND PHARMACODYNAMICS

Chemical Structure

Vitamin E is a lipid-soluble, chain-breaking antioxidant that prevents the propagation of free radicals. Synthesized by plants alone, vitamin E exists in eight different forms: four tocopherols and four tocotrienols. The positions and numbers of the methyl groups attached to the chromanol ring designate each form as α, β, γ, or δ. Tocopherols have a saturated phytyl tail, whereas tocotrienols contain an unsaturated side chain. The antioxidant properties of vitamin E is due entirely to the chroman head, whereas the phytyl tail largely determines mobility [43]. The structure of each form governs its biological activity.

Absorption, Transport, and Distribution

Dietary vitamin E is solubilized into mixed micelles in the intestinal lumen, absorbed in the small intestine via passive diffusion, and packaged into chylomicrons. A

TABLE 12.1
Randomized Controlled Trials on the Biochemical and Histological Effects of Antioxidant Therapy in Biopsy-Proven NAFLD/NASH

Author	n	Antioxidant	Comparator	ALT	Steatosis	Inflammation	Ballooning	Fibrosis
Lavine et al. 2011 (46)	173	Vitamin E (800 IU daily for 96 weeks)	Metformin; placebo	—	—	—	↓	—
Sanyal et al. 2010 (47)	247	Vitamin E (800 IU daily for 96 weeks)	Pioglitazone; placebo	↓	↓	↓	↓	—
Abdelmalek et al. 2009 (48)	55	Betaine (20 g daily for 12 months)	Placebo	—	↓	—	—	—
Dufour et al. 2006 (49)	48	Vitamin E (800 IU daily) plus UDCA (12–15 mg/kg/day) for 2 years	UDCA + placebo; placebo + placebo	↓	↓	—	NA	—
Sanyal et al. 2004 (50)	20	Vitamin E (400 IU daily) plus pioglitazone (30 mg daily) for 6 months	Vitamin E	—	—	↓	↓	—
Harrison et al. 2003 (51)	49	Vitamin E (1000 IU daily) plus vitamin C (1000 mg daily) for 6 months	Placebo	—	NA	—	NA	↑

Note: ALT, alanine aminotransferase; NAFLD, nonalcoholic fatty liver disease; NASH, nonalcoholic steatohepatitis; UDCA, ursodeoxycholic acid.

recent study, however, has suggested the role of scavenger receptor class B type 1 (SR-BI) in mediating vitamin E transport across the enterocytes [44]. On entry into the circulation via the lymphatic system, chylomicrons are hydrolyzed by lipoprotein lipase (LPL), and as a result, a fraction of vitamin E is released and taken up by extrahepatic tissues via the postulated LPL-dependent bridging mechanism [45]. The transformed chylomicron remnant is taken up by the liver mainly via receptor-mediated endocytosis.

In the hepatocytes, the α-tocopherol form of vitamin E is preferentially bound to α-tocopherol transfer protein (α-TTP) for resecretion into the circulation [46]. Defects in human α-TTP gene leads to vitamin E deficiency [47]. Similar manifestation has also been demonstrated in mice with deletion of α-TTP gene [48]. Hence, α-TTP essentially maintains the levels of α-tocopherol in plasma and tissues, whereas other vitamin E forms are preferentially metabolized by microsomal P450 or excreted into the bile [49,50].

It has been proposed previously that secretion of α-tocopherol from the hepatocytes is dependent on VLDL assembly and secretion [51]. However, a Golgi-independent mechanism not directly coupled to VLDL secretion has been indicated to facilitate α-tocopherol secretion into the plasma [52]. This is supported by a recent study in mice that showed no reduction in α-tocopherol content in peripheral tissues in the absence of VLDL due to lack of microsomal triglyceride transfer protein [53]. The process whereby α-tocopherol is acquired from endosomes by α-TTP, transferred, and released to the plasma membrane to be acquired by lipoproteins has been suggested [54]. Alternatively, ATP-binding cassette protein A1 (ABCA 1) has been described to participate in α-tocopherol secretion in cultured hepatocytes [55].

In the plasma, lipoproteins are considered to be major carriers of α-tocopherol, serving as efficient sources for peripheral tissue uptake. The plasma phospholipid transfer protein enhances the transfer of vitamin E between lipoproteins and cells [56]. Although LDL receptor may modulate uptake of α-tocopherol to tissues, it has been found to be nonessential in maintaining steady-state tissue levels of vitamin E in vivo [57,58]. Interestingly, the role of SR-BI, a cell surface receptor, in the peripheral distribution of HDL-associated α-tocopherol has been increasingly recognized. In vivo studies in SR-BI–deficient mice have shown decreased α-tocopherol levels in several peripheral organs [59].

Antioxidant Properties

During the initiation phase of lipid peroxidation, free radicals extract hydrogen atom from the susceptible polyunsaturated fatty acid (PUFA) within biological membranes, resulting in the formation of a lipid radical (ROOH). Oxygen then reacts with the unstable lipid radical forming a peroxyl radical (ROO·), a chain-carrying radical that is able to attack another PUFA, thus propagating a chain reaction. Vitamin E intercepts the propagation of peroxyl radical more rapidly than PUFA by donating its phenolic hydrogen to the radical and converting it to a hydroperoxide product [43]. Consequently, the formation of tocopheroxyl radical reacts with another peroxyl radical, thereby forming nonradical products. In humans and experimental animals, vitamin E suppresses the production of isoprostanes, an index of lipid peroxidation [60,61]. By protecting against peroxidation, vitamin E becomes consumed rapidly.

The cytoplasmic antioxidant cycling network, which includes vitamin C and thiol antioxidants such as glutathione and lipoic acid, regenerates back vitamin E to its reduced form [62,63].

Vitamin E in NASH Clinical Trials

The levels of plasma α-tocopherol are found to be decreased in NASH patients compared with healthy controls, forming a theoretical basis for its use in the treatment of NASH [39]. More recently, two large multicenter randomized controlled trials were conducted by NASH Clinical Research Network to evaluate the efficacy of vitamin E for ameliorating NASH in adults and children (PIVENS and TONIC), respectively. The PIVENS trial included 247 nondiabetic and noncirrhotic adults with NASH who received vitamin E (800 IU/day), pioglitazone (30 mg/day), or placebo for 96 weeks [64]. The primary outcome was improvement in histological features, as assessed by standardized scores for steatosis, inflammation, hepatocellular ballooning, and fibrosis. The study design was to compare the treatment group (vitamin E or pioglitazone) versus the placebo group with less than 0.025 considered as statistical significance for multiple comparisons. Compared with placebo, vitamin E therapy demonstrated a robust improvement in NASH (43% versus 19%, p = 0.001), whereas pioglitazone did not reach statistical significance (34% versus 19%, p = 0.04). Although significant reduction in hepatic steatosis, lobular inflammation, and hepatocellular ballooning was observed, no significant improvement in fibrosis score was associated in both treatment groups. Interestingly, combination therapy of vitamin E and pioglitazone in a small pilot study was superior to vitamin E alone by demonstrating not only a significant decrease in steatosis, cytologic ballooning, Mallory's hyaline, and inflammation but also a significant reduction in pericellular fibrosis [65].

In the Treatment of Nonalcoholic Fatty Liver Disease in Children (TONIC) trial, 173 children were randomized to receive vitamin E (400 IU twice daily), metformin (500 mg twice daily), or placebo for 96 weeks [66]. Neither agent was superior to placebo in attaining the primary outcome, a reduction in ALT level 50% or less of the baseline or 40 U/L or less at each visit from 48 to 96 weeks. Resolution of NASH was significantly greater for vitamin E treatment group, as compared with placebo, which was attributed mainly to the significant improvement in hepatocellular ballooning. Unlike in PIVENS, no significant reduction in steatosis and inflammation was observed. Similarly, both trials showed no improvement in fibrosis.

Recently, a comprehensive analysis of metabolomic profiles quantified by mass spectrometry was performed by Cheng et al. in vitamin E responders, vitamin E nonresponders, and placebo responders in the PIVENS trial [67]. At baseline, phenyl-propionic acid and indole-propionic acid levels, two intestinal microbiome-derived metabolites, were directly associated with a subsequent histological response to vitamin E treatment. After adjusting for baseline, the end of treatment levels of γ-glutamyl leucine and γ-glutamyl valine were significantly lower in vitamin E responders compared with nonresponders. This is an indication of decreased glutathione turnover and improved oxidative stress. This study provides evidence of the existing differences in the circulating metabolomic profiles of subjects with NASH who will or will not respond to vitamin E treatment and among those who are responding to treatment versus those who are not.

Vitamin E Safety

Concerns about the safety of vitamin E supplementation have been raised because of its implications in increased overall mortality and the development of hemorrhagic stroke and prostate cancer. Although some meta-analyses suggested that the use of high-dose vitamin E (>400 IU/day) increased all-cause mortality, others failed to show such an association [68–71]. Another meta-analysis that includes nine trials indicated that vitamin E might increase the risk for hemorrhagic stroke [72]. More recently, an extended follow-up of a large RCT observed an increased prostate cancer incidence in healthy men taking vitamin E (400 IU/day) over 7 years [73].

OTHER ANTIOXIDANTS IN NAFLD

SILYMARIN AND SILIBININ

Silymarin (milk thistle) is capable of scavenging free radicals, and it is also known to have hepatoprotective, anti-inflammatory, and anti-fibrotic properties [74]. It has been shown to increase expression of superoxide dismutase in lymphocytes in alcoholic cirrhosis [75]. Silibinin, an active component comprising 50%–60% of silymarin, has also been studied in liver diseases [74]. The therapeutic efficacy of silymarin and silibinin in NAFLD has been reported in experimental and human studies. Several studies in experimental NASH models have suggested their potential utility in preventing progression of liver injury by modulating hepatic lipid homoestasis and suppressing oxidative stress-induced lipotoxicity, NF-κB activation, and hepatic stellate cell activation [76–78]. Silymarin treatment has been shown to reduce serum aminotransferases and ultrasonographic liver steatosis in patients with NAFLD [79,80]. In another study, conjugation of silibinin with vitamin E and phospholipids has resulted in significant improvement in hepatic steatosis as assessed by ultrasound [81].

α-LIPOIC ACID

α-Lipoic acid is considered a "universal" antioxidant, as it functions both in the membranous and aqueous phases [82]. Its antioxidant properties include quenching a variety of ROS as well as in recycling other antioxidants. It has been shown to be beneficial in several animal models of NAFLD not only by reducing oxidative stress but also by acting through multiple mechanisms, including modulation of mitochondrial function and reduction in hepatic lipid accumulation, immune activation, inflammation, and ER stress [83–86]. However, published studies on the effects of α-lipoic acid in human NAFLD are scant.

VITAMIN C

As an electron donor, vitamin C is a potent water-soluble antioxidant in humans [87]. In addition, it also acts by enhancing regeneration of vitamin E [88]. Several clinical trials have investigated the utility of vitamin C in NAFLD, but they are conducted in combination with other agents. Vitamin C combined with vitamin E has been shown to decrease serum aminotransferases compared with ursodeoxycholic acid in NAFLD [89]. In a randomized controlled trial, the same antioxidant combination therapy has resulted in significant improvement in fibrosis score, but without improvement in ALT or necro-inflammatory activity in subjects with NASH [90]. Recently, atorvastin (10 mg/day) plus vitamin C (1 g/day) and vitamin E (1000 IU/day) has been demonstrated to lower hepatic steatosis as detected by liver spleen ratio on computed tomography scans after 4 years of therapy [91].

N-ACETYLCYSTEINE

N-Acetylcysteine (NAC) provides the substrate cysteine for the synthesis of GSH. In rat models of NASH, NAC therapy has been shown to attenuate hepatocellular injury by reducing oxidative stress, specifically by increasing GSH levels and decreasing lipid peroxidation products [92,93]. In NAFLD, 3 months of oral NAC therapy (600 mg every 12 h) has led to significant improvement in serum alanine aminotransferase compared with vitamin C (1000 mg every 12 h) [94]. However, the absence of histological data is a limitation of this study. In a prospective pilot study involving 20 consecutive NASH patients, the combination of NAC (1.2 g/day) and metformin (850–1000 mg/day) given for 12 months has resulted in improved liver enzymes and histological liver steatosis and fibrosis, although there was no effect on hepatocyte ballooning or inflammation [95].

S-ADENOSYLMETHIONINE AND BETAINE

Like NAC, both S-adenosylmethionine (SAMe) and betaine attenuate oxidative stress by augmenting GSH synthesis. This is achieved by serving as methyl donors in the methionine cycle [96]. Although evidence is available supporting a therapeutic role of SAMe in experimental NAFLD or liver injury, no studies to date have used SAMe in human NAFLD [97–99]. A prospective cohort study has supported the use of betaine in NASH by improving liver function tests and histology [100]. In a randomized controlled trial, 55 patients with biopsy-proven NASH receiving betaine therapy (20 g/day) has shown improvement in hepatic steatosis, but without improvement in the NAFLD activity score or fibrosis [101].

PROBOCUL

Probocul is a lipid-lowering agent that also exhibits strong antioxidant property [102]. In a double-blind randomized controlled study, probocul (500 mg daily for 6 months) therapy in NASH subjects has been demonstrated to significantly decrease ALT levels [103]. The same group has subsequently evaluated the histological changes of 10 NASH patients following 1 year of probocul treatment [104]. Although this study is able to demonstrate reduction in histological steatosis and inflammation, the sample size is too small to make a definitive conclusion. Recently, an open-label study has reported improved NAFLD activity score in Japanese NASH patients with dyslipidema receiving probocul (500 mg/day) for 1 year [105].

CONCLUSION

The therapeutic efficacy of antioxidants has been difficult to demonstrate despite overwhelming evidence linking oxidative stress to NAFLD pathogenesis. The only convincing evidence currently available is the use of vitamin E in patients with active NASH who do not have diabetes as recommended by recent AASLD guidelines. However, caution should be exercised when using vitamin E as long-term adverse outcomes were reported. Thus, studies with larger number of patients and longer treatment duration would be helpful to assess its long-term safety and clinical outcomes, particularly liver-related and cardiovascular outcomes. Since NAFLD is considered a multifactorial disease, combining antioxidants with other agents is also a potential approach to treatment. Clearly, well-designed studies with histological end points are much needed to validate the role of antioxidants in NAFLD.

REFERENCES

1. Lazo M, Clark JM. The epidemiology of nonalcoholic fatty liver disease: a global perspective. *Semin Liver Dis* 2008;28:339–350.
2. Angulo P. Nonalcoholic fatty liver disease. *N Engl J Med* 2002;346:1221–1231.
3. Rafiq N, Bai C, Fang Y, Srishord M, McCullough A, Gramlich T, Younossi ZM. Long-term follow-up of patients with nonalcoholic fatty liver. *Clin Gastroenterol Hepatol* 2009;7:234–238.
4. Lazo M, Hernaez R, Bonekamp S, Kamel IR, Brancati FL, Guallar E, Clark JM. Non-alcoholic fatty liver disease and mortality among US adults: prospective cohort study. *BMJ* 2011;343:d6891.
5. Soderberg C, Stal P, Askling J, Glaumann H, Lindberg G, Marmur J, Hultcrantz R. Decreased survival of subjects with elevated liver function tests during a 28-year follow-up. *Hepatology* 2010;51:595–602.
6. Day CP, James OF. Steatohepatitis: a tale of two "hits"? *Gastroenterology* 1998;114: 842–845.
7. Rolo AP, Teodoro JS, Palmeira CM. Role of oxidative stress in the pathogenesis of non-alcoholic steatohepatitis. *Free Radic Biol Med* 2012;52:59–69.
8. Yang S, Zhu H, Li Y, Lin H, Gabrielson K, Trush MA, Diehl AM. Mitochondrial adaptations to obesity-related oxidant stress. *Arch Biochem Biophys* 2000;378:259–268.
9. Leclercq IA, Farrell GC, Field J, Bell DR, Gonzalez FJ, Robertson GR. CYP2E1 and CYP4A as microsomal catalysts of lipid peroxides in murine nonalcoholic steatohepatitis. *J Clin Invest* 2000;105:1067–1075.
10. Hardwick RN, Fisher CD, Canet MJ, Lake AD, Cherrington NJ. Diversity in antioxidant response enzymes in progressive stages of human nonalcoholic fatty liver disease. *Drug Metab Dispos* 2010;38:2293–2301.
11. Lirussi F, Azzalini L, Orando S, Orlando R, Angelico F. Antioxidant supplements for non-alcoholic fatty liver disease and/or steatohepatitis. *Cochrane Database Syst Rev* 2007:CD004996.
12. Chalasani N, Younossi Z, Lavine JE, Diehl AM, Brunt EM, Cusi K, Charlton M et al. The diagnosis and management of non-alcoholic fatty liver disease: practice guideline by the American Association for the Study of Liver Diseases, American College of Gastroenterology, and the American Gastroenterological Association. *Hepatology* 2012;55:2005–2023.

13. Oliveira CP, da Costa Gayotto LC, Tatai C, Della Bina BI, Janiszewski M, Lima ES, Abdalla DS et al. Oxidative stress in the pathogenesis of nonalcoholic fatty liver disease, in rats fed with a choline-deficient diet. *J Cell Mol Med* 2002;6:399–406.

14. Hensley K, Kotake Y, Sang H, Pye QN, Wallis GL, Kolker LM, Tabatabaie T et al. Dietary choline restriction causes complex I dysfunction and increased H(2)O(2) generation in liver mitochondria. *Carcinogenesis* 2000;21:983–989.

15. Chalasani N, Deeg MA, Crabb DW. Systemic levels of lipid peroxidation and its metabolic and dietary correlates in patients with nonalcoholic steatohepatitis. *Am J Gastroenterol* 2004;99:1497–1502.

16. Yesilova Z, Yaman H, Oktenli C, Ozcan A, Uygun A, Cakir E, Sanisoglu SY et al. Systemic markers of lipid peroxidation and antioxidants in patients with nonalcoholic fatty liver disease. *Am J Gastroenterol* 2005;100:850–855.

17. Begriche K, Igoudjil A, Pessayre D, Fromenty B. Mitochondrial dysfunction in NASH: causes, consequences and possible means to prevent it. *Mitochondrion* 2006;6:1–28.

18. Pessayre D, Mansouri A, Fromenty B. Nonalcoholic steatosis and steatohepatitis. V. Mitochondrial dysfunction in steatohepatitis. *Am J Physiol Gastrointest Liver Physiol* 2002;282:G193–G199.

19. Haouzi D, Lekehal M, Tinel M, Vadrot N, Caussanel L, Letteron P, Moreau A et al. Prolonged, but not acute, glutathione depletion promotes Fas-mediated mitochondrial permeability transition and apoptosis in mice. *Hepatology* 2001;33:1181–1188.

20. Fernandez-Checa JC, Kaplowitz N. Hepatic mitochondrial glutathione: transport and role in disease and toxicity. *Toxicol Appl Pharmacol* 2005;204:263–273.

21. Serviddio G, Bellanti F, Tamborra R, Rollo T, Capitanio N, Romano AD, Sastre J et al. Uncoupling protein-2 (UCP2) induces mitochondrial proton leak and increases susceptibility of non-alcoholic steatohepatitis (NASH) liver to ischaemia-reperfusion injury. *Gut* 2008;57:957–965.

22. Radi R, Cassina A, Hodara R, Quijano C, Castro L. Peroxynitrite reactions and formation in mitochondria. *Free Radic Biol Med* 2002;33:1451–1464.

23. Dasarathy S, Yang Y, McCullough AJ, Marczewski S, Bennett C, Kalhan SC. Elevated hepatic fatty acid oxidation, high plasma fibroblast growth factor 21, and fasting bile acids in nonalcoholic steatohepatitis. *Eur J Gastroenterol Hepatol* 2011;23:382–388.

24. Perez-Carreras M, Del Hoyo P, Martin MA, Rubio JC, Martin A, Castellano G, Colina F et al. Defective hepatic mitochondrial respiratory chain in patients with nonalcoholic steatohepatitis. *Hepatology* 2003;38:999–1007.

25. Caldwell SH, Swerdlow RH, Khan EM, Iezzoni JC, Hespenheide EE, Parks JK, Parker WD, Jr. Mitochondrial abnormalities in non-alcoholic steatohepatitis. *J Hepatol* 1999;31:430–434.

26. Pirola CJ, Gianotti TF, Burgueno AL, Rey-Funes M, Loidl CF, Mallardi P, Martino JS et al. Epigenetic modification of liver mitochondrial DNA is associated with histological severity of nonalcoholic fatty liver disease. *Gut* 2013;62:1356–1363.

27. Santamaria E, Avila MA, Latasa MU, Rubio A, Martin-Duce A, Lu SC, Mato JM et al. Functional proteomics of nonalcoholic steatohepatitis: mitochondrial proteins as targets of S-adenosylmethionine. *Proc Natl Acad Sci USA* 2003;100:3065–3070.

28. Sanyal AJ, Campbell-Sargent C, Mirshahi F, Rizzo WB, Contos MJ, Sterling RK, Luketic VA et al. Nonalcoholic steatohepatitis: association of insulin resistance and mitochondrial abnormalities. *Gastroenterology* 2001;120:1183–1192.

29. Koek GH, Liedorp PR, Bast A. The role of oxidative stress in non-alcoholic steatohepatitis. *Clin Chim Acta* 2011;412:1297–1305.

30. Chalasani N, Gorski JC, Asghar MS, Asghar A, Foresman B, Hall SD, Crabb DW. Hepatic cytochrome P450 2E1 activity in nondiabetic patients with nonalcoholic steatohepatitis. *Hepatology* 2003;37:544–550.

31. Weltman MD, Farrell GC, Hall P, Ingelman-Sundberg M, Liddle C. Hepatic cytochrome P450 2E1 is increased in patients with nonalcoholic steatohepatitis. *Hepatology* 1998;27:128–133.
32. Emery MG, Fisher JM, Chien JY, Kharasch ED, Dellinger EP, Kowdley KV, Thummel KE. CYP2E1 activity before and after weight loss in morbidly obese subjects with nonalcoholic fatty liver disease. *Hepatology* 2003;38:428–435.
33. Malaguarnera M, Di Rosa M, Nicoletti F, Malaguarnera L. Molecular mechanisms involved in NAFLD progression. *J Mol Med (Berl)* 2009;87:679–695.
34. Reddy JK, Mannaerts GP. Peroxisomal lipid metabolism. *Annu Rev Nutr* 1994;14:343–370.
35. Collins JC, Scheinberg IH, Giblin DR, Sternlieb I. Hepatic peroxisomal abnormalities in abetalipoproteinemia. *Gastroenterology* 1989;97:766–770.
36. Hardwick JP, Osei-Hyiaman D, Wiland H, Abdelmegeed MA, Song BJ. PPAR/RXR regulation of fatty acid metabolism and fatty acid omega-hydroxylase (CYP4) isozymes: implications for prevention of lipotoxicity in fatty liver disease. *PPAR Res* 2009;2009:952734.
37. Videla LA, Rodrigo R, Orellana M, Fernandez V, Tapia G, Quinones L, Varela N et al. Oxidative stress-related parameters in the liver of non-alcoholic fatty liver disease patients. *Clin Sci (Lond)* 2004;106:261–268.
38. Watson AM, Poloyac SM, Howard G, Blouin RA. Effect of leptin on cytochrome P-450, conjugation, and antioxidant enzymes in the ob/ob mouse. *Drug Metab Dispos* 1999;27:695–700.
39. Erhardt A, Stahl W, Sies H, Lirussi F, Donner A, Haussinger D. Plasma levels of vitamin E and carotenoids are decreased in patients with Nonalcoholic Steatohepatitis (NASH). *Eur J Med Res* 2011;16:76–78.
40. Namikawa C, Shu-Ping Z, Vyselaar JR, Nozaki Y, Nemoto Y, Ono M, Akisawa N et al. Polymorphisms of microsomal triglyceride transfer protein gene and manganese superoxide dismutase gene in non-alcoholic steatohepatitis. *J Hepatol* 2004;40:781–786.
41. Fromenty B, Robin MA, Igoudjil A, Mansouri A, Pessayre D. The ins and outs of mitochondrial dysfunction in NASH. *Diabetes Metab* 2004;30:121–138.
42. Schulze-Osthoff K, Bakker AC, Vanhaesebroeck B, Beyaert R, Jacob WA, Fiers W. Cytotoxic activity of tumor necrosis factor is mediated by early damage of mitochondrial functions. Evidence for the involvement of mitochondrial radical generation. *Annu Rev Nutr* 1990;10:357–382.
43. Burton GW, Traber MG. Vitamin E: antioxidant activity, biokinetics, and bioavailability. *Annu Rev Nutr* 1990;10:357–382.
44. Reboul E, Klein A, Bietrix F, Gleize B, Malezet-Desmoulins C, Schneider M, Margotat A et al. Scavenger receptor class B type I (SR-BI) is involved in vitamin E transport across the enterocyte. *J Biol Chem* 2006;281:4739–4745.
45. Rigotti A. Absorption, transport, and tissue delivery of vitamin E. *Mol Aspects Med* 2007;28:423–436.
46. Kaempf-Rotzoll DE, Traber MG, Arai H. Vitamin E and transfer proteins. *Curr Opin Lipidol* 2003;14:249–254.
47. Ouahchi K, Arita M, Kayden H, Hentati F, Ben Hamida M, Sokol R, Arai H et al. Ataxia with isolated vitamin E deficiency is caused by mutations in the alpha-tocopherol transfer protein. *Nat Genet* 1995;9:141–145.
48. Yokota T, Igarashi K, Uchihara T, Jishage K, Tomita H, Inaba A, Li Y et al. Delayed-onset ataxia in mice lacking alpha-tocopherol transfer protein: model for neuronal degeneration caused by chronic oxidative stress. *Proc Natl Acad Sci USA* 2001;98:15185–15190.
49. Brigelius-Flohe R, Traber MG. Vitamin E: function and metabolism. *FASEB J* 1999;13:1145–1155.

50. Parker RS, Sontag TJ, Swanson JE, McCormick CC. Discovery, characterization, and significance of the cytochrome P450 omega-hydroxylase pathway of vitamin E catabolism. *Ann NY Acad Sci* 2004;1031:13–21.
51. Traber MG, Burton GW, Hughes L, Ingold KU, Hidaka H, Malloy M, Kane J et al. Discrimination between forms of vitamin E by humans with and without genetic abnormalities of lipoprotein metabolism. *J Lipid Res* 1992;33:1171–1182.
52. Arita M, Nomura K, Arai H, Inoue K. Alpha-tocopherol transfer protein stimulates the secretion of alpha-tocopherol from a cultured liver cell line through a brefeldin A-insensitive pathway. *Proc Natl Acad Sci USA* 1997;94:12437–12441.
53. Minehira-Castelli K, Leonard SW, Walker QM, Traber MG, Young SG. Absence of VLDL secretion does not affect alpha-tocopherol content in peripheral tissues. *J Lipid Res* 2006;47:1733–1738.
54. Horiguchi M, Arita M, Kaempf-Rotzoll DE, Tsujimoto M, Inoue K, Arai H. pH-dependent translocation of alpha-tocopherol transfer protein (alpha-TTP) between hepatic cytosol and late endosomes. *Genes Cells* 2003;8:789–800.
55. Shichiri M, Takanezawa Y, Rotzoll DE, Yoshida Y, Kokubu T, Ueda K, Tamai H et al. ATP-binding cassette transporter A1 is involved in hepatic alpha-tocopherol secretion. *J Nutr Biochem* 2010;21:451–456.
56. Kostner GM, Oettl K, Jauhiainen M, Ehnholm C, Esterbauer H, Dieplinger H. Human plasma phospholipid transfer protein accelerates exchange/transfer of alpha-tocopherol between lipoproteins and cells. *Biochem J* 1995;305:659–667.
57. Cohn W, Kuhn H. The role of the low density lipoprotein receptor for alpha-tocopherol delivery to tissues. *Ann NY Acad Sci* 1989;570:61–71.
58. Cohn W, Goss-Sampson MA, Grun H, Muller DP. Plasma clearance and net uptake of alpha-tocopherol and low-density lipoprotein by tissues in WHHL and control rabbits. *Biochem J* 1992;287:247–254.
59. Mardones P, Strobel P, Miranda S, Leighton F, Quinones V, Amigo L, Rozowski J et al. Alpha-tocopherol metabolism is abnormal in scavenger receptor class B type I (SR-BI)-deficient mice. *J Nutr* 2002;132:443–449.
60. Pratico D, Tangirala RK, Rader DJ, Rokach J, Fitz-Gerald GA. Vitamin E suppresses isoprostane generation in vivo and reduces atherosclerosis in ApoE-deficient mice. *Nat Med* 1998;4:1189–1192.
61. Davi G, Alessandrini P, Mezzetti A, Minotti G, Bucciarelli T, Costantini F, Cipollone F et al. In vivo formation of 8-Epi-prostaglandin F2 alpha is increased in hypercholesterolemia. *Arterioscler Thromb Vasc Biol* 1997;17:3230–3235.
62. Constantinescu A, Han D, Packer L. Vitamin E recycling in human erythrocyte membranes. *J Biol Chem* 1993;268:10906–10913.
63. Packer L, Weber SU, Rimbach G. Molecular aspects of alpha-tocotrienol antioxidant action and cell signalling. *J Nutr* 2001;131:369S–373S.
64. Sanyal AJ, Chalasani N, Kowdley KV, McCullough A, Diehl AM, Bass NM, Neuschwander-Tetri BA et al. Pioglitazone, vitamin E, or placebo for nonalcoholic steatohepatitis. *N Engl J Med* 2010;362:1675–1685.
65. Sanyal AJ, Mofrad PS, Contos MJ, Sargeant C, Luketic VA, Sterling RK, Stravitz RT et al. A pilot study of vitamin E versus vitamin E and pioglitazone for the treatment of nonalcoholic steatohepatitis. *Clin Gastroenterol Hepatol* 2004;2:1107–1115.
66. Lavine JE, Schwimmer JB, Van Natta ML, Molleston JP, Murray KF, Rosenthal P, Abrams SH et al. Effect of vitamin E or metformin for treatment of nonalcoholic fatty liver disease in children and adolescents: the TONIC randomized controlled trial. *JAMA* 2011;305:1659–1668.
67. Cheng J, Joyce A, Yates K, Aouizerat B, Sanyal AJ. Metabolomic profiling to identify predictors of response to vitamin E for non-alcoholic steatohepatitis (NASH). *PLoS One* 2012;7:e44106.

68. Miller ER, 3rd, Pastor-Barriuso R, Dalal D, Riemersma RA, Appel LJ, Guallar E. Meta-analysis: high-dosage vitamin E supplementation may increase all-cause mortality. *Ann Intern Med* 2005;142:37–46.
69. Bjelakovic G, Nikolova D, Gluud LL, Simonetti RG, Gluud C. Mortality in random-ized trials of antioxidant supplements for primary and secondary prevention: systematic review and meta-analysis. *JAMA* 2007;297:842–857.
70. Berry D, Wathen JK, Newell M. Bayesian model averaging in meta-analysis: vitamin E supplementation and mortality. *Clin Trials* 2009;6:28–41.
71. Gerss J, Kopcke W. The questionable association of vitamin E supplementation and mortality—inconsistent results of different meta-analytic approaches. *Cell Mol Biol (Noisy-le-grand)* 2009;55 Suppl:OL1111–1120.
72. Schurks M, Glynn RJ, Rist PM, Tzourio C, Kurth T. Effects of vitamin E on stroke sub-types: meta-analysis of randomised controlled trials. *BMJ* 2010;341:c5702.
73. Klein EA, Thompson IM, Jr., Tangen CM, Crowley JJ, Lucia MS, Goodman PJ, Minasian LM et al. Vitamin E and the risk of prostate cancer: the Selenium and Vitamin E Cancer Prevention Trial (SELECT). *JAMA* 2011;306:1549–1556.
74. Abenavoli L, Capasso R, Milic N, Capasso F. Milk thistle in liver diseases: past, present, future. *Phytother Res* 2010;24:1423–1432.
75. Pradhan SC, Girish C. Hepatoprotective herbal drug, silymarin from experimental phar-macology to clinical medicine. *Indian J Med Res* 2006;124:491–504.
76. Haddad Y, Vallerand D, Brault A, Haddad PS. Antioxidant and hepatoprotective effects of silibinin in a rat model of nonalcoholic steatohepatitis. *Evid Based Complement Alternat Med* 2011;2011:nep164.
77. Kim M, Yang SG, Kim JM, Lee JW, Kim YS, Lee JI. Silymarin suppresses hepatic stel-late cell activation in a dietary rat model of non-alcoholic steatohepatitis: analysis of isolated hepatic stellate cells. *Int J Mol Med* 2012;30:473–479.
78. Salamone F, Galvano F, Cappello F, Mangiameli A, Barbagallo I, Li Volti G. Silibinin modulates lipid homeostasis and inhibits nuclear factor kappa B activation in experi-mental nonalcoholic steatohepatitis. *Transl Res* 2012;159:477–486.
79. Hajiaghamohammadi AA, Ziaee A, Oveisi S, Masroor H. Effects of metformin, pio-glitazone, and silymarin treatment on non-alcoholic fatty liver disease: a randomized controlled pilot study. *Hepat Mon* 2012;12:e6099.
80. Cacciapuoti F, Scognamiglio A, Palumbo R, Forte R, Cacciapuoti F. Silymarin in non alcoholic fatty liver disease. *World J Hepatol* 2013;5:109–113.
81. Loguercio C, Federico A, Trappoliere M, Tuccillo C, de Sio I, Di Leva A, Niosi M et al. The effect of a silybin-vitamin e-phospholipid complex on nonalcoholic fatty liver disease: a pilot study. *Dig Dis Sci* 2007;52:2387–2395.
82. Packer L, Witt EH, Tritschler HJ. Alpha-Lipoic acid as a biological antioxidant. *Free Radic Biol Med* 1995;19:227–250.
83. Valdecantos MP, Perez-Matute P, Gonzalez-Muniesa P, Prieto-Hontoria PL, Moreno-Aliaga MJ, Martinez JA. Lipoic acid improves mitochondrial function in nonalcoholic steatosis through the stimulation of sirtuin 1 and sirtuin 3. *Obesity (Silver Spring)* 2012;20:1974–1983.
84. Jung TS, Kim SK, Shin HJ, Jeon BT, Hahm JR, Roh GS. Alpha-lipoic acid prevents non-alcoholic fatty liver disease in OLETF rats. *Liver Int* 2012;32:1565–1573.
85. Min AK, Kim MK, Kim HS, Seo HY, Lee KU, Kim JG, Park KG et al. Alpha-lipoic acid attenuates methionine choline deficient diet-induced steatohepatitis in C57BL/6 mice. *Life Sci* 2012;90:200–205.
86. Valdecantos MP, Perez-Matute P, Gonzalez-Muniesa P, Prieto-Hontoria PL, Moreno-Aliaga MJ, Martinez JA. Lipoic acid administration prevents nonalcoholic steatosis linked to long-term high-fat feeding by modulating mitochondrial function. *J Nutr Biochem* 2012;23:1676–1684.

87. Padayatty SJ, Katz A, Wang Y, Eck P, Kwon O, Lee JH, Chen S et al. Vitamin C as an antioxidant: evaluation of its role in disease prevention. *J Am Coll Nutr* 2003;22:18–35.

88. Chan AC. Partners in defense, vitamin E and vitamin C. *Can J Physiol Pharmacol* 1993;71:725–731.

89. Ersoz G, Gunsar F, Karasu Z, Akay S, Batur Y, Akarca US. Management of fatty liver disease with vitamin E and C compared to ursodeoxycholic acid treatment. *Turk J Gastroenterol* 2005;16:124–128.

90. Harrison SA, Torgerson S, Hayashi P, Ward J, Schenker S. Vitamin E and vitamin C treatment improves fibrosis in patients with nonalcoholic steatohepatitis. *Am J Gastroenterol* 2003;98:2485–2490.

91. Foster T, Budoff MJ, Saab S, Ahmadi N, Gordon C, Guerci AD. Atorvastatin and antioxidants for the treatment of nonalcoholic fatty liver disease: the St Francis Heart Study randomized clinical trial. *Am J Gastroenterol* 2011;106:71–77.

92. Thong-Ngam D, Samuhasaneeto S, Kulaputana O, Klaikeaw N. N-acetylcysteine attenuates oxidative stress and liver pathology in rats with non-alcoholic steatohepatitis. *World J Gastroenterol* 2007;13:5127–5132.

93. Baumgardner JN, Shankar K, Hennings L, Albano E, Badger TM, Ronis MJ. N-acetylcysteine attenuates progression of liver pathology in a rat model of nonalcoholic steatohepatitis. *J Nutr* 2008;138:1872–1879.

94. Khoshbaten M, Aliasgarzadeh A, Masnadi K, Tarzamani MK, Farhang S, Babaei H, Kiani J et al. N-acetylcysteine improves liver function in patients with non-alcoholic fatty liver disease. *Hepat Mon* 2010;10:12–16.

95. de Oliveira CP, Stefano JT, de Siqueira ER, Silva LS, de Campos Mazo DF, Lima VM, Furuya CK et al. Combination of N-acetylcysteine and metformin improves histological steatosis and fibrosis in patients with non-alcoholic steatohepatitis. *Hepatol Res* 2008;38:159–165.

96. Bottiglieri T. S-Adenosyl-L-methionine (SAMe): from the bench to the bedside—molecular basis of a pleiotrophic molecule. *Am J Clin Nutr* 2002;76:1151S–1157S.

97. Lieber CS, Leo MA, Cao Q, Mak KM, Ren C, Ponomarenko A, Wang X et al. The combination of S-adenosylmethionine and dilinoleoylphosphatidylcholine attenuates non-alcoholic steatohepatitis produced in rats by a high-fat diet. *Nutr Res* 2007;27:565–573.

98. Oz HS, Im HJ, Chen TS, de Villiers WJ, McClain CJ. Glutathione-enhancing agents protect against steatohepatitis in a dietary model. *J Biochem Mol Toxicol* 2006;20:39–47.

99. Anstee QM, Day CP. S-Adenosylmethionine (SAMe) therapy in liver disease: a review of current evidence and clinical utility. *J Hepatol* 2012;57:1097–1109.

100. Mukherjee S. Betaine and nonalcoholic steatohepatitis: back to the future? *World J Gastroenterol* 2011;17:3663–3664.

101. Abdelmalek MF, Sanderson SO, Angulo P, Soldevila-Pico C, Liu C, Peter J, Keach J et al. Betaine for nonalcoholic fatty liver disease: results of a randomized placebo-controlled trial. *Hepatology* 2009;50:1818–1826.

102. Liu GX, Ou DM, Liu JH, Huang HL, Liao DF. Probucol inhibits lipid peroxidation of macrophage and affects its secretory properties. *Acta Pharmacol Sin* 2000;21:637–640.

103. Merat S, Malekzadeh R, Sohrabi MR, Sotoudeh M, Rakhshani N, Sohrabpour AA, Naserimoghadam S. Probucol in the treatment of non-alcoholic steatohepatitis: a double-blind randomized controlled study. *J Hepatol* 2003;38:414–418.

104. Merat S, Aduli M, Kazemi R, Sotoudeh M, Sedighi N, Sohrabi M, Malekzadeh R. Liver histology changes in nonalcoholic steatohepatitis after one year of treatment with probucol. *Dig Dis Sci* 2008;53:2246–2250.

105. Ishitobi T, Hyogo H, Tokumo H, Arihiro K, Chayama K. Efficacy of probucol for the treatment of non-alcoholic steatohepatitis with dyslipidemia: An open-label pilot study. *Hepatol Res* 2014;44:429–435.

APPENDIX: CONFLICT OF INTEREST DISCLOSURE

Arun J. Sanyal, MD, as of January 2014 (based on incomes over last 24 months)

Company	Stock	Employment	Speaker	Consulting Advisor	Research Grants	Travel Grants	Intellectual Property	Royalties
Abbott	A	A	A	B	A	A	A	A
Exhalenz	A	A	A	A	A	A	A	A
Conatus	A	A	A	A	C[a]	A	A	A
Genentech	A	A	A	B[b]	A	A	A	A
GenFit	A	A	A	A[c]	A	A	A	A
Gilead	A	A	A	B	F	A	A	A
Echosens-Sandhill	A	A	A	A[c]	A[d]	A	A	A
Ikaria	A	A	A	B	E	A	A	A
Immuron	A	A	A	A[e]	A	A	A	A
Intercept	A	A	A	A[c]	A	A	A	A
Merck	A	A	A	B	A	A	A	A
Norgine	A	A	A	B	A	A	A	A
Roche	A	A	A	B	A	A	A	A
Salix	A	A	A	C	E	A	A	A
Uptodate	A	A	A	A	A	A	A	C
Takeda	A	A	A	B	D	A	A	A
Astellas	A	A	A	A	D	A	A	A
Novartis	A	A	A	A[f]	E	A	A	A
Nimbus	A	A	A	B	A	A	A	A
Galectin	A	A	A	A[f]	E	A	A	A
Nitto Denko	A	A	A	B	A	A	A	A
Sequana	A	A	A	A[c]	A	A	A	A
Bristol Myers	A	A	A	B	A	A	A	A

Source: Dr. Arun Sanyal is a consultant at Genentech regarding NASH and fibrosis (no remuneration received as of January 2014). Research grants listed above for Salix, Gore, Gilead, and Exhalenz represent the site budgets for VCU clinical trials involving these companies and do not support Dr. Arun J. Sanyal directly. Research collaborations without any funding from the commercial entity include Regulus, CSL Behring, Ferring, ZoraLipidomics, and Metabolon.

Note: A, No interest; B, <$5000; C, $5001–10,000; D, $10,001–$50,000; E, $50,001–100,000; F, > $100,000. Research grants listed above for Salix, Gilead and Exhalenz represent the site budgets for VCU clinical trials involving these companies and do not support me directly. Research collaborations without any funding from the commercial entity: Regulus, CSL Behring, Ferring, Zora Lipidomics, and Metabolon.

[a] They will provide drug and lab costs for a NIAAA sponsored study of a caspase inhibitor for alcoholic hepatitis. I have no personal financial conflict of interest.

[b] I am consulting with Genentech re Nash and fibrosis.

[c] I am a consultant but have divested myself- I have no financial conflict of interest.

[d] Echosens has provided a fibroscan machine for dedicated research use for NASH related studies via NIDDK NASH CRN.

[e] I will be the PI of the Immuron upcoming trial for alcoholic hepatitis as part of NIAAA funded TREAT consortium. Immuron will provide drug and no additional funding.

[f] Have provided advice but not taken any personal remuneration.

13 ω-3 Fatty Acids and Nonalcoholic Fatty Liver Disease

Christopher M. Depner, Kelli A. Lytle,
Sasmita Tripathy, and Donald B. Jump

CONTENTS

INTRODUCTION

Nonalcoholic fatty liver disease (NAFLD) is defined as excess accumulation of liver fat (hepatosteatosis), mainly as neutral lipids consisting of triacylglycerol (TAG), cholesterol ester (CE), and diacylglycerol (DAG). NAFLD ranges from benign hepatosteatosis to nonalcoholic steatohepatitis (NASH) (Angulo, 2002), which is defined as hepatosteatosis with inflammation and hepatic injury (Chalasani et al., 2012) (Figure 13.1). Although simple hepatosteatosis is considered clinically benign, NASH is the progressive form of the disease and can lead to significant changes in hepatic morphology (hepatocyte ballooning) and injury (cell death and fibrosis). NASH can progress to cirrhosis, hepatocellular carcinoma, and end-stage liver disease (McCullough, 2006). Liver biopsy is the only accurate method of diagnosing NASH (Chalasani et al., 2012). Histologically, NASH is indistinguishable from alcoholic liver disease (Ludwig et al., 1980). Thus, the diagnosis of NAFLD requires ruling out significant alcohol consumption and all other potential causes of chronic fatty liver disease, such as viral infections (Chalasani et al., 2012).

The incidence of NAFLD has increased in parallel with the obesity epidemic. The prevalence of NAFLD in the general population is estimated to range from 6% to 33%, depending on the method of analysis and population studied (Vernon et al., 2011). Approximately 30% to 40% of individuals with hepatic steatosis progress to NASH (McCullough, 2006), and the prevalence of NASH ranges from 3% to 5% in the general population (Vernon et al., 2011). NAFLD and NASH have high prevalence (≥60%) in the type 2 diabetic (T2D) population (Prashanth et al., 2009). Of patients undergoing bariatric surgery, 93% had NAFLD; of those, 26% had NASH (Ong et al., 2005). NASH patients have higher mortality rates than NAFLD patients, and both are higher than in the general population (Soderberg et al., 2010; Ekstedt et al., 2006; Adams et al., 2005). Over a 10-year period, cirrhosis and liver-related death occurs in 20% and 12% of NASH patients, respectively (McCullough, 2004). Given the increasing prevalence of NASH and its clinical outcome, NASH is rapidly becoming a significant public health burden. Because NASH can progress to cirrhosis, hepatocellular cancer, and liver failure, it is currently the third most common cause for liver transplantation. By 2020, NASH is projected to be the leading cause of liver transplantation in the United States (McCullough, 2011).

THE "THREE-HIT" HYPOTHESIS FOR THE DEVELOPMENT OF NASH

The original model for NASH was proposed to follow a two-hit hypothesis (Day and James, 1998), followed by the other hypotheses (LaBrecque et al., 2012; Tilg and Moschen, 2010) (Figure 13.1). The World Gastroenterology Organization Global Guidelines recently described a "three-hit" mechanism (LaBrecque et al., 2012). The "first hit" involves excessive neutral lipid accumulation in the liver, which sensitizes the liver to the "second hit." This "second hit" is characterized by hepatic inflammation, oxidative stress, and insulin resistance. These events lead to hepatocellular injury resulting in cell death and necrosis (necro-inflammation) and the induction of fibrosis, i.e., the "third hit." Fibrosis is mediated by hepatic stellate cell activation and myofibrillar cell infiltration of the liver; these cells are involved in excessive production of extracellular proteins, like collagen (Friedman, 2008). If not corrected, NASH can progress to cirrhosis, hepatocellular cancer, and liver failure. These hypotheses provide a framework to further evaluate factors contributing to NASH development and progression and assess how therapeutic interventions impact specific steps in NASH progression.

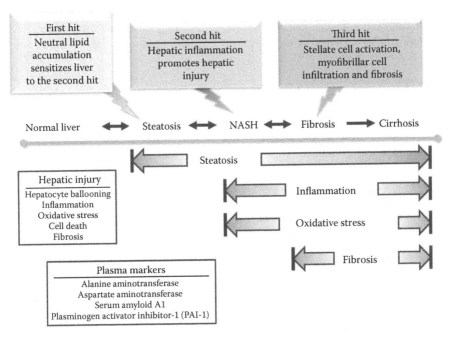

FIGURE 13.1 The "three-hit hypothesis" for NASH development.

Hepatosteatosis develops because of an imbalance of hepatic lipid metabolism leading to the accumulation of neutral lipids as TAG, DAG, and CE. Fatty acid sources of hepatic TAG and CE include nonesterified fatty acids (NEFAs) mobilized from adipose tissue, de novo lipogenesis (DNL), and the diet via the portal circulation. Hepatic fatty acid oxidation (FAO) and very-low-density lipoprotein (VLDL) assembly and secretion represent two pathways for removal of fatty acids from the liver. Hepatosteatosis develops when lipid storage exceeds lipid export or oxidation (Matherly and Puri, 2012). In humans with NAFLD, ~60% of the fatty acids appearing in the liver are derived from circulating NEFA mobilized from adipose tissue: 26% are from DNL and 15% from diet (Donnelly et al., 2005). Both hepatic and peripheral insulin resistance are key factors contributing to the disruption of these pathways and to the development of hepatosteatosis (Matherly and Puri, 2012).

Dietary (fat, cholesterol, and fructose), metabolic (hepatic or plasma NEFA, hepatic ceramide), endocrine (insulin and leptin), gut (endotoxemia), and genetic factors (patatin-like phospholipase domain–containing 3 [PNPLA3] polymorphisms) have been suggested as triggers for NASH (Abdelmalek et al., 2010; Guturu and Duchini, 2012; Wouters et al., 2008; Pagadala et al., 2012; Harte et al., 2010; Hooper et al., 2011). In all likelihood, it is a combination of these factors that are involved in hepatosteatosis and NASH progression. The development of new therapies for NASH requires a more complete understanding of the disease process than is currently available. Recent research has focused on understanding the genetic and environmental factors contributing to NASH in humans and animal models. Human studies, however, are limited in their capacity to define the mechanism. Rodent models that recapitulate many of the features of human NAFLD and NASH have been very useful in identifying mechanisms associated with disease onset and progression. The outcome of these studies should enable investigators to tailor strategies for the prevention and treatment of NAFLD and NASH.

ENVIRONMENTAL AND GENETIC FACTORS CONTRIBUTING TO NAFLD AND NASH

Both the type and amount of dietary fat ingested contributes to NAFLD and NASH. In mice, it is well established that long-term high-fat diet (HFD; ≥45% kcal) feeding induces hepatosteatosis with minimal inflammation and liver damage (Schattenberg and Galle, 2010). Although there are fewer studies in humans, HFD have been reported to induce hepatosteatosis independent of weight change (Cortez-Pinto et al., 2006; Westerbacka et al., 2005). The type of fat ingested is also important. Fat consumed by NASH patients has a lower ratio of polyunsaturated fatty acid (PUFA) to saturated fatty acid (SFA) when compared with the general population (Toshimitsu et al., 2007; Musso et al., 2003). Consumption of a low ratio of ω-3 PUFA to ω-6 PUFA is also associated with NAFLD development, whereas increased consumption of dietary long-chain ω-3 PUFA decreases hepatic steatosis (Capanni et al., 2006; Cortez-Pinto et al., 2006; Levy et al., 2004).

Recently, Pachikian et al. (2011) established that removal of all ω-3 PUFA from the diet of mice significantly affected whole-body metabolism. After 3 months on the ω-3 PUFA-deficient diet, mice developed hepatosteatosis and insulin resistance. The mechanism was linked to a major decline in hepatic α-linolenic acid (ALA, 18:3,ω-3), eicosapentaenoic acid (EPA, 20:5,ω-3), and docosahexaenoic acid (DHA, 22:6,ω-3), but no change in hepatic linoleic acid (LA, 18:2,ω-6) and arachidonic acid (ARA, 20:4,ω-6) levels. Depletion of hepatic ω-3 PUFA lowered FAO, a peroxisome proliferator–activated receptor α (PPAR-α)–regulated mechanism, and increased fatty acid synthesis and triglyceride accumulation; sterol regulatory element-binding protein 1 (SREBP-1), carbohydrate regulatory element–binding protein (ChREBP), max-like factor X (MLX)–regulated mechanisms. PPAR-α, SREBP-1, and the ChREBP/MLX heterodimer are well-established targets of C_{20-22} ω-3 PUFA control (Jump et al., 2013).

Although *trans*-fatty acid (TFA) consumption is associated with insulin resistance and cardiovascular disease, the impact of TFA consumption on NAFLD in humans is less clear (Zelber-Sagi et al., 2011). Studies utilizing mice suggest that TFA consumption is associated with hepatic steatosis and injury (Tetri et al., 2008; Lottenberg et al., 2012).

Dietary cholesterol plays a role in NASH (Yasutake et al., 2009). The effect of dietary cholesterol hepatosteatosis is mixed, the effect of dietary cholesterol on hepatic inflammation and damage is clear (Wouters et al., 2008; Wouters et al., 2010; Teratani et al., 2012; Depner et al., 2012). High hepatic cholesterol content likely contributes to NASH progression. In the *LDLR$^{-/-}$* mouse model, high-fat/high-cholesterol (HFHC) diets promote NASH (Walenbergh et al., 2013). Kupffer cells, i.e., resident hepatic macrophage, become engorged with oxidized LDL (ox-LDL), which induces inflammatory cytokine secretion. These locally secreted cytokines act on other hepatic cells and induce cell injury. Kupffer cells also secrete chemokines (monocyte chemoattractant protein 1, MCP1) that recruit monocytes to the liver and amplify the inflammatory process. Controlling hepatic inflammation is an obvious target for NASH therapy.

Dietary monounsaturated fatty acids (MUFAs) have beneficial effects on the plasma lipids in humans when MUFA replace dietary carbohydrate (Mensink et al., 2003). However, similar observations exist for both PUFA and SFA, bringing to question the role of MUFA in NAFLD. A recent study suggest diets containing medium chain fatty acids also reduced NAFLD (Ronis et al., 2013). Patients diagnosed with NAFLD do not have different MUFA consumption compared with healthy controls (Zelber-Sagi et al., 2007). Moreover, there is no compelling data to suggest MUFA play a role in human NAFLD development.

Excessive consumption of sugar is clearly involved in hepatosteatosis and NASH progression. Over the last 30 years, there has been a dramatic increase in obesity and NAFLD in the United States; total fat consumption has remained steady while carbohydrate and total caloric intake have dramatically increased (Marriott et al., 2010a, b; Chun et al., 2010; Chanmugam et al., 2003; Lee et al., 2007). As such, elevated carbohydrate, specifically fructose consumption, has been linked to NAFLD and NASH progression (Vos et al., 2008; Lim et al., 2010; Bizeau and Pagliassotti, 2005). Fructose consumption has more than doubled in the last 30 years, and fructose is the monosaccharide most elevated with the increased carbohydrate consumption.

The liver expresses glucose transporter 5 (GLUT5), a fructose-specific transporter. Moreover, the liver is responsible for metabolizing up to 70% of dietary fructose (Bizeau and Pagliassotti, 2005; Lim et al., 2010). Fructose metabolism is independent of insulin. When compared with glucose, fructose more readily enters the pathway for fatty acid synthesis (DNL) and is assimilated into TAG. Fructose promotes all aspects of metabolic syndrome (MetS) including hepatosteatosis, insulin resistance, dyslipidemia, hyperglycemia, obesity, hypertension, and endotoxinemia. These metabolic features can explain why dietary fructose is highly implicated in NAFLD and NASH progression (Leclercq et al., 2000).

The majority of fructose enters the liver independent of insulin and bypasses the glucokinase step; fructose is phosphorylated by fructokinase and is subsequently converted to pyruvate through glycolysis. Once pyruvate is converted to acetyl-CoA, it enters the Krebs cycle. A large fructose bolus will generate sufficient acetyl-CoA to overwhelm the Krebs cycle leading to citrate export to the cytosol via the citrate shuttle. Cytosolic citrate is converted to acetyl-CoA by ATP-citrate lyase and used as a substrate for DNL and cholesterol synthesis. Increased substrate availability drives fatty acid and cholesterol synthesis providing substrates for triglyceride and cholesterol ester synthesis and storage. Malonyl-CoA, an intermediate in DNL, accumulates with elevated fatty acid synthesis and inhibits carnitine palmitoyl transferase 1 (CPT-1), a rate-limiting enzyme of FAO. Elevated DNL and reduced FAO resulting from high fructose consumption results in rapid development of hepatosteatosis (Bizeau and Pagliassotti, 2005).

In contrast to fructose, hepatic glucose metabolism is well regulated by insulin; glucose is also converted to glycogen for storage. Excess glucose consumption does not promote hepatosteatosis as aggressively as excess fructose consumption. Fructose also affects several biochemical events that exacerbate NASH development, including formation of reactive oxygen species (ROS), methylglyoxal and advanced glycation end products (Schalkwijk et al., 2004; Bunn and Higgins, 1981; Bose and Chakraborti, 2008; Wei et al., 2013).

A confounding issue in human NAFLD and NASH is that only a fraction of NAFLD patients progress to NASH. A recent review suggest that genetic variation is one potential factor explaining why some patients develop NASH and others do not (Hooper et al., 2011). The well-studied example is the PNPLA3 (also known as adiponutrin) gene. Single nucleotide polymorphisms (SNP) in PNPLA3 gene have been associated with NAFLD and fibrosis (Daly et al., 2011). Hispanics, for example, are more susceptible to NAFLD; this population expresses the PNPLA3 (rs738409[G]) allele, which is associated with higher hepatic lipid and inflammation levels (Romeo et al., 2008). African Americans, in contrast, have the lowest risk of NAFLD and commonly express the PNPLA3 (rs6006460[T]) allele; this allele is associated with lower hepatic lipid accumulation (Romeo et al., 2008). Although PNPLA3 gene polymorphisms are well characterized with respect to NAFLD, how these polymorphisms contribute to NAFLD, hepatic lipid metabolism and inflammation is less clear.

CURRENT TREATMENT OPTIONS FOR NAFLD AND NASH PATIENTS

Currently, there are no specific treatments for NAFLD or NASH. The standard of care for patients diagnosed with NAFLD or NASH is to treat the associated comorbidities including obesity, MetS, T2D, hyperlipidemia, and hypertension (Chalasani et al., 2012; Lam and Younossi, 2009; Musso et al., 2010; Mahady and George, 2012). More than 200 registered clinical trials are investigating NAFLD or NASH, and over half of these are focused on potential treatments (Table 13.1). A wide range of treatment approaches are being assessed including, but not limited to, metformin, farnesoid X receptor (FXR) ligands (obeticholic acid), PPAR-γ ligands (pioglitazone), statins, exercise versus diet, antioxidants (vitamin E), probiotics, and ω-3 fatty acids. This wide range of potential treatments stems from the complexity of abnormalities associated with NAFLD and NASH. Most trials completed to date are either observational or do not have histological end points. As such, effective treatments have yet to be identified.

Both calorie restriction and specific diets such as fat restriction, carbohydrate restriction, ketogenic diets, and high-protein diets have been evaluated as therapies for NAFLD and NASH (Mahady and George, 2012). To date, no one specific diet has been identified as superior for NASH treatment. It is well accepted that weight loss should be gradual and avoiding specific foods rather than calorie restriction will likely be more successful in the long run (Mahady and George, 2012; Andersen et al., 1991). Some diets or dietary components are hypothesized to have potential benefit for NAFLD and NASH patients such as the Mediterranean diet (Ryan et al., 2013) or ω-3 PUFA (Scorletti et al., 2013). NAFLD patients have lower consumption of ω-3 PUFA versus ω-6 PUFA, and long-chain ω-3 PUFA have known benefits on the control of both lipid metabolism and inflammation (Mahady and George, 2012; Jump, 2002; Calder, 2012). Recent clinical studies suggested that dietary C_{20-22} ω-3 PUFA have the potential to reduce hepatic lipid content in both children and adults (Nobili et al., 2011; Sofi et al., 2011; Bulchandani et al., 2011; Oya et al., 2011; Kishino et al., 2011).

ANIMAL MODELS FOR NAFLD AND NASH

Liver biopsies are required to accurately diagnose NAFLD and NASH. Such invasive procedures are not without risk to the patient. In efforts to better define the disease process and to develop better strategies for treatment, animal models are used. These models provide a powerful approach to investigate mechanisms involved in the onset and progression of disease and to assess new approaches for prevention and treatment. Both genetic and nutritional models have been used to study NAFLD and NASH.

Genetic Models of NAFLD and NASH

Mice with defective leptin signaling are frequently used to study mechanisms of obesity and obesity-linked diseases, such as NAFLD. The *ob/ob* and the *db/db* mouse models have defective leptin signaling. In the mice models, the *ob/ob* mice fail to produce leptin, whereas the *db/db* mice lack a functional leptin receptor. These mice are characterized by hyperphagia, obesity, inactivity, hyperglycemia, insulin resistance, and hyperinsulinemia (Bray and York, 1979); the phenotype resembles human MetS. Although leptin-deficient mice develop hepatosteatosis, they do not progress to NASH. Fibrosis is a detrimental clinical aspect of NASH, and these studies implicated leptin as essential for the development of hepatic fibrosis in chronic liver injury (Leclercq et al., 2002).

Two genetic models of defective cholesterol metabolism have been used to study NAFLD. In the apolipoprotein E2 (APOE2) knockin mouse (APOE2ki), the endogenous mouse *APOE* gene is replaced by the human *APOE2* allele (Sullivan et al., 1998). Human *APOE2* has reduced affinity for low-density lipoprotein receptor (LDLR) and APOE2ki mice fed a HFD develop a plasma lipoprotein profile that closely resembles human type III hyperlipoproteinemia (Sullivan et al., 1998). APOE2ki mice fed a HFD develop hepatosteatosis and inflammation. However, the inflammation resolves with prolonged feeding, thus limiting the use of this model in the study of NASH (Tous et al., 2006).

Mice with global ablation of the LDLR (LDLR$^{-/-}$) develop hypercholesteremia due to elevated plasma VLDL and LDL (Ishibashi et al., 1993). Historically, these mice were used as a model to study atherosclerosis. When fed HFHC diets, these mice develop hepatosteatosis with hepatic inflammation, injury, and fibrosis (Saraswathi et al., 2007, 2009; Depner et al., 2012, 2013a). *LDLR$^{-/-}$* mice fed a low-fat chow diet develop mild hepatosteatosis after an overnight fast, but do not develop hepatic inflammation, oxidative stress, or fibrosis (Depner et al., 2013a). As such, both diet and disrupted cholesterol metabolism are required for NASH development in this model. Since humans and *LDLR$^{-/-}$* mice develop NAFLD and NASH in a similar context, these mice are a useful model to investigate the development of NAFLD and NASH in the context of MetS.

Nutritional Models of NAFLD and NASH

A common nutritional model of NAFLD and NASH is the methionine–choline-deficient (MCD) diet. Methionine and choline are essential nutrients for β-oxidation, phospholipid synthesis, and hepatic VLDL export. The MCD diet induces rapid hepatosteatosis with elevated oxidative stress that causes hepatic inflammation and fibrosis (George et al., 2003). Although this is a severe NASH-like phenotype, rodents fed the MCD diet have reduced body weight, white adipose tissue, and plasma TAG, with elevated systemic insulin sensitivity (Rinella et al., 2008; Rinella and Green, 2004). Although this model is useful to study some facets of NASH, e.g., inflammation and fibrosis, NASH does not develop in the context of MetS. Therefore, conclusions drawn from studies using the MCD model have limited applicability to humans.

HFD (≥45% calories as fat) are commonly used to induce hepatosteatosis. Feeding rodents a HFD induces obesity, insulin resistance, dyslipidemia, hepatosteatosis with mild oxidative stress, inflammation, and fibrosis (Omagari et al., 2008; Varela-Rey et al., 2009; Matsuzawa et al., 2007; Schattenberg and Galle, 2010; Depner et al., 2012). The NASH-like phenotype in the HFD-fed mouse is less severe and takes longer (~12 weeks) to develop than the fatty liver phenotype in MCD fed mice. The pathophysiology associated with HFD feeding, however, closely resembles human MetS and NAFLD. As such, HFD models are commonly used to study NAFLD and are often combined with either genetic or other dietary modifications to induce a phenotype with severe hepatic inflammation and fibrosis.

Classic HFD manipulations used in atherosclerosis studies include increased dietary cholesterol, cholic acid, fructose, and sucrose, and these same manipulation are used to study NAFLD. These dietary manipulations induce a NASH phenotype resembling human NASH, i.e., with fibrosis and inflammation (Matsuzawa et al., 2007; Wouters et al., 2008; Jeong et al., 2005; Spruss et al., 2009; Depner et al., 2013a). These studies support the notion that multiple dietary components are responsible for the development of NAFLD or NASH.

Models of overnutrition in rodents have also been used to induce insulin resistance and NAFLD. In humans, the most common cause of these metabolic ailments is overnutrition, or chronic energy intake exceeding energy expenditure (Farrell and Larter, 2006). Rodents, however, metabolically adapt to a HFD and fail to develop metabolic abnormalities associated with NASH (Romestaing et al., 2007). To circumvent this metabolic adaptation, rodents can be force-fed by gavage or with a gastrostomy tube. Forced overnutrition in rodents results in obesity, hyperglycemia, hyperinsulinemia, hyperleptinemia, glucose intolerance, hepatic inflammation, damage, and fibrosis (Deng et al., 2005). These overnutrition models develop a similar pathophysiology as human NAFLD and NASH. The technical procedures associated with these models, however, are complex and time intensive. As such, overfeeding models are less frequently used compared with other approaches that resemble the human pathophysiology of NAFLD.

RATIONALE FOR THE USE OF ω-3 FATTY ACIDS IN NASH THERAPY

ω-3 PUFAs are currently being evaluated for treatment of fatty liver diseases (Table 13.1). Several recent clinical studies suggested that dietary C_{20-22} ω-3 PUFA may reduce hepatic lipid content in children and adults (Nobili et al., 2011; Sofi et al., 2011; Bulchandani et al., 2011; Oya et al., 2011; Kishino et al., 2011). Moreover, a recent review on the topic supports further research on ω-3 PUFA and NAFLD (Scorletti and Byrne, 2013). As an aid to future human studies, we recently assessed the capacity of

TABLE 13.1

Clinical Trials on Fatty Liver Disease and ω-3 Fatty Acids

	Total Trials	ω-3 Fatty Acid Trials
Fatty liver disease	404	42
Alcoholic fatty liver disease	9	–
NAFLD	202	12
NASH	183	8
Viral-induced fatty liver disease	38	2
Cirrhosis	785	4

Source: http://www.clinicaltrials.gov/ct2/results?term=fatty+liver+disease& Search=Search; http://www.clinicaltrials.gov/ct2/results?term=fatty+ liver+disease+and+omega-3+fatty+acids&Search=Search; http://www .clinicaltrials.gov/ct2/results?term=alcoholic+fatty+liver+disease+& Search=Search; http://www.clinicaltrials.gov/ct2/results?term=NAFL D&Search=Search; http://www.clinicaltrials.gov/ct2/results?term= NAFLD+and+omega-3+fatty+acids&Search=Search; http://www .clinicaltrials.gov/ct2/results?term=NASH&Search=Search; http://www .clinicaltrials.gov/ct2/results?term=virus+induced+fatty+liver+ disease&Search=Search; http://www.clinicaltrials.gov/ct2/results?term =virus+induced+fatty+liver+disease+and+omega+3+fatty+acids& Search=Search;http://www.clinicaltrials.gov/ct2/results?term=cirrhosis &Search=Search; http://www.clinicaltrials.gov/ct2/results?term= cirrhosis+and+omega-3+fatty+acids&Search=Search.

ω-3 PUFA to prevent HFHC diet–induced NASH in *LDLR*$^{-/-}$ mice. The outcome of these studies provides key information on capacity and limitations of dietary ω-3 PUFA to control the various aspects of diet-induced NASH (Depner et al., 2012, 2013a).

ω-3 PUFA represents one of two major classes of dietary long-chain PUFA. The major dietary ω-3 PUFA include ALA, EPA, and DHA (Figure 13.2). The major dietary ω-6 PUFA include LA and γ-linolenic acid (GLA, 18:3,ω-6). LA, however, is the predominant PUFA in Western diets (WDs). LA and ALA are essential fatty acids; they cannot be synthesized de novo in humans (Spector, 1999). These two fatty acids are precursors for C_{20-22} ω-6 and ω-3 PUFA found in all cells of the body. LA, ARA, and DHA are the major PUFA accumulating in all tissues.

Considerable interest in the health benefits of C_{20-22} ω-3 PUFA originated in the 1970s when Greenl and Inuits were found to have reduced rates of myocardial infarction when compared with individuals in Western countries (Bang et al., 1971, 1976; Bang and Dyerberg, 1972; Dyerberg et al., 1975; O'Keefe and Harris, 2000; Harris et al., 2009; Jump et al., 2012). These effects were linked to high dietary intake of C_{20-22} ω-3 PUFA, resulting in enrichment of blood lipids with C_{20-22} ω-3 PUFA and reduced fasting triglycerides (Bang et al., 1971; Dyerberg et al., 1975, 1978). The beneficial effects of C_{20-22} ω-3 PUFA on cardiovascular disease extend beyond effects on blood lipids and involve control of several other mechanisms, such heart

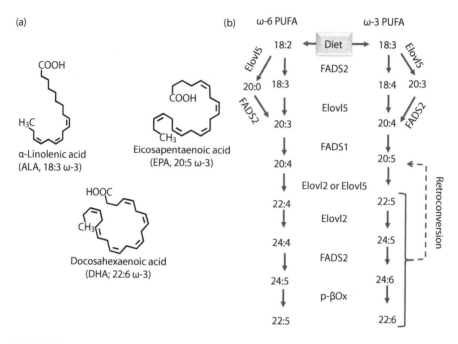

FIGURE 13.2 ω-3 PUFA: (a) structures of ω-3 PUFA and (b) pathway for PUFA synthesis.

rate (arrhythmia), inflammation, and endothelial function (Mozaffarian and Wu, 2011; Jump et al., 2012). Over 500 clinical trials have been carried out on ω-3 PUFA; these trials have examined effects of ω-3 PUFA on cardiovascular disease, MetS, diabetes, obesity, inflammation, dyslipidemia, liver disease, hypertension, visual acuity, cognitive development and decline, cancer prevention, and total mortality (Harris et al., 2009). Thus, these fatty acids have been well tested and found to be safe.

To prevent deficiency systems, humans require ALA at levels ~10% of LA, i.e., at ≥1.5 g/day (Gebauer et al., 2006). Humans, however, convert <10% of ingested ALA to DHA (Brenna, 2002; Plourde and Cunnane, 2007; Hussein et al., 2005; Rapoport et al., 2011). The basis for the inefficient conversion of ALA to DHA in humans is due to low Fads2 activity and high levels of dietary LA relative to ALA. Despite this low level of conversion, ALA does not accumulate in blood or most cells; ALA is channeled to β-oxidization or adipose storage (Brenna, 2002; Pawlosky et al., 2001). To increase cellular EPA or DHA to levels above those achieved with ALA intake alone requires the consumption of foods or supplements containing EPA or DHA. Food sources include fatty fish such as salmon and anchovies; dietary supplements are derived from fish, krill, algae, and genetically engineered yeast (Jump et al., 2012). Consumption of ~500 mg/day of EPA and DHA (combined) is recommended to lower the risk for cardiovascular disease (Kris-Etherton et al., 2002, 2003a, b; Mozaffarian and Wu, 2011; Lee et al., 2009; Gebauer et al., 2006; Saravanan et al., 2010; Harris et al., 2009). Lovaza™ (GSK), a pharmaceutical grade of ω-3 fatty acids (EPA and DHA ethyl esters), is prescribed at 4 g/day to treat patients with hypertriglyceridemia (Davidson et al., 2007).

PUFA Metabolism

ALA and LA are precursors to ω-3 and ω-6 C_{20-22} PUFA, i.e., DHA and ARA, respectively (Figure 13.2b). These fatty acids play structural roles in cells and serve as substrates for β-oxidation and energy production. They also regulate many physiological processes affecting human health, as NEFA, esterified (membrane-associated) fatty acids, or oxidized fatty acids. As such, both the dietary supply of these fatty acids and their metabolism is important for their effects on cell function (Jump, 2002; Jump et al., 2013).

The pathway for conversion of the essential fatty acids, LA and ALA to C_{20-22} ω-6 and ω-3 PUFA involves two fatty acid desaturases (Fads1 and Fads2) and two fatty acid elongases (Elovl2 and Elovl5) (Figure 13.2b). The final step in DHA (22:6,ω-3) synthesis requires peroxisomal β-oxidation (p-βOx) of 24:6,ω-3 (Jump, 2008; Sprecher, 2000). ARA and DHA are the major products of this pathway. DHA is the major ω-3 PUFA accumulating in cells, whereas LA and ARA are the major ω-6 PUFA accumulating in cells.

An unusual feature of C_{20-22} PUFA metabolism is that the C_{22} PUFA are retroconverted to C_{20} PUFA in the peroxisome (Sprecher, 2000). This reaction occurs in humans and mice; it involves p-βOx and the reduction of a double bond to generate EPA from DHA (Figure 13.3) (Sprecher, 2000; Jump et al., 2012). This reaction is apparent for DHA, but not for docosapentaenoic acid (22:5,ω-6), because there are few dietary sources with sufficient 22:5,ω-6 to promote this reaction; 22:5,ω-6 is typically seen at very low levels in cells and tissues.

The expression of enzymes involved in PUFA synthesis are regulated by transcriptional mechanisms by at least two transcription factors, PPAR-α and sterol regulatory element-binding protein 1 (SREBP-1) (Wang et al., 2005, 2006; Matsuzaka et al., 2002; Matsuzaka and Shimano, 2009). The expression of these enzymes is modestly sensitive to regulation by changes in blood insulin, a key regulator of SREBP-1 nuclear abundance. In contrast, elevated levels of dietary C_{20-22} ω-3 PUFA or fibrates (hypolipemic drugs) significantly activate PPAR-α (Ren et al., 1997) and induce expression of the desaturases and elongases. C_{20-22} ω-3 PUFAs are robust suppressors of Elovl5, FADS1, and FADS2 expression (Wang et al., 2005; Depner et al., 2013a). As such, C_{20-22} ω-3 PUFA are negative feedback inhibitors of PUFA synthesis. This feedback mechanism affects both ω-3 and ω-6 PUFA synthesis. As such, elevated consumption of dietary C_{20-22} ω-3 PUFA suppresses ARA production and increase cellular content of EPA and DHA (Depner et al., 2012, 2013a).

ω-3 PUFA are Pleiotropic Regulators of Cell Function

The products and some intermediates of the pathway for PUFA synthesis are assimilated into complex lipids as phosphoglycerolipids and neutral lipids; there is little nonesterified fatty acid in cells (usually <0.1% of total fatty acid). Once these fatty acids are assimilated into membrane lipids, they have the capacity to affect membrane structure,and serve as a reservoir of substrates for the generation of bioactive oxidized lipids, like eicosanoids (C_{20} PUFA) and docosanoids (C_{22} PUFA).

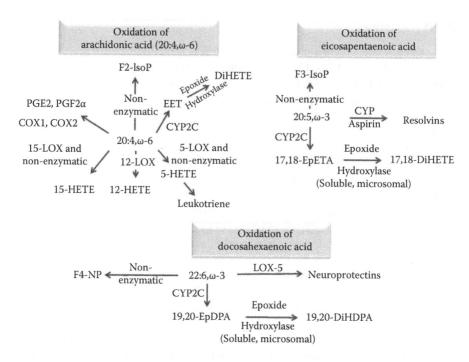

FIGURE 13.3 Generation of oxidized PUFA. PUFA ω-3 and ω-6 are subjected to enzymatic and nonenzymatic oxidation, and many of these oxidized lipids are biologically active. COX, cyclooxygenase; LOX, lipoxygenase; PGE2, prostaglandin E2; EET, epoxyeicosatrienoic acid; DiHETE, dihydroxyeicosatrienoic; HETE, hydroxyeicosatrienoic acid; EpETA, epoxyeicosa-tetraenoic acid; EpDPA, epoxydocosapentaenoic acid; DiHDPA, dihydroxydocosapentaenoic acid; CYP, cytochrome P450; F2-IsoP, F2-isoprostanes; F3-IsoP, F3-isoprostanes; F4-NP, F4-neuroprostanes.

Membrane Effects of ω-3 PUFA

Assimilation of ω-3 PUFA into membrane phospholipids have major effects on cell signaling by altering membrane fluidity, lipid raft structure, and substrate availability for the synthesis of bioactive oxidized fatty acids (Jump, 2002). DHA, for example, is a highly unsaturated fatty acid that alters membrane fluidity, membrane choles-terol content, and lipid raft organization (Stillwell, 2008). Some plasma membrane receptor systems affected by membrane DHA content include the toll-like receptors (TLR2 and TLR4) (Hsueh et al., 2011; Lee et al., 2003, 2010) and Src family kinases (Fyn, c-Yes) (Stulnig et al., 1998; Chen et al., 2005, 2007). Disruption of raft struc-ture alters downstream signaling events, such as nuclear factor κB (NF-κB), a major transcription factor controlling the expression of multiple genes encoding inflam-matory cytokines, chemokines, adhesion molecules, and cyclooxygenase 2 (COX2) (Vallabhapurapu and Karin, 2009). The attenuation of expression of these genes rep-resents one mechanism for the anti-inflammatory actions of ω-3 PUFA (Jump, 2002).

Fatty acids bind G-protein–coupled receptors (GPR) (Nilsson et al., 2003; Brown et al., 2005); these receptors control cellular levels of second messengers (cAMP and intracellular Ca^{+2}), and these receptors are expressed in a tissue-specific fashion. GRP120 was recently described as a ω-3 PUFA receptor and is expressed in macrophages and adipocytes. Ligand binding to GRP120 inhibits inflammatory events, including the control of NF-κB and c-Jun N-terminal kinase (JNK) and reverses insulin resistance in obese mice (Oh et al., 2011).

Oxidation of ω-3 and ω-6 PUFA

C_{20-22} ω-3 and ω-6 PUFAs are oxidized by enzymatic and nonenzymatic mechanisms (Figure 13.3). C_{20-22} PUFAs are preferentially assimilated into the sn2 position of membrane phospholipids. These fatty acids are excised from phospholipids by cellular phospholipase A2 (cPLA2), and the excised fatty acid serves as substrate for COX1 (constitutive), COX2 (inducible), lipoxygenases (LOX-5, LOX-12, and LOX-15), and cytochrome P450 (subtypes CYP2C and CYP4) enzymes. Eicosanoids derived from the COX and LOX pathways (Wada et al., 2007) regulate GPR as described above. Although EPA and DHA are poor substrates for COX and LOX, these enzymes generate series 3 and series 5 eicosanoids from EPA, respectively. These ω-3 PUFA–derived products are poor activators of eicosanoid receptors when compared with the ω-6 PUFA–derived products of COX and LOX (Smith, 2008; Wada et al., 2007; Calder, 2006).

Resolvins and protectins have attracted considerable attention because of their involvement in the resolution of inflammation (Spite and Serhan, 2010). The E-series resolvins (from EPA) and D-series resolvins (from DHA) are formed by the action of COX2 plus aspirin, whereas neuroprotectin D1 is formed by the action of LOX-5. Resolvins and neuroprotectins regulate inflammatory mechanisms (Serhan et al., 2009; Zhang and Bazan, 2010).

Non-esterified C_{20-22} ω-3 and ω-6 PUFA are substrates for cytochrome P450 enzymes (e.g., CYP2C and CYP4A/4F subtypes). This is a major mechanism for generating oxidized fatty acids in cells lacking COX 1 or COX2 activity, like hepatic parenchymal cells. CYP2C/2J, for example, synthesize regioisomeric epoxides of ARA, EPA, and DHA, i.e., 14,15-epoxyeicosatrienoic acid (14,15-EpET), 17,18-epoxy-eicosatetraenoic acid (17,18-EpET), and 19,20-epoxydoc-osapentaenoic acid (19,20-EpDP), respectively (Arnold et al., 2010a, b). These epoxides are converted to dihydroxy fatty acids (diols) by soluble or microsomal epoxide hydrolases. The EPA-derived epoxide, 17,18-EpET, for example, has anti-arrhythmic effects in neonatal cardiomyocytes (Falck et al., 2012). These CYP450-dependent metabolites of EPA and DHA are found in the heart, and they may play a role in C_{20-22} ω-3 PUFA-linked cardioprotection (Arnold et al., 2010a, b). They have also been found in the liver, but their hepatic function is unknown (Arnold et al., 2010a, b).

The C_{20-22} ω-3 and ω-6 PUFA are also subject to nonenzymatic oxidation. For example, ARA, EPA, and DHA are oxidized to F2-isoprostanes (F2-IsoP), F3-isoprostanes (F3-IsoP), and F4-neuroprostanes (F4-NP), respectively, by nonenzymatic processes (Milne et al., 2008, 2011; Saraswathi et al., 2007, 2009). C_{20-22} PUFA are susceptible to free radical attack when oxidative stress is increased in cells. Lipid peroxidation is a hallmark of oxidative stress; excessive production of lipid peroxides has been implicated in the pathogenesis of human diseases. The free radical–mediated (hydroxy-radicals, alkoxyl-radicals, peroxyl-radicals, or peroxyni-trate) lipid peroxidation chain reaction generates products found in membrane lipids and NEFA and in cells, blood, and urine. Formation of these oxidized lipids in mem-branes likely affects membrane fluidity and the function of membrane-associated proteins. F2-IsoP are bioactive, they activate thromboxane and prostaglandin F2α (PGF2α) receptors; they also induce vasoconstriction in vascular smooth muscle cells. In contrast, F3-IsoP do not regulate these receptors or smooth muscle vaso-constriction (Milne et al., 2011; Song et al., 2009). Whether the F3-IsoP and F4-NP have anti-inflammatory properties such as series 3 and 5 eicosanoids has not been established.

Nuclear Effects of ω-3 PUFA

NEFAs bind to and regulate the activity of several nuclear receptors including, PPAR (α, β/δ, γ), LXR (α, β), RXR, and HNF4α (Jump, 2013). Of these, fatty acid regula-tion of the PPAR family has been most extensively studied. In primary rat hepa-tocytes, EPA significantly induces PPAR-α–regulated target genes, which include genes involved in FAO. Although DHA modestly induces these same genes, ALA and DPA are ineffective. Analysis of hepatocyte NEFA following fatty acid treat-ment revealed that addition of DHA to cells increases esterified and nonesterified EPA through retroconversion, and EPA is the most potent ω-3 PUFA activator of PPAR-α in liver (Pawar and Jump, 2003). Co-crystals of PPARβ/δ-EPA, but not PPAR-DHA, have been described (Xu et al., 1999).

Dietary PUFA inhibits hepatic fatty acid synthesis by suppressing the expression of enzymes involved in DNL. This is achieved by PUFA suppression of the nuclear abundance of several transcription factors involved in hepatic carbohydrate and lipid metabolism, including SREBP-1, ChREBP, and MLX (Jump, 2013). Dietary PUFA control the nuclear abundance of SREBP-1 by regulating transcription of the SREBP-1c gene and the turnover of the SREBP-1 mRNA. DHA suppresses SREBP-1 nuclear abundance through these same mechanisms but also induces proteasomal degradation of nuclear SREBP-1 (Botolin et al., 2006).

C_{20-22} ω-3 PUFA suppresses inflammation, at least in part, by suppressing the nuclear abundance of NF-κB, a major transcription factor regulating expression of multiple genes encoding proteins involved in inflammation (Ben-Neriah and Karin, 2011). Some NF-κB target genes include COX2, cytokines (e.g., TNF-α, IL-1β), and chemokines (e.g., monocyte chemoattractant protein, MCP1). NF-κB nuclear abun-dance is typically regulated by controlling the interaction of NF-κB subunits (p50 and p65) with IκB subtypes (α, β, ε, ζ). IκB sequesters p50/p65 in the cytosol; phos-phorylation of IκB by IκB kinase promotes IκB dissociation from p50/p65, IκB is degraded in the proteasome, and p50/p65 accumulates in nuclei. IκB kinase activ-ity is regulated by its phosphorylation status; two kinases controlling IκB kinase phosphorylation status include Akt and transforming growth factor activated kinase 1 (TAK1). The NF-κB subunits bind promoters as heterodimers of p50/p65 and homodimers of p50; p65 can heterodimerizes with other transcription factors, like c/EBPα.

The regulation of NF-κB nuclear content by C_{20-22} ω-3 PUFA is achieved through several mechanisms, including (1) ω-3-PUFA inhibition of membrane receptor systems, e.g., TLRs, that activate the NF-κB pathway (Lee et al., 2003); (2) activated PPAR-α negatively affects NF-κB nuclear abundance by inducing IκBα; (3) PPAR-γ binds and sequesters NF-κB; and (4) ω-3 PUFA selectively suppresses p50 versus p65 nuclear abundance (Jump, 2013).

DIETARY C_{20-22} ω-3 PUFAs PREVENT HFD-INDUCED NASH IN *LDLR$^{-/-}$* MICE

C_{20-22} ω-3 PUFA are pleiotropic regulators of cell function. Because of their effects on fatty acid metabolism and inflammation, they would appear to be ideal nutrients to prevent NAFLD and NASH. Few studies, however, have actually determined the capacity of these fatty acids to prevent hepatosteatosis or inflammation in mouse models of HFD-induced NAFLD or NASH (Fedor et al., 2012; Kajikawa et al., 2011; Ishii et al., 2009; Takayama et al., 2010; Vemuri et al., 2007). Although human studies suggest ω-3 PUFA lower hepatosteatosis (Nobili et al., 2011; Sofi et al., 2011; Bulchandani et al., 2011; Oya et al., 2011; Kishino et al., 2011), there is no information on whether these treatments controlled hepatic inflammation or fibrosis.

To address this question, we first developed a mouse model of NASH that recapitulates many of the clinical features of human NASH. We fed wild-type (WT) and *LDLR$^{-/-}$* mice (C57BL/6J background) a HFD or a HFHC diet for 12 weeks. The HFD is typically used to induce insulin resistance in mice is obtained from Research Diets (New Brunswick, NJ) (D12492C$_{20-}$); it consists of 60% energy as fat (primarily as lard), 20% carbohydrate (starch/sucrose = 2:1), and 20% protein (casein and L-cystine). The HFHC is used to induce NASH with oxidative stress (Saraswathi et al., 2007). This is a custom diet from Research Diets, with 54% energy as fat, 27% energy as carbohydrate, 19% energy as protein, and 0.5 g% cholesterol.

The HFD and HFHC diet induced hepatosteatosis in WT and *LDLR$^{-/-}$* mice when compared with WT and *LDLR$^{-/-}$* mice fed a chow diet (Depner et al., 2012). The change in gene expression markers of hepatic inflammation (MCP1), fibrosis (procollagen 1A1, proCol1A1), and oxidative stress (hemeoxygenase 1, Hmox1) was low in WT and *LDLR$^{-/-}$* mice fed the HFDs but significantly higher in the *LDLR$^{-/-}$* mice fed the HFHC diet. Interestingly, feeding the *LDLR$^{-/-}$* mice the HFHC diet lowered urinary F2-IsoPs, suggesting a decline in whole-body oxidative stress. This diet also significantly increased hepatic and plasma ARA content, but suppressed hepatic and plasma C_{20-22} ω-3 PUFA content. These effects on hepatic PUFA content were explained by the induction of hepatic Elovl5 and Fads2 expression (Depner et al., 2012). More importantly, these findings correlated with those found in NAFLD patients (Araya et al., 2004, 2010; Kishino et al., 2011; Zheng et al., 2012). Thus, increased dietary precursors such as LA, coupled with increased capacity to synthesize ARA, accounts for increased hepatic and plasma ARA in mice and humans.

We next assessed the capacity of dietary ω-3 PUFA to restore hepatic C_{20-22} ω-3 PUFA, lower hepatosteatosis, and attenuate hepatic inflammation. WT and *LDLR$^{-/-}$* mice were fed the HFHC diet supplemented with menhaden oil (HFHC-M), a rich source of EPA and DHA (Depner et al., 2012). Total EPA and DHA in the HFHC-M diet was at 2% total energy; a dose comparable to that used to treat patients with dyslipidemia (Lovaza™; GSK) (Davidson et al., 2007). The HFHC diet was supplemented with olive oil (HFHC + O) to keep the diets isocaloric. When compared with

WT or $LDLR^{-/-}$ mice fed the HFHC + O diet, mice fed the HFHC + M diet had a significant reduction in many NASH markers, including hepatosteatosis and markers of hepatic inflammation and fibrosis. The HFHC + M diet, however, did not suppress hepatic HMOX1, a marker of hepatic oxidative stress.

The HFHC + M diet induced whole-body oxidative stress as evidence by increased urinary F2-IsoP. The HFHC + M diet also increased urinary levels of C_{20-22} ω-3 PUFA-derived isoprostanes, i.e., F3-IsoP and F4-NP (Depner et al., 2012). Since EPA and DHA are highly peroxidizable, their accumulation in tissues, coupled with elevated oxidative stress in tissues induced by the HFHC + O diet, was expected to promote lipid peroxidation. Feeding mice the HFHC + M diet also lowered plasma and hepatic ARA but increased EPA and DHA.

Nonenzymatic oxidation products of LA are increased in plasma of patients with NASH (Feldstein et al., 2010; Puri et al., 2009). The induction of oxidative stress in NASH patients (Ndisang and Jadhav, 2010; Yu et al., 2010; Nicolai et al., 2009; Abraham et al., 2008; Paine et al., 2011; Inoue et al., 2011) has led to several clinical studies assessing the impact of dietary antioxidants as potential NASH therapies (Sanyal et al., 2010; Lavine et al., 2011; Zein et al., 2012; Di Minno et al., 2012). Since increased oxidative stress, i.e., urinary F2-IsoP, is typically correlated with increased tissue damage, our finding that dietary C_{20-22} ω-3 PUFA increased urinary isoprostanes may raise concerns for their use in NAFLD and NASH therapy. Our study, however, shows that C_{20-22} ω-3 PUFA induction of F3-IsoP and F4-NP is associated with decreased hepatic injury, not increased hepatic injury, in response to the HFHC + M diet. Although the biological activity of F2-IsoPs has been established, it is unclear if the F3-IsoP and F4-NP have any biological activity (Milne et al., 2011; Song et al., 2009). Defining the biological function of F3-IsoP and F4-NP is important to determine if these isoprostanes are hepatoprotective or benign markers of ω-3 PUFA status.

DHA ATTENUATES WD–INDUCED NASH IN $LDLR^{-/-}$ MICE

Our previous study suggested that dietary ω-3 PUFA can protect against diet-induced NASH (Depner et al., 2012). Previous studies from our lab, however, suggested that EPA and DHA have differential effects on hepatic function (reviewed by Jump, 2013). Moreover, the level of NASH developed in the HFHC-fed $LDLR^{-/-}$ mouse model was a mild form of disease. To access specific ω-3 PUFA and test the limits of ω-3 PUFA to prevent diet-induced NASH, we used the WD.

The WD (D12079B; Research Diets; 40% energy as fat, mainly milk fat; 43% energy as carbohydrate, 29% energy is sucrose; 17% energy as protein [casein + methionine]; 0.21 g% cholesterol) is specifically designed to recapitulate a high-fat/high-sugar diet consumed by a large segment of westernized countries populaces. In contrast to the HFD and HFHC diet, $LDLR^{-/-}$ mice fed the WD developed a robust NASH phenotype that is characterized by severe hepatosteatosis, hepatic inflammation, oxidative stress, and fibrosis. The robust NASH phenotype in these mice was attributed to the duration of feeding (16 versus 12 weeks) and the high sucrose, fat, and cholesterol in the WD (Depner et al., 2013a).

To assess prevention, the WD was supplemented with either olive oil (WD + O), EPA (WD + E), DHA (WD + D), or EPA + DHA (WD + ED). As above, all ω-3 PUFA supplements were isocaloric, i.e., at 2% total calories. Inclusion of EPA, DHA, or EPA + DHA in the WD attenuated multiple markers of inflammation, oxidative stress, and fibrosis, without significant reduction of hepatosteatosis. Accordingly, the suppressive effects of EPA and DHA on hepatic pathology did not require a significant reduction of hepatic lipid content. As such, EPA and DHA preferentially act at the level of the "second and third hits" (Figure 13.1). This outcome may be particularly advantageous to the obese patient who presents with NASH (Depner et al., 2013a).

Hepatic Lipid Metabolism

Feeding *LDLR*$^{-/-}$ mice the WD leads to a massive accumulation of hepatic SFA and MUFA (Figure 13.4a). This is due to the high dietary content of SFA and MUFA as well as the induction of enzymes involved in DNL (fatty acid synthase) and MUFA (stearoyl CoA desaturase 1) synthesis and the high substrate (glucose and fructose) in the WD. The WD diet also significantly increases hepatic ARA and lowered hepatic EPA and DHA (Depner et al., 2013a). Like the HFHC diet, the WD also induced expression of Elovl5 and Fads2, key enzymes involved in PUFA synthesis (Figure 13.2b). These changes in hepatic PUFA synthesis in *LDLR*$^{-/-}$ mice paralleled changes in PUFA metabolism seen in patients with NAFLD (Araya et al., 2004, 2010). The consequence of the change in hepatic ω-3 and ω-6 PUFA content is a major change in the ratio of ω-6/ω-3 PUFA (Figure 13.4b). ω-6 PUFA are precursors for the synthesis of proinflammatory bioactive lipids, whereas the ω-3 PUFA are precursors for anti-inflammatory bioactive lipids (Figures 13.3 and 13.4).

Feeding *LDLR*$^{-/-}$ mice the WD containing EPA and/or DHA suppressed hepatic ARA content. DHA, however, was more effective than EPA in suppressing both ARA and the expression of enzymes involved in PUFA synthesis (Elovl2, Elovl5, Fads1, and Fads2). Thus, DHA was very effective at lowering the ω-6:ω-3 PUFA ratio in liver (Figure 13.4b). In addition, DHA is retroconverted to EPA, leading to a significant accumulation of hepatic EPA and DPA. Although dietary EPA significantly increased hepatic EPA and DPA, dietary EPA does not significantly increase DHA (Depner et al., 2013a).

Because of these major changes in hepatic ARA, EPA, and DHA, we were surprised to find that WD + E or WD + D did not induce acyl CoA oxidase (AOX) or other enzymes involved in FAO (carnitine palmitoyl transferase 1 [CPT1 and CPT2]). These enzymes are targets of PPAR-α and EPA activates PPAR-α (Ren et al., 1997; Pawar and Jump, 2003). Recent studies, however, have established that interleukin (IL) 1β signaling interferes with PPAR-α signaling (Stienstra et al., 2010). Hepatic IL-1β is induced in mice fed the WD + O and repressed in mice fed the WD + EPA or WD + DHA diets (Figure 13.5a). The WD, regardless of the absence or presence of EPA or DHA, induces hepatic FAO, as reflected by increased blood levels of β-hydroxybutyrate. Although dietary DHA is the most effective treatment for reducing hepatic SFA and MUFA content, it is not sufficient to return neutral lipids to levels found in control mice (Figure 13.4a). This failure to induce FAO may

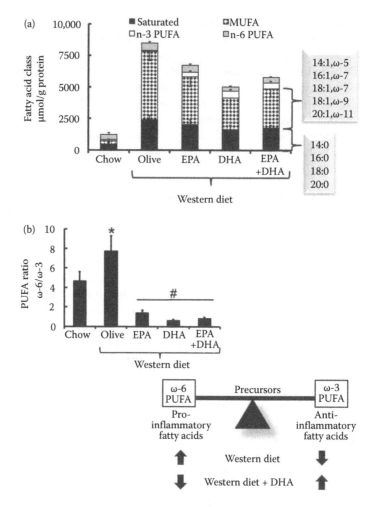

FIGURE 13.4 Effects of the WD, EPA, and DHA on hepatic fatty acid composition. *LDLR$^{-/-}$* mice were fed a chow or the WD supplemented with olive oil, EPA, DHA of EPA + DHA for 16 weeks. After 16 weeks on the WD, the WD-fed mice were obese, dyslipidemic, and expressed multiple markers of NASH. (a) Hepatic fatty acid content was quantified and expressed as total SFA, MUFA, ω-3 PUFA, or ω-6 PUFA as μmol of fatty acid/g hepatic protein (mean ± SD, n = 8). (b) Using data from (a), results are expressed as the molar ratio of total ω-6 versus ω-3 PUFA. *p ≤ 0.05 versus chow; #p ≤ 0.05 versus WD + olive oil. (From Depner, C.M. et al., *J Nutr*, 143, 315–323, 2013.)

be one explanation for the limited suppression of hepatosteatosis in WD containing EPA and/or DHA.

Hepatic Inflammation

Although dietary EPA or DHA did not return hepatic neutral lipids to normal levels, histological scoring of inflammation, coupled with hepatic gene expression analysis established that the WD + O induced inflammation was significantly attenuated by

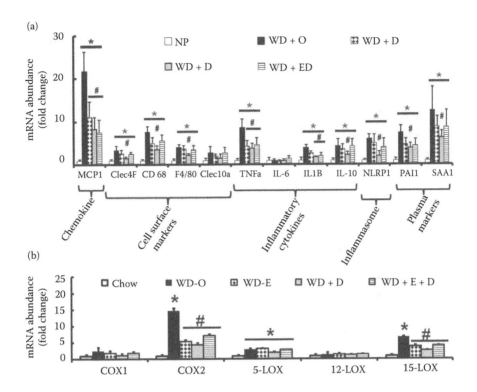

FIGURE 13.5 Effects of the WD, EPA, and DHA on multiple gene expression markers of inflammation. Hepatic abundance of mRNAs encoding proteins involved in inflammation was quantified as described. (a) Gene markers for chemokines, Kupffer cell, and macrophage surface markers; inflammatory cytokines, inflammasome proteins; plasma markers of inflammation expressed in liver. (b) Gene markers for enzymes involved in generating oxidized PUFA. COX, cyclooxygenase; LOX, lipoxygenase. *$p \leq 0.05$ versus chow; #$p \leq 0.05$ versus WD + olive oil. Results are expressed as fold change (mean ± SD, n = 8). (From Depner, C.M. et al., *J Nutr*, 143, 315–323, 2013.)

WD + E and WD + E (Figure 13.5). In no case was WD + E more effective than WD + D; in many cases, WD + D was more effective than WD + E. DHA attenuated WD + O induction of chemokines proteins (Mcp1), cell surface markers associated with macrophage (Clec4f, CD68, and F4/80), inflammatory cytokines (IL-1β and TNF-α), inflammasome-associated proteins (NLRP1), hepatic-generated plasma proteins linked to inflammation (SAA and PAI1). In addition, TLR2, TLR4, and TLR9 and associated proteins (CD14) were most significantly suppressed by DHA. The impact of WD + D on both TLR (2, 4, and 9) and inflammasome components (NLRP1) is significant because each is linked to the development of NASH and insulin resistance (Miura et al., 2013; Vandanmagsar et al., 2011).

Since oxidized bioactive PUFA are involved in hepatic inflammation, we assessed the impact of diet on this pathway by measuring the expression of hepatic COX1, COX2, 5-LOX, 12-LOX, and 15-LOX (Figure 13.5b). COX1 and 12-LOX mRNA levels were not affected by diet. In contrast, COX2, 5-LOX, and 15-LOX were induced ≥2-fold by WD + O. The expression of COX2 and 15-LOX was suppressed by WD containing EPA or DHA, whereas 5-LOX was suppressed by DHA only.

Hepatic abundance of these transcripts (Figure 13.5b) is regulated by mechanisms controlling NF-κB nuclear abundance. Although the WD + O induced the accumulation of NF-κB (p50 and p65) in hepatic nuclei, WD + D attenuated this response. DHA, however, only suppressed NF-κB p50 nuclear content. WD + E, in contrast, did not suppress hepatic nuclear abundance of NF-κB p50 or p65. These results suggest that DHA is the major ω-3 PUFA controlling NF-κB-dependent mechanisms (Depner et al., 2013a).

Source of the Inflammatory Signal

A key unanswered question in our previous study was the source of the inflammatory signal(s) inducing hepatic inflammation (Depner et al., 2013a). Two sources of inflammatory signals have been described; oxidized LDL (ox-LDL) (Walenbergh et al., 2013) and endotoxin (Cani et al., 2007; Harte et al., 2010). The role of ox-LDL in cardiovascular disease and inflammation is well established (Lusis, 2000). Endotoxin originates from the gut either by increased gut permeability or cotransport with chylomicron (Erridge et al., 2007; Harte et al., 2010; Laugerette et al., 2011). Other factors such as products from hepatocellular death may exacerbate hepatic inflammation (Tilg and Moschen, 2010; Marra et al., 2008).

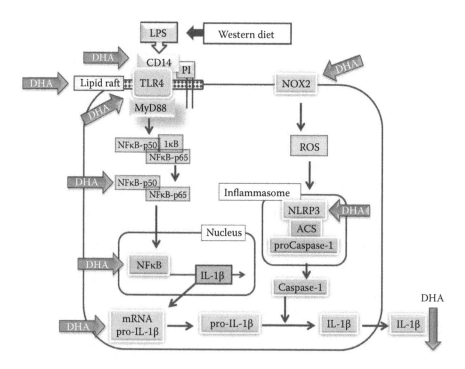

FIGURE 13.6   Pleiotropic effects of DHA on hepatic inflammation.

We quantified plasma levels of endotoxin and found that feeding $LDLR^{-/-}$ mice the WD + O for 16 weeks increased plasma endotoxin 15-fold. None of the ω-3 PUFA–supplemented WD lowered plasma endotoxin (Depner et al., 2013b) or hepatic cholesterol (Depner et al., 2013a). These outcomes suggest that dietary ω-3 PUFA does not attenuate hepatic inflammation by regulating the source of this inflammatory agent (endotoxin or cholesterol). We suggest that DHA functions by controlling the cellular response to endotoxin or inflammatory cytokines (Figure 13.6). DHA suppresses expression of CD14, the endotoxin receptor, as well as TLR4 (Akira and Takeda, 2004). TLR4 function requires a defined lipid raft structure (Fessler and Parks, 2011), and DHA is a well-established disruptor of lipid rafts (Wassall and Stillwell, 2009; Soni et al., 2008). The downstream targets of TLR4 include NF-κB, and the vast network of NF-κB target genes involved in inflammation (Akira and Takeda, 2004). DHA suppresses the accumulation of NF-κB p50 in the nucleus and the expression of multiple chemokines, cell surface markers, inflammatory cytokines IL-1β, inflammasome components (NLRP3), and plasma markers linked to inflammation (Figures 13.5 and 13.6) (Depner et al., 2013a). DHA is a pleiotropic regulator of hepatic inflammation.

Hepatic Oxidative Stress

We examined multiple markers of hepatic oxidative stress; including hepatic nuclear content of nuclear factor E2–related factor 2 (Nrf2) and the expression of several genes involved in oxidative stress (HMOX1, glutathione S-transferase α1 [Gstα1], and NADPH oxidase [NOX] subunits). Nrf2 is a key transcription factor involved in the antioxidant response; it regulates the expression of several genes including HMOX1 and Gstα1. Although the WD + O induced hepatic nuclear Nrf2 content and HMOX1 expression (>2-fold, $p < 0.05$), the WD + D diet did not attenuate this response (Depner et al., 2013a).

We also examined the effect of diet on multiple transcripts linked to the NOX pathway, including Nox1, Nox2 (gp91), Nox4, Noxa1, Noxo1, RAS-related C3 botulinum substrate 1 (Rac1), cytochrome b-245 light chain (P22phox), neutrophil cytosolic factor 4 (P40phox), neutrophil cytosolic factor 1 (P47phox), and neutrophil cytosolic factor 2 (P67phox). Of these, Nox2, P22phox, P40phox, P47phox, and P67phox were well induced (4- to 6-fold; $p < 0.05$) in mice fed WD + O compared with chow-fed mice. Feeding WD + D was more effective than the WD + E in attenuating the WD + O induction of these transcripts. NOX is important for the generation of reactive oxygen species, and its role in NASH progression, especially fibrosis, has been well established (De Minicis and Brenner, 2007; Paik et al., 2011; Cui et al., 2011).

Hepatic Fibrosis

We assessed hepatic fibrosis by histological examination of livers stained with trichrome and measurement of gene expression markers of fibrosis and activated stellate cells, i.e., proCol1α1 (procollagen1α1), tissue inhibitor metalloprotease 1 (TIMP-1) and BMP, and activin membrane–bound inhibitor a TGFβ pseudo-receptor (BAMBI) (Teratani et al., 2012; Hernandez-Gea and Friedman, 2011). ProCol1α1 and TIMP-1 mRNAs were induced ~20- and ~40-fold, respectively, whereas BAMBI was not induced by WD + O (Figure 13.7). Of the collagen subtypes examined, Col1A1 was

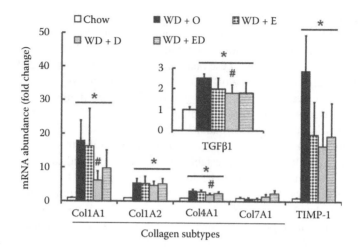

FIGURE 13.7 Effect of the WD, EPA, and DHA on hepatic fibrosis. Hepatic abundance of mRNAs encoding proteins involved in hepatic fibrosis was quantified as described. Results are expressed as fold change (mean ± SD, n = 8). *p ≤ 0.05 versus chow; #p ≤ 0.05 versus WD + olive oil. (From Depner, C.M. et al., *J Nutr*, 143, 315–323, 2013.)

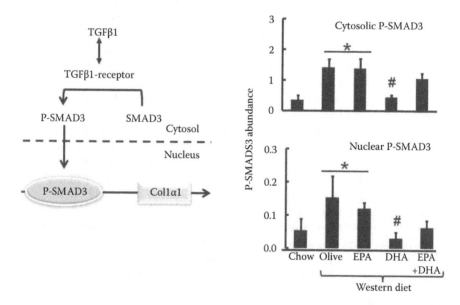

FIGURE 13.8 Effect of the WD, EPA, and DHA on phospho-SMAD3 cytosolic and nuclear abundance. Cytosolic and nuclear proteins were isolated from livers of mice fed chow or the WD supplement with EPA and/or DHA, as described. Both phospho-SMAD2 and phospho-SMAD3 were quantified by immunoblot and normalized to loading controls: Na,K-ATPase for cytosolic proteins and TATA-binding protein (TBP) for nuclear proteins. Only phospho-SMAD3 was regulated by these diets. Results are expressed as the ratio of phospho-SMAD3/Na,K-ATPase (cytosolic) and phospho-SMAD3/TBP (nuclear) proteins (mean ± SD, n = 8). *p ≤ 0.05 versus chow; #p ≤ 0.05 versus WD + olive oil. (From Depner, C.M. et al., *J Nutr*, 143, 315–323, 2013.)

the most affected by diet. DHA was superior to EPA in the attenuation of proCol1A1 expression, whereas EPA and DHA were equivalent in the attenuation of TIMP1 expression. This novel effect of DHA on fibrosis was not only evident in effects on collagen gene expression but also on hepatic collagen content as quantified by tri-chrome staining of liver (Depner et al., 2013a).

The mechanism for the DHA effect on collagen was linked to changes in SMAD-3 (mother against DPP homologue 3) nuclear content. SMAD-3 is a key transcription factor regulating collagen 1A1 transcription (Matsuzaki, 2012). Activated TGFβ1 receptor phosphorylates SMAD-3, leading to P-SMAD-3 accumulation in nuclei where it binds the proCol1A1 promoter (Figure 13.8). DHA, but not EPA, lowers phospho-SMAD-3 in the cytosol and nucleus. As such, DHA likely inhibits transcription of the proCol1A1 gene by interfering with TGFβ1 signaling and SMAD-3 control of proCol1A1 expression.

SUMMARY AND FUTURE STUDIES

Our studies have established that C_{20-22} ω-3 fatty acids in menhaden oil, when included in a HFHC diet at a physiologically relevant level (2% total calories), effectively attenuates multiple markers of NAFLD and NASH including hepatosteatosis, inflammation, and fibrosis but not oxidative stress (Depner et al., 2012). This outcome was encouraging and provided evidence for the use of C_{20-22} ω-3 PUFA supplements in the control of mild forms of NAFLD/NASH.

The WD, in contrast, induced a severe form of NASH in *LDLR*$^{-/-}$ mice, and supplementing the WD with EPA and/or DHA attenuated hepatic inflammation (TLR4, TLR9, NF-κB p50, and multiple NF-κB target genes) and fibrosis (proCol1A1 expression and SMAD-3 phosphorylation) and selectively suppressed oxidative stress (NOX2 and its subunits), but it did not prevent hepatosteatosis. DHA, however, did lower hepatic SFA and MUFA content (Figure 13.4). This outcome indicates that a major reduction in hepatic lipid content is not required to significantly attenuate expression of NASH markers, specifically inflammation, oxidative stress (NOX pathway), and fibrosis.

Dietary DHA was equal or superior to EPA in regulating every NASH parameter examined. DHA has robust anti-inflammatory and anti-fibrotic actions (Figures 13.5 to 13.8). Much of this effect was directed at TLR4 and NF-κB signaling, where DHA suppressed the expression of multiple components of the TLR4 pathway as well as multiple NF-κB target genes. DHA also suppressed expression of an inflammasomes component (NLRP1) and multiple NOX subunits. Since DHA is retroconverted to EPA, EPA-dependent mechanisms can be activated such as PPAR-α regulation of FAO. However, neither EPA nor DHA significantly induced hepatic FAO. EPA, however, is poorly converted to DHA, and the anti-fibrotic action of DHA through control of SMAD-3 phosphorylation and nuclear abundance would not be achieved with dietary EPA alone. In fact, our results suggest that the combination of EPA + DHA or fish oil would provide less suppression of fibrosis than that seen with dietary DHA alone (Figures 13.7 and 13.8) (Depner et al., 2013a). These outcomes suggest that DHA supplementation may be more efficacious for abrogating human NASH. The effects of ω-3 PUFA on liver function and composition were achieved without

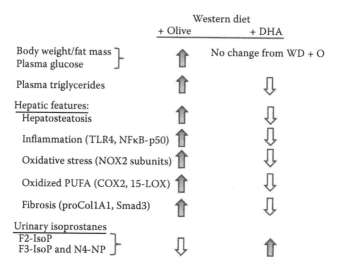

FIGURE 13.9 Summary of WD and DHA effects on markers of MetS and NASH. The markers of MetS are body weight, body composition, fasting blood glucose, and triglycerides. The markers of NASH include hepatosteatosis, inflammation, oxidative stress, and fibrosis. Arrows for the WD + olive oil group indicate direction of change relative to the chow-fed group. Arrows for the WD + DHA group represent the direction of change relative to the WD + olive oil group for continuity.

significant weight loss, change in food consumption, body composition (% fat mass), or blood glucose (Figure 13.9) (Depner et al., 2012, 2013a). The pleiotropic properties of DHA make it an attractive dietary supplement in the management of NASH.

Our studies raise several unanswered questions. Particularly relevant is the elevation of urinary isoprostanes by dietary ω-3 PUFA (Depner et al., 2012). The increase in urinary F2-IsoP, F3-IsoP, and F4-NP was associated with improved liver parameters. A further study is required to establish whether F3-IsoP and F4-NP have hepatoprotective activities. Similarly, the analysis of the COX and LOX subtypes suggest significant changes in the oxidized fatty acid composition of the liver. A lipidomic analysis focused on these metabolites and the CYP-dependent metabolites may reveal the formation of hepatoprotective oxidized lipids, such as resolvins, protectins, EpETA, or EpDPA, in animals fed DHA. Finally, our analysis was designed to prevent diet-induced NASH. Future studies are needed to assess the molecular and metabolic events associated with the onset and progression of NASH as well as whether DHA supplementation can reverse NASH once it has developed.

ACKNOWLEDGMENTS

This work was supported by the National Institute of Food and Agriculture grant (2009-65200-05846) and the National Institutes of Health grant (DK94600).

REFERENCES

Abdelmalek, M. F., A. Suzuki, C. Guy et al. 2010. Increased fructose consumption is associated with fibrosis severity in patients with nonalcoholic fatty liver disease. *Hepatology* 51:1961–71.

Abraham, N. G., and A. Kappas. 2008. Pharmacological and clinical aspects of heme oxygenase. *Pharmacol Rev* 60:79–127.

Adams, L. A., J. F. Lymp, J. St Sauver et al. 2005. The natural history of nonalcoholic fatty liver disease: a population-based cohort study. *Gastroenterology* 129:113–21.

Akira, S., and K. Takeda. 2004. Toll-like receptor signalling. *Nat Rev Immunol* 4:499–511.

Andersen, T., C. Gluud, M. B. Franzmann, and P. Christoffersen. 1991. Hepatic effects of dietary weight loss in morbidly obese subjects. *J Hepatol* 12:224–9.

Angulo, P. 2002. Nonalcoholic fatty liver disease. *N Engl J Med* 346:1221–31.

Araya, J., R. Rodrigo, L. Pettinelli, V. Araya, J. Poniachik, and L. A. Videla. 2010. Decreased liver fatty acid delta-6 and delta-5 desaturase activity in obese patients. *Obesity* 18:1460–3.

Araya, J., R. Rodrigo, L. A. Videla, L. Thielemann, M. Orellana, P. Pettinelli, and J. Poniachik. 2004. Increase in long-chain polyunsaturated n-6/n-3 ration in relation to hepatic steatosis in patients with non-alcoholic fatty liver disease. *Clin Sci* 106:635–43.

Arnold, C., A. Konkel, R. Fischer, and W.-H. Schunck. 2010a. Cytochrome P450-dependent metabolism of omega-6 and omega-3 long-chain polyunsaturated fatty acids. *Pharma Rep* 62:536–47.

Arnold, C., M. Markovic, K. Blossey, G. Wallukat, R. Fisher, R. Dechend, A. Konkel, C. Von Schaky, F. C. Luft, D. N. Muller, M. Rothe, and W.-H. Schunck. 2010b. Arachidonic acid-metabolizing cytochrome P450 enzymes are targets of omega-3 fatty acids. *J Biol Chem* 285:32720–33.

Bang, H. O., and J. Dyerberg. 1972. Plasma lipids and lipoproteins in Greenlandic west coast Eskimos. *Acta Med Scand* 192:85–94.

Bang, H. O., J. Dyerberg, and N. Hjoorne. 1976. The composition of food consumed by Greenland Eskimos. *Acta Med Scand* 200:69–73.

Bang, H. O., J. Dyerberg, and A. B. Nielsen. 1971. Plasma lipid and lipoprotein pattern in Greenlandic West-coast Eskimos. *Lancet* 1:1143–5.

Ben-Neriah, Y., and M. Karin. 2011. Inflammation meets cancer, with NF-kappaB as the matchmaker. *Nat Immunol* 12:715–23.

Bizeau, M. E., and M. J. Pagliassotti. 2005. Hepatic adaptations to sucrose and fructose. *Metabolism* 54:1189–201.

Bose, T., and A. S. Chakraborti. 2008. Fructose-induced structural and functional modifications of hemoglobin: implication for oxidative stress in diabetes mellitus. *Biochim Biophys Acta* 1780:800–8.

Botolin, D., Y. Wang, B. Christian, and D. B. Jump. 2006. Docosahexaneoic acid (22:6,n-3) regulates rat hepatocyte SREBP-1 nuclear abundance by Erk- and 26S proteasome-dependent pathways. *J Lipid Res* 47:181–92.

Bray, G. A., and D. A. York. 1979. Hypothalamic and genetic obesity in experimental animals: an autonomic and endocrine hypothesis. *Physiol Rev* 59:719–809.

Brenna, J. T. 2002. Efficiency of conversion of alpha-linolenic acid to long chain n-3 fatty acids in man. *Curr Opin Clin Nutr Metab Care* 5:127–32.

Brown, A. J., S. Jupe, and C. P. Briscoe. 2005. A family of fatty acid binding receptors. *DNA Cell Biol* 24:54–61.

Bulchandani, D. G., J. S. Nachnani, A. Nookala et al. 2011. Treatment with omega-3 fatty acids but not exendin-4 improves hepatic steatosis. *Eur J Gastroenterol Hepatol* 22:1245–52.

Bunn, H. F., and P. J. Higgins. 1981. Reaction of monosaccharides with proteins: possible evolutionary significance. *Science* 213:222–4.

Calder, P. C. 2006. n-3 polyunsaturated fatty acids, inflammation, and inflammatory diseases. *Am J Clin Nutr* 83:1505S–1519S.

Calder, P. C. 2012. Mechanisms of action of (n-3) fatty acids. *J Nutr* 142:592S–599S.

Cani, P. D., J. Amar, M. A. Iglesias et al. 2007. Metabolic endotoxemia initiates obesity and insulin resistance. *Diabetes* 56:1761–72.

Capanni, M., F. Calella, M. R. Biagini et al. 2006. Prolonged n-3 polyunsaturated fatty acid supplementation ameliorates hepatic steatosis in patients with non-alcoholic fatty liver disease: a pilot study. *Aliment Pharmacol Ther* 23:1143–51.

Chalasani, N., Z. Younossi, J. E. Lavine et al. 2012. The diagnosis and management of non-alcoholic fatty liver disease: practice guideline by the American Gastroenterological Association, American Association for the Study of Liver Diseases, and American College of Gastroenterology. *Gastroenterology* 142:1592–609.

Chanmugam, P., J. F. Guthrie, S. Cecilio, J. F. Morton, P. P. Basiotis, and R. Anand. 2003. Did fat intake in the United States really decline between 1989–1991 and 1994–1996? *J Am Diet Assoc* 103:867–72.

Chen, W., W. J. Esselman, D. B. Jump, and J. V. Busik. 2005. Anti-inflammatory effect of docosahexaenoic acid on cytokine-induced adhesion molecule expression in human retinal vascular endothelial cells. *Invest Ophthalmol Vis Sci* 46:4342–7.

Chen, W., D. B. Jump, W. J. Esselman, and J. V. Busik. 2007. Inhibition of cytokine signaling in human retinal endothelial cells through modification of caveolae/lipid rafts by docosahexaenoic acid. *Invest Ophthalmol Vis Sci* 48:18–26.

Chun, O. K., C. E. Chung, Y. Wang, A. Padgitt, and W. O. Song. 2010. Changes in intakes of total and added sugar and their contribution to energy intake in the U.S. *Nutrients* 2:834–54.

ClinicalTrials.gov. http://www.clinicaltrials.gov/ct2/results?term=fatty+liver+disease&Search=Search (accessed June 30, 2014).

ClinicalTrials.gov. http://www.clinicaltrials.gov/ct2/results?term=fatty+liver+disease+and+omega-3+fatty+acids&Search=Search (accessed June 30, 2014).

ClinicalTrials.gov. http://www.clinicaltrials.gov/ct2/results?term=alcoholic+fatty+liver+disease+&Search=Search (accessed June 30, 2014).

ClinicalTrials.gov. http://www.clinicaltrials.gov/ct2/results?term=NAFLD&Search=Search (accessed June 30, 2014).

ClinicalTrials.gov. http://www.clinicaltrials.gov/ct2/results?term=NAFLD+and+omega-3+fatty+acids&Search=Search (accessed June 30, 2014).

ClinicalTrials.gov. http://www.clinicaltrials.gov/ct2/results?term=NASH&Search=Search (accessed June 30, 2014).

ClinicalTrials.gov. http://www.clinicaltrials.gov/ct2/results?term=virus+induced+fatty+liver+disease&Search=Search (accessed June 30, 2014).

ClinicalTrials.gov. http://www.clinicaltrials.gov/ct2/results?term=virus+induced+fatty+liver+disease+and+omega+3+fatty+acids&Search=Search (accessed June 30, 2014).

ClinicalTrials.gov. http://www.clinicaltrials.gov/ct2/results?term=cirrhosis&Search=Search (accessed June 30, 2014).

ClinicalTrials.gov. http://www.clinicaltrials.gov/ct2/results?term=cirrhosis+and+omega-3+fatty+acids&Search=Search (accessed June 30, 2014).

Cortez-Pinto, H., L. Jesus, H. Barros, C. Lopes, M. C. Moura, and M. E. Camilo. 2006. How different is the dietary pattern in non-alcoholic steatohepatitis patients? *Clin Nutr* 25:816–23.

Cui, W., K. Matsuno, K. Iwata et al. 2011. NOX1/nicotinamide adenine dinucleotide phosphate, reduced form (NADPH) oxidase promotes proliferation of stellate cells and aggravates liver fibrosis induced by bile duct ligation. *Hepatology* 54:949–58.

Daly, A. K., S. Ballestri, L. Carulli, P. Loria, and C. P. Day. 2011. Genetic determinants of susceptibility and severity in nonalcoholic fatty liver disease. *Expert Rev Gastroenterol Hepatol* 5:253–63.

Davidson, M. H., E. A. Stein, H. E. Bays et al. 2007. Efficacy and tolerability of adding pre-scription omega-3 fatty acids 4 g/d to simvastatin 40 mg/d in hypertriglyceridemic patients: an 8-week, randomized, double-blind, placebo-controlled study. *Clin Ther* 29:1354–67.

Day, C. P., and O. F. James. 1998. Steatohepatitis: a tale of two "hits"? *Gastroenterology* 114:842–5.

De Minicis, S., and D. A. Brenner. 2007. NOX in liver fibrosis. *Arch Biochem Biophys* 462:266–72.

Deng, Q. G., H. She, J. H. Cheng et al. 2005. Steatohepatitis induced by intragastric overfeed-ing in mice. *Hepatology* 42:905–14.

Depner, C. M., M. Torres-Gonzalez, S. Tripathy, G. Milne, and D. B. Jump. 2012. Menhaden oil decreases high-fat diet-induced markers of hepatic damage, steatosis, inflammation, and fibrosis in obese Ldlr-/- mice. *J Nutr* 142:1495–503.

Depner, C. M., K. A. Philbrick, and D. B. Jump. 2013a. Docosahexaenoic acid attenuates hepatic inflammation, oxidative stress, and fibrosis without decreasing hepatosteatosis in a Ldlr(-/-) mouse model of Western diet–induced nonalcoholic steatohepatitis. *J Nutr* 143:315–23.

Depner, C. M., M. G. Traber, G. Bobe, E. Kensicki, K. M. Bohren, G. Milne, and D. B. Jump. 2013b. A metabolomic analysis of omega-3 fatty acid-mediated attenuation of western diet-induced nonalcoholic steatohepatitis in LDLR-/- mice. *PLoS One* 17:e83756.

Di Minno, M. N., A. Russolillo, R. Lupoli, P. Ambrosino, A. Di Minno, and G. Tarantino. 2012. Omega-3 fatty acids for the treatment of non-alcoholic fatty liver disease. *World J Gastroenterol* 18:5839–47.

Donnelly, K. L., C. I. Smith, S. J. Schwarzenberg, J. Jessurun, M. D. Boldt, and E. J. Parks. 2005. Sources of fatty acids stored in liver and secreted via lipoproteins in patients with nonalcoholic fatty liver disease. *J Clin Invest* 115:1343–51.

Dyerberg, J., H. O. Bang, and N. Hjorne. 1975. Fatty acid composition of the plasma lipids in Greenland Eskimos. *Am J Clin Nutr* 28:958–66.

Dyerberg, J., H. O. Bang, E. Stoffersen, S. Moncada, and J. R. Vane. 1978. Eicosapentaenoic acid and prevention of thrombosis and atherosclerosis? *Lancet* 2:117–9.

Ekstedt, M., L. E. Franzen, U. L. Mathiesen et al. 2006. Long-term follow-up of patients with NAFLD and elevated liver enzymes. *Hepatology* 44:865–73.

Erridge, C., T. Attina, C. M. Spickett, and D. J. Webb. 2007. A high-fat meal induces low-grade endotoxemia: evidence of a novel mechanism of postprandial inflammation. *Am J Clin Nutr* 86:1286–92.

Falck, J. R., G. Wallukat, N. Puli et al. 2012. 17(R),18(S)-epoxyeicosatetraenoic acid, a potent eicosapentaenoic acid (EPA) derived regulator of cardiomyocyte contraction: structure-activity relationships and stable analogues. *J Med Chem* 54:4109–18.

Farrell, G. C., and C. Z. Larter. 2006. Nonalcoholic fatty liver disease: from steatosis to cir-rhosis. *Hepatology* 43:S99–S112.

Fedor, D. M., Y. Adkins, B. E. Mackey, and D. S. Kelley. 2012. Docosahexaenoic acid pre-vents *trans*-10, *cis*-12-conjugated linoleic acid-induced nonalcoholic fatty liver disease in mice by altering expression of hepatic genes regulating fatty acid synthesis and oxida-tion. *Metab Syndr Relat Disord* 10:175–80.

Feldstein, A. E., R. Lopez, T. A.-R. Tamimi, L. Yerian, Y.-M. Chung, M. Berk, R. Zhang, T. M. McIntyre, and S. L. Hazen. 2010. Mass spectrometric profiling of oxidized lipidprod-ucts in human nonalcoholic fatty liver disease and nonalcoholic steatohepatitis. *J Lipid Res* 51:3046–54.

Fessler, M. B., and J. S. Parks. 2011. Intracellular lipid flux and membrane microdomains as organizing principles in inflammatory cell signaling. *J Immunol* 187:1529–35.

Friedman, S. L. 2008. Mechanisms of hepatic fibrogenesis. *Gastroenterology* 134:1655–69.

Gebauer, S. K., T. L. Psota, W. S. Harris, and P. M. Kris-Etherton. 2006. n-3 fatty acid dietary recommendations and food sources to achieve essentiality and cardiovascular benefits. *Am J Clin Nutr* 83:1526S–1535S.

George, J., N. Pera, N. Phung, I. Leclercq, J. Yun Hou, and G. Farrell. 2003. Lipid peroxidation, stellate cell activation and hepatic fibrogenesis in a rat model of chronic steatohepatitis. *J Hepatol* 39:756–64.

Guturu, P., and A. Duchini. 2012. Etiopathogenesis of nonalcoholic steatohepatitis: role of obesity, insulin resistance and mechanisms of hepatotoxicity. *Int J Hepatol* 2012:212865.

Harris, W. S., D. Mozaffarian, M. Lefevre et al. 2009. Towards establishing dietary reference intakes for eicosapentaenoic and docosahexaenoic acids. *J Nutr* 139:804S–19S.

Harte, A. L., N. F. da Silva, S. J. Creely et al. 2010. Elevated endotoxin levels in non-alcoholic fatty liver disease. *J Inflamm (Lond)* 7:15.

Hernandez-Gea, V., and S. L. Friedman. 2011. Pathogenesis of liver fibrosis. *Annu Rev Pathol* 6:425–56.

Hooper, A. J., L. A. Adams, and J. R. Burnett. 2011. Genetic determinants of hepatic steatosis in man. *J Lipid Res* 52:593–617.

Hsueh, H. W., Z. Zhou, J. Whelan et al. 2011. Stearidonic and eicosapentaenoic acids inhibit interleukin-6 expression in *ob/ob* mouse adipose stem cells via Toll-like receptor-2-mediated pathways. *J Nutr* 141:1260–6.

Hussein, N., E. Ah-Sing, P. Wilkinson, C. Leach, B. A. Griffin, and D. J. Millward. 2005. Long-chain conversion of [13C]linoleic acid and alpha-linolenic acid in response to marked changes in their dietary intake in men. *J Lipid Res* 46:269–80.

Inoue, M., S. Tazuma, K. Kanno, H. Hyogo, K. Igarashi, and K. Chayama. 2011. Bach1 gene ablation reduces steatohepatitis in mouse MCD diet model. *J Clin Biochem Nutr* 48:161–6.

Ishibashi, S., M. S. Brown, J. L. Goldstein, R. D. Gerard, R. E. Hammer, and J. Herz. 1993. Hypercholesterolemia in low density lipoprotein receptor knockout mice and its reversal by adenovirus-mediated gene delivery. *J Clin Invest* 92:883–93.

Ishii, H., Y. Horie, S. Ohshima et al. 2009. Eicosapentaenoic acid ameliorates steatohepatitis and hepatocellular carcinoma in hepatocyte-specific Pten-deficient mice. *J Hepatol* 50:562–71.

Jeong, W. I., D. H. Jeong, S. H. Do et al. 2005. Mild hepatic fibrosis in cholesterol and sodium cholate diet-fed rats. *J Vet Med Sci* 67:235–42.

Jump, D. B. 2002. The biochemistry of n-3 polyunsaturated fatty acids. *J Biol Chem* 277:8755–8.

Jump, D. B. 2008. N-3 polyunsaturated fatty acid regulation of hepatic gene transcription. *Curr Opin Lipidol* 19:242–7.

Jump, D. B., C. M. Depner, and S. Tripathy. 2012. Omega-3 fatty acid supplementation and cardiovascular disease. *J Lipid Res* 53:2525–45.

Jump, D. B., S. Tripathy, and C. M. Depner. 2013. Fatty acid-regulated transcription factors in the liver. *Annu Rev Nutr* 33:249–69.

Kajikawa, S., K. Imada, T. Takeuchi et al. 2011. Eicosapentaenoic acid attenuates progression of hepatic fibrosis with inhibition of reactive oxygen species production in rats fed methionine- and choline-deficient diet. *Dig Dis Sci* 56:1065–74.

Kishino, T., H. Ohnishi, K. Ohtsuka et al. 2011. Low concentrations of serum n-3 polyunsaturated fatty acids in non-alcoholic fatty liver disease patients with liver injury. *Clin Chem Lab Med* 49:159–62.

Kris-Etherton, P. M., W. S. Harris, and L. J. Appel. 2002. Fish consumption, fish oil, omega-3 fatty acids, and cardiovascular disease. *Circulation* 106:2747–57.

Kris-Etherton, P. M., W. S. Harris, and L. J. Appel. 2003a. Fish consumption, fish oil, omega-3 fatty acids, and cardiovascular disease. *Arterioscler Thromb Vasc Biol* 23:e20–30.

Kris-Etherton, P. M., W. S. Harris, and L. J. Appel. 2003b. Omega-3 fatty acids and cardiovascular disease: new recommendations from the American Heart Association. *Arterioscler Thromb Vasc Biol* 23:151–2.

LaBrecque, D., Z. Abbas, F. Anania, P. Ferenci, A. Gahafoor Kahn, K.-L. Goh, S. S. Hamid, V. Isakov, M. Lizarzabal, M. Mojica Pernaranda, J. F. Rivera Ramos, S. Sarin, D. Stimak, A. B. R. Thomson, M. Umar, J. Krabshuis, and A. LeMair. 2012. Nonalcoholic fatty liver disease and nonalcoholic steatohepatitis. *World Gastroentrol Org Global Guidelines* June:1–29.

Lam, B. P., and Z. M. Younossi. 2009. Treatment regimens for non-alcoholic fatty liver disease. *Ann Hepatol* 8 Suppl 1:S51–9.

Laugerette, F., C. Vors, A. Geloen et al. 2011. Emulsified lipids increase endotoxemia: possible role in early postprandial low-grade inflammation. *J Nutr Biochem* 22:53–9.

Lavine, J. E., J. B. Schwimmer, M. L. Van Natta et al. 2011. Effect of vitamin E or metformin for treatment of nonalcoholic fatty liver disease in children and adolescents: the TONIC randomized controlled trial. *J Amer Med Assoc* 305:1659–68.

Leclercq, I. A., G. C. Farrell, R. Schriemer, and G. R. Robertson. 2002. Leptin is essential for the hepatic fibrogenic response to chronic liver injury. *J Hepatol* 37:206–13.

Leclercq, I. A., J. Field, A. Enriquez, G. C. Farrell, and G. R. Robertson. 2000. Constitutive and inducible expression of hepatic CYP2E1 in leptin-deficient *ob/ob* mice. *Biochem Biophys Res Commun* 268:337–44.

Lee, J. Y., A. Plakidas, W. H. Lee et al. 2003. Differential modulation of Toll-like receptors by fatty acids: preferential inhibition by n-3 polyunsaturated fatty acids. *J Lipid Res* 44:479–86.

Lee, J. Y., L. Zhao, and D. H. Hwang. 2010. Modulation of pattern recognition receptor-mediated inflammation and risk of chronic diseases by dietary fatty acids. *Nutr Rev* 68:38–61.

Lee, J. H., J. H. O'Keefe, C. J. Lavie, and W. S. Harris. 2009. Omega-3 fatty acids: cardiovascular benefits, sources and sustainability. *Nat Rev Cardiol* 12:753–8.

Lee, S., L. Harnack, D. R. Jacobs, Jr., L. M. Steffen, R. V. Luepker, and D. K. Arnett. 2007. Trends in diet quality for coronary heart disease prevention between 1980–1982 and 2000–2002: The Minnesota Heart Survey. *J Am Diet Assoc* 107:213–22.

Levy, J. R., J. N. Clore, and W. Stevens. 2004. Dietary n-3 polyunsaturated fatty acids decrease hepatic triglycerides in Fischer 344 rats. *Hepatology* 39:608–16.

Lim, J. S., M. Mietus-Snyder, A. Valente, J. M. Schwarz, and R. H. Lustig. 2010. The role of fructose in the pathogenesis of NAFLD and the metabolic syndrome. *Nat Rev Gastroenterol Hepatol* 7:251–64.

Lottenberg, A. M., S. Afonso Mda, M. S. Lavrador, R. M. Machado, and E. R. Nakandakare. 2012. The role of dietary fatty acids in the pathology of metabolic syndrome. *J Nutr Biochem* 23:1027–40.

Ludwig, J., T. R. Viggiano, D. B. McGill, and B. J. Oh. 1980. Nonalcoholic steatohepatitis: Mayo Clinic experiences with a hitherto unnamed disease. *Mayo Clin Proc* 55:434–8.

Lusis, A. J. 2000. Atherosclerosis. *Nature* 407:233–41.

Mahady, S. E., and J. George. 2012. Management of nonalcoholic steatohepatitis: an evidence-based approach. *Clin Liver Dis* 16:631–45.

Marra, F., A. Gastaldelli, G. S. Baroni, G. Tell, and C. Tiribelli. 2008. Molecular basis and mechanisms of progression of non-alcoholic steatohepatitis. *Trends Mol Med* 14:72–81.

Marriott, B. P., L. Olsho, L. Hadden, and P. Connor. 2010a. Intake of added sugars and selected nutrients in the United States, National Health and Nutrition Examination Survey (NHANES) 2003–2006. *Crit Rev Food Sci Nutr* 50:228–58.

Marriott, B. P., L. Olsho, L. Hadden, and P. Connor. 2010b. Intake of added sugars in the United States: what is the measure? *Am J Clin Nutr* 94:1652–3; author reply 1653.

Matherly, S. C., and P. Puri. 2012. Mechanisms of simple hepatic steatosis: not so simple after all. *Clin Liver Dis* 16:505–24.

Matsuzaka, T. and H. Shimano. 2009. Elovl6: a new player in fatty acid metabolism and insulin sensitivity. *J Mol Med* 87:379–84.

Matsuzaka, T., H. Shimano, N. Yahagi et al. 2002. Dual regulation of mouse Delta(5)- and Delta(6)-desaturase gene expression by SREBP-1 and PPARalpha. *J Lipid Res* 43:107–14.

Matsuzaki, K. 2012. Smad phosphoisoform signals in acute and chronic liver injury: similarties and differences between epithelial and mesenchymal cells. *Cell Tissue Res* 347:225–43.

Matsuzawa, N., T. Takamura, S. Kurita et al. 2007. Lipid-induced oxidative stress causes steatohepatitis in mice fed an atherogenic diet. *Hepatology* 46:1392–403.

McCullough, A. J. 2011. Epidemiology of the metabolic syndrome in the USA. *J Dig Dis* 12:333–40.

McCullough, A. J. 2004. The clinical features, diagnosis and natural history of nonalcoholic fatty liver disease. *Clin Liver Dis* 8:521–33, viii.

McCullough, A. J. 2006. Pathophysiology of nonalcoholic steatohepatitis. *J Clin Gastroenterol* 40 Suppl 1:S17–29.

Mensink, R. P., P. L. Zock, A. D. Kester, and M. B. Katan. 2003. Effects of dietary fatty acids and carbohydrates on the ratio of serum total to HDL cholesterol and on serum lipids and apolipoproteins: a meta-analysis of 60 controlled trials. *Am J Clin Nutr* 77:1146–55.

Milne, G. L., H. Yin, K. D. Hardy, S. S. Davies, and L. J. Roberts, 2nd. 2011. Isoprostane generation and function. *Chem Rev* 111:5973–96.

Milne, G. L., H. Yin, and J. D. Morrow. 2008. Human biochemistry of the isoprostane pathway. *J Biol Chem* 283:15533–7.

Miura, K., L. Yang, N. van Rooijen, D. A. Brenner, H. Ohnishi, and E. Seki. 2013. TLR2 and palmitic acid cooperatively contribute to the development of nonalcoholic steatohepatitis through inflammasome activation. *Hepatology* 57:577–89.

Mozaffarian, D. and J. H. Y. Wu. 2011. Omega-3 fatty acids and cardiovascular disease. Effects of risk factor, molecular pathways and clinical events. *J Am Coll Cardio* 58:2047–67.

Musso, G., R. Gambino, F. De Michieli et al. 2003. Dietary habits and their relations to insulin resistance and postprandial lipemia in nonalcoholic steatohepatitis. *Hepatology* 37:909–16.

Musso, G., R. Gambino, and M. Cassader. 2010. Non-alcoholic fatty liver disese from pathogenesis to management: an update. *Obes Rev* 11:430–45.

Ndisang, J. F. and A. Jadhav. 2010. Up-regulating the hemeoxygenase system enhances insulin sensitivity and improves glucose metabolism in insulin-resistant diabetes in Goto-Kakizaki rats. *Endocrinology* 150:2627–36.

Nicolai, A., M. Li, D. H. Kim et al. 2009. Heme oxygenase-1 induction remodels adipose tissue and improves insulin sensitivity in obesity-induced diabetic rats. *Hypertension* 53:508–15.

Nilsson, N. E., K. Kotarsky, C. Owman, and B. Olde. 2003. Identification of a free fatty acid receptor, FFA2R, expressed on leukocytes and activated by short-chain fatty acids. *Biochem Biophys Res Commun* 303:1047–52.

Nobili, V., G. Bedogni, A. Alisi et al. 2011. Docosahexaenoic acid supplementation decreases liver fat content in children with non-alcoholic fatty liver disease: double-blind randomised controlled clinical trial. *Arch Dis Child* 96:350–3.

O'Keefe, J. H., Jr., and W. S. Harris. 2000. From Inuit to implementation: omega-3 fatty acids come of age. *Mayo Clin Proc* 75:607–14.

Oh, D. Y., S. Talukdar, E. J. Bae et al. 2011. GPR120 is an omega-3 fatty acid receptor mediating potent anti-inflammatory and insulin-sensitizing effects. *Cell* 142:687–98.

Omagari, K., S. Kato, K. Tsuneyama et al. 2008. Effects of a long-term high-fat diet and switching from a high-fat to low-fat, standard diet on hepatic fat accumulation in Sprague-Dawley rats. *Dig Dis Sci* 53:3206–12.

Ong, J. P., H. Elariny, R. Collantes et al. 2005. Predictors of nonalcoholic steatohepatitis and advanced fibrosis in morbidly obese patients. *Obes Surg* 15:310–5.

Oya, J., T. Nakagami, S. Sasaki et al. 2011. Intake of n-3 polyunsaturated fatty acids and non-alcoholic fatty liver disease: a cross-sectional study in Japanese men and women. *Eur J Clin Nutr* 64:1179–85.

Pachikian, B. D., A. Essaghir, J. B. Demoulin et al. 2011. Hepatic n-3 polyunsaturated fatty acid depletion promotes steatosis and insulin resistance in mice: genomic analysis of cellular targets. *PLoS One* 6:e23365.

Pagadala, M., T. Kasumov, A. J. McCullough, N. N. Zein, and J. P. Kirwan. 2012. Role of ceramides in nonalcoholic fatty liver disease. *Trends Endocrinol Metab* 23:365–71.

Paik, Y. H., K. Iwaisako, E. Seki et al. 2011. The nicotinamide adenine dinucleotide phosphate oxidase (NOX) homologues NOX1 and NOX2/gp91(phox) mediate hepatic fibrosis in mice. *Hepatology* 53:1730–41.

Paine, A., B. Eiz-Vesper, R. Blasczyk, and S. Immenschuh. 2011. Signaling to heme oxygenase-1 and its anti-inflammatory therapeutic potential. *Biochem Pharmacol* 80:1895–903.

Pawar, A., and D. B. Jump. 2003. Unsaturated fatty acid regulation of peroxisome proliferator–activated receptor alpha activity in rat primary hepatocytes. *J Biol Chem* 278:35931–9.

Pawlosky, R. J., J. R. Hibbeln, J. A. Novotny, and N. Salem, Jr. 2001. Physiological compartmental analysis of alpha-linolenic acid metabolism in adult humans. *J Lipid Res* 42:1257–65.

Plourde, M., and S. C. Cunnane. 2007. Extremely limited synthesis of long chain polyunsaturates in adults: implications for their dietary essentiality and use as supplements. *Appl Physiol Nutr Metab* 32:619–34.

Prashanth, M., H. K. Ganesh, M. V. Vima et al. 2009. Prevalence of nonalcoholic fatty liver disease in patients with type 2 diabetes mellitus. *J Assoc Physicians India* 57:205–10.

Puri, P., M. M. Wiest, O. Cheung et al. 2009. The plasma lipidomic signature of nonalcoholic steatohepatitis. *Hepatology* 50:1827–38.

Rapoport, S. I., M. Igarashi, and F. Gao. 2011. Quantitative contributions of diet and liver synthesis to docosahexaenoic acid homeostasis. *Prostaglandins Leukot Essent Fatty Acids* 82:273–6.

Ren, B., A. P. Thelen, J. M. Peters, F. J. Gonzalez, and D. B. Jump. 1997. Polyunsaturated fatty acid suppression of hepatic fatty acid synthase and S14 gene expression does not require peroxisome proliferator–activated receptor alpha. *J Biol Chem* 272:26827–32.

Rinella, M. E., M. S. Elias, R. R. Smolak, T. Fu, J. Borensztajn, and R. M. Green. 2008. Mechanisms of hepatic steatosis in mice fed a lipogenic methionine choline-deficient diet. *J Lipid Res* 49:1068–76.

Rinella, M. E., and R. M. Green. 2004. The methionine-choline deficient dietary model of steatohepatitis does not exhibit insulin resistance. *J Hepatol* 40:47–51.

Romeo, S., J. Kozlitina, C. Xing et al. 2008. Genetic variation in PNPLA3 confers susceptibility to nonalcoholic fatty liver disease. *Nat Genet* 40:1461–5.

Romestaing, C., M. A. Piquet, E. Bedu et al. 2007. Long term highly saturated fat diet does not induce NASH in Wistar rats. *Nutr Metab (Lond)* 4:4.

Ronis, M. J., J. N. Baumgardner, N. Sharma et al. 2013. Medium chain triglycerides dose-dependently prevent liver pathology in a rat model of non-alcoholic fatty liver disease. *Exp Biol Med (Maywood)* 238:151–62.

Ryan, M. C., C. Itsiopoulos, T. Thodis et al. 2013. The Mediterranean diet improves hepatic steatosis and insulin sensitivity in individuals with non-alcoholic fatty liver disease. *J Hepatol* 59:138–43.

Sanyal, A. J., N. Chalasani, K. V. Kowdley et al. 2010. Pioglitazone, vitamin E, or placebo for nonalcoholic steatohepatitis. *N Engl J Med* 362:1675–85.

Saraswathi, V., L. Gao, J. D. Morrow, A. Chait, K. D. Niswender, and A. H. Hasty. 2007. Fish oil increases cholesterol storage in white adipose tissue with concomitant decreases in inflammation, hepatic steatosis, and atherosclerosis in mice. *J Nutr* 137:1776–82.

Saraswathi, V., J. D. Morrow, and A. H. Hasty. 2009. Dietary fish oil exerts hypolipidemic effects in lean and insulin sensitizing effect in obese LDLR$^{-/-}$ mice. *J Nutr* 139:2380–6.

Saravanan, P., N. C. Davidson, E. B. Schmidt, and P. C. Calder. 2010. Cardiovascular effects of marine omega-3 fatty acids. *Lancet* 375:540–50.

Schalkwijk, C. G., C. D. Stehouwer, and V. W. van Hinsbergh. 2004. Fructose-mediated non-enzymatic glycation: sweet coupling or bad modification. *Diabetes Metab Res Rev* 20:369–82.

Schattenberg, J. M., and P. R. Galle. 2010. Animal models of non-alcoholic steatohepatitis: of mice and man. *Dig Dis* 28:247–54.

Scorletti, E. and C. D. Byrne. 2013. Omega-3 fatty acids, hepatic lipid metabolism and non-alcoholic fatty liver disease. *Ann Rev Nutr* 33:231–48.

Serhan, C. N., R. Yang, K. Martinod et al. 2009. Maresins: novel macrophage mediators with potent antiinflammatory and proresolving actions. *J Exp Med* 206:15–23.

Smith, W. L. 2008. Nutritionally essential fatty acids and biologically indispensable cyclooxygenases. *Trends Biochem Sci* 33:27–37.

Soderberg, C., P. Stal, J. Askling et al. 2010. Decreased survival of subjects with elevated liver function tests during a 28-year follow-up. *Hepatology* 51:595–602.

Sofi, F., I. Giangrandi, F. Cesari et al. 2011. Effects of a 1-year dietary intervention with n-3 polyunsaturated fatty acid-enriched olive oil on non-alcoholic fatty liver disease patients: a preliminary study. *Int J Food Sci Nutr* 61:792–802.

Song, W. L., G. Paschos, S. Fries et al. 2009. Novel eicosapentaenoic acid-derived F3-isoprostanes as biomarkers of lipid peroxidation. *J Biol Chem* 284:23636–43.

Soni, S. P., D. S. LoCascio, Y. Liu et al. 2008. Docosahexaenoic acid enhances segregation of lipids between: 2H-NMR study. *Biophys J* 95:203–14.

Spector, A. A. 1999. Essentiality of fatty acids. *Lipids* 34:S1–S4.

Spite, M., and C. N. Serhan. 2010. Novel lipid mediators promote resolution of acute inflammation: impact of aspirin and statins. *Circ Res* 107:1170–84.

Sprecher, H. 2000. Metabolism of highly unsaturated n-3 and n-6 fatty acids. *Biochim Biophys Acta* 1486:219–31.

Spruss, A., G. Kanuri, S. Wagnerberger, S. Haub, S. C. Bischoff, and I. Bergheim. 2009. Toll-like receptor 4 is involved in the development of fructose-induced hepatic steatosis in mice. *Hepatology* 50:1094–104.

Stienstra, R., F. Saudale, C. Duval et al. 2010. Kupffer cells promote hepatic steatosis via interleukin-1beta-dependent suppression of peroxisome proliferator–activated receptor alpha activity. *Hepatology* 51:511–22.

Stillwell, W. 2008. Docosahexaenoic acid: a most unusual fatty acid. *Chem Phys Lipids* 153:1–2.

Stulnig, T. M., M. Berger, T. Sigmund, D. Raederstorff, H. Stockinger, and W. Waldhausl. 1998. Polyunsaturated fatty acids inhibit T cell signal transduction by modification of detergent-insoluble membrane domains. *J Cell Biol* 143:637–44.

Sullivan, P. M., H. Mezdour, S. H. Quarfordt, and N. Maeda. 1998. Type III hyperlipoproteinemia and spontaneous atherosclerosis in mice resulting from gene replacement of mouse Apoe with human Apoe*2. *J Clin Invest* 102:130–5.

Takayama, F., K. Nakamoto, N. Totani et al. 2010. Effects of docosahexaenoic acid in an experimental rat model of nonalcoholic steatohepatitis. *J Oleo Sci* 59:407–14.

Teratani, T., K. Tomita, T. Suzuki et al. 2012. A high-cholesterol diet exacerbates liver fibrosis in mice via accumulation of free cholesterol in hepatic stellate cells. *Gastroenterology* 142:152–164 e10.

Tetri, L. H., M. Basaranoglu, E. M. Brunt, L. M. Yerian, and B. A. Neuschwander-Tetri. 2008. Severe NAFLD with hepatic necroinflammatory changes in mice fed *trans* fats and a high-fructose corn syrup equivalent. *Am J Physiol Gastrointest Liver Physiol* 295:G987–95.

Tilg, H., and A. R. Moschen. 2010. Evolution of inflammation in nonalcoholic fatty liver disease: the multiple parallel hits hypothesis. *Hepatology* 52:1836–46.

Toshimitsu, K., B. Matsuura, I. Ohkubo et al. 2007. Dietary habits and nutrient intake in nonalcoholic steatohepatitis. *Nutrition* 23:46–52.

Tous, M., N. Ferre, A. Rull et al. 2006. Dietary cholesterol and differential monocyte chemoattractant protein-1 gene expression in aorta and liver of apo E-deficient mice. *Biochem Biophys Res Commun* 340:1078–84.

Vallabhapurapu, S., and M. Karin. 2009. Regulation and function of NF-kappaB transcription factors in the immune system. *Annu Rev Immunol* 27:693–733.

Vandanmagsar, B., Y. H. Youm, A. Ravussin et al. 2011. The NLRP3 inflammasome instigates obesity-induced inflammation and insulin resistance. *Nat Med* 17:179–88.

Varela-Rey, M., N. Embade, U. Ariz, S. C. Lu, J. M. Mato, and M. L. Martinez-Chantar. 2009. Non-alcoholic steatohepatitis and animal models: understanding the human disease. *Int J Biochem Cell Biol* 41:969–76.

Vemuri, M., D. S. Kelley, B. E. Mackey, R. Rasooly, and G. Bartolini. 2007. Docosahexaenoic acid (DHA) but not eicosapentaenoic acid (EPA) prevents *trans*-10, *cis*-12 conjugated linoleic acid (CLA)-induced insulin resistance in mice. *Metab Syndr Relat Disord* 5:315–22.

Vernon, G., A. Baranova, and Z. M. Younossi. 2011. Systematic review: the epidemiology and natural history of non-alcoholic fatty liver disease and non-alcoholic steatohepatitis in adults. *Aliment Pharmacol Ther* 34:274–85.

Vos, M. B., J. E. Kimmons, C. Gillespie, J. Welsh, and H. M. Blanck. 2008. Dietary fructose consumption among US children and adults: the Third National Health and Nutrition Examination Survey. *Medscape J Med* 10:160.

Wada, M., C. J. DeLong, Y. H. Hong et al. 2007. Enzymes and receptors of prostaglandin pathways with arachidonic acid-derived versus eicosapentaenoic acid-derived substrates and products. *J Biol Chem* 282:22254–66.

Walenbergh, S. M. A., G. H. Koek, V. Bieghs, and R. Shiri-Sverdlov. 2013. Non-alcoholic steatohepatitis: the role of oxidized low-density lipoproteins. *J Hepatol* 58:801–20.

Wang, Y., D. Botolin, B. Christian, J. Busik, J. Xu, and D. B. Jump. 2005. Tissue-specific, nutritional, and developmental regulation of rat fatty acid elongases. *J Lipid Res* 46:706–15.

Wang, Y., D. Botolin, J. Xu et al. 2006. Regulation of hepatic fatty acid elongase and desaturase expression in diabetes and obesity. *J Lipid Res* 47:2028–41.

Wassall, S. R., and W. Stillwell. 2009. Polyunsaturated fatty acid-cholesterol interactions: Domain formation in membranes. *Biochim Biophys Acta* 1788:24–32.

Wei, Y., D. Wang, G. Moran, A. Estrada, and M. J. Pagliassotti. 2013. Fructose-induced stress signaling in the liver involves methylglyoxal. *Nutr Meta (Lond)* 10:32–8.

Westerbacka, J., K. Lammi, A. M. Hakkinen et al. 2005. Dietary fat content modifies liver fat in overweight nondiabetic subjects. *J Clin Endocrinol Metab* 90:2804–9.

Wouters, K., M. van Bilsen, P. J. van Gorp et al. 2010. Intrahepatic cholesterol influences progression, inhibition and reversal of non-alcoholic steatohepatitis in hyperlipidemic mice. *FEBS Lett* 584:1001–5.

Wouters, K., P. J. van Gorp, V. Bieghs et al. 2008. Dietary cholesterol, rather than liver steatosis, leads to hepatic inflammation in hyperlipidemic mouse models of nonalcoholic steatohepatitis. *Hepatology* 48:474–86.

Xu, H. E., M. H. Lambert, V. G. Montana et al. 1999. Molecular recognition of fatty acids by peroxisome proliferator–activated receptors. *Mol Cell* 3:397–403.

Yasutake, K., M. Nakamuta, Y. Shima et al. 2009. Nutritional investigation of non-obese patients with non-alcoholic fatty liver disease: the significance of dietary cholesterol. *Scand J Gastroenterol* 44:471–7.

Yu, J., E. S. Chu, R. Wang, S. Wang, C. W. Wu, V. W. Wong, H. L. Chan, G. C. Farrell, and J. J. Sung. 2010. Heme oxygenase-1 protects against steatohepatitis in both cultured hepatocytes and mice. *Gastroenterology* 138:694–704.

Zein, C. O., R. Lopez, J. P. Kirwan et al. 2012. Pentoxifylline decreases oxidized lipid prod-
    ucts in nonalcoholic steatohepatitis: New evidence on the potential therapeutic mecha-
    nism. *Hepatology* 56:1291–9.
Zelber-Sagi, S., D. Nitzan-Kaluski, R. Goldsmith et al. 2007. Long term nutritional intake
    and the risk for non-alcoholic fatty liver disease (NAFLD): a population based study.
    J Hepatol 47:711–7.
Zelber-Sagi, S., V. Ratziu, and R. Oren. 2011. Nutrition and physical activity in NAFLD: an
    overview of the epidemiological evidence. *World J Gastroenterol* 17:3377–89.
Zhang, C., and N. G. Bazan. 2010. Lipid-mediated cell signaling protects agains injury and
    neurodegeneration. *J Nutr* 140:858–63.
Zheng, J. S., A. Xu, T. Huang, X. Yu, and D. Li. 2012. Low docosahexaenoic acid content in
    plasma phospholipids is associated with increased non-alcoholic fatty liver disease in
    China. *Lipids* 47:549–56.

14 Nutraceuticals in the Prevention and Treatment of Fatty Liver Disease

Anna Aronis

CONTENTS

NATURAL COMPOUNDS IN MODERN RESEARCH

Natural compounds have been used in traditional medicine for thousands of years, and a variety of evidence of their efficiency has been accumulated. The role of the modern research is to reveal the relevance of those evidence for treatment and prevention of diseases and the ways of their integration with the conventional medicine. According to the Dietary Supplement, Health and Education Act, dietary supplements are products intended to supplement the diet that bears or contains one or more of the following dietary ingredients: a vitamin, a mineral, an herb or other botanical, an amino acid, a dietary substance for use by man to supplement the diet by increasing the total daily intake, or a concentrate, metabolite, constituent, extract, or combinations of these ingredients (Chauhan et al., 2013). Safety and efficiency issues have been arisen along with reports of toxicity of specific nutraceuticals, requiring from regulatory bodies to define indications, limitations, and claims for each dietary supplement (Chauhan et al., 2013).

This chapter is discussing accumulated research evidence regarding the role of nutraceuticals in fatty liver disease. As this area of research is relatively modern, evidence from human studies are yet limited. Fatty liver mostly is observed as a part of obesity, diabetes, metabolic syndrome, or polycystic ovary syndrome (Schuppan and Schattenberg, 2013; Karoli et al., 2013; Asrih and Jornayvaz, 2013) or as a part of alcoholic (Crawford, 2012) or viral disease (Roingeard, 2013); therapeutic strategies developed for those conditions are also possible to reverse partly the symptoms of fatty liver and improve liver function. However, the aim of this chapter was to screen nutraceuticals that are specific for fatty liver disease and not only for the conditions initiating it.

The effects of ω-3 fatty acids and antioxidants in liver disease are described in Chapter 13 in this book, and for this reason, this chapter does not focus on them.

MICROBIOTA

ROLE OF MICROBIOTA IN ETIOLOGY OF FATTY LIVER DISEASE

Alimentary tract is populated by more than 500 species of microorganisms composed of bacteria, Archaea, yeasts, and viruses. Although the major portion of microbiota is found in the large intestine, smaller amounts are distributed all over the lumen, ranging from 10^3/g content in the stomach, 10^4–10^7 in the small intestine, and up to 10^{12}/g in the large intestine (Prakash et al., 2011). Microbiota's role in the digestive tract is diverse and includes strengthening of physical intestinal barriers, competition with pathogenic strains, excretion of antimicrobial peptides, regulation of innate and adaptive immunity, stimulation of villus mucrovasculature, and production of short chain fatty acids (Li et al., 2013).

Recent studies shed light on changes in composition of gut microbiota in metabolic syndrome, nonalcoholic fatty liver disease (NAFLD), and high-fat diet. Those conditions are characterized by increase in Firmicutes and decrease in Bacteriodetes (Sweeney and Morton, 2013; de Wit et al., 2012; Machado and Cortez-Pinto, 2012). Treatment with probiotics, modifying the ratio of microbiotic strains toward a non-obese individual profile, also improves metabolic markers of nonalcoholic steatohepatitis (NASH). Wong et al. (2013a) demonstrated that probiotic treatment–induced fecal microbiota changes in 16 NASH patients has correlated with changes in intrahepatic triglycerides (IHTG) at month 6 of the treatment. At the phylum level, a reduction in IHTG has been accompanied by a reduction in the abundance of Firmicutes and an increase in Bacteroidetes. Improvement in hepatic steatosis has been also associated with reduced abundance of the class Clostridia, the order Clostridiales, and the genus *Faecalibacterium*. In contrast, reduced IHTG level has been associated with increased abundance of the class Bacteroidia and the order Bacteroidales (Wong et al., 2013a).

The portal vein delivers bacterial toxins LPS, peptidoglycans, and bacterial DNA to the liver, where they stimulate proinflammatory Toll-like receptors (TLRs), TLR2, TLR4, and TLR9, and induce elevation of plasma tumor necrosis factor (TNF) α, interleukin (IL) 1, and IL-6 (Li et al., 2013). Several studies demonstrated changes in composition of the intestinal flora in individuals with different features of metabolic syndrome and NAFLD (Spencer et al., 2011). Currently, the hypothesis of development of NAFLD and subsequent steatohepatitis following exposure to bacterial endotoxins is being strengthened by accumulating evidence in animals and humans (Spencer et al., 2011; Henao-Mejia et al., 2012; Raman et al., 2013). Moreover, there are clinical trials that have found that transplantation of human microbiota from lean donors to obese subjects induced an improvement in peripheral insulin sensitivity and a trend to improvement (p = 0.08) in hepatic insulin sensitivity (Vrieze et al., 2012, 2013).

PROBIOTIC SUPPLEMENTATION IN FATTY LIVER DISEASE

Probiotics are live microorganisms that, when administered in adequate amounts, confer a health benefit on the host. In FAO/WHO guidelines, probiotics are a food matter and refer to beneficial microorganisms contained in foods; whereas the use of beneficial bacteria in subjects affected by pathological conditions must be considered as a therapeutic matter (Morelli and Capurso, 2012). Therapeutic effects of probiotics are being widely studied in gastrointestinal disorders, and the measure of their benefit has been described in several reviews and meta-analysis (Johnston et al., 2011; Caselli et al., 2013; Salari et al., 2012; Guandalini, 2011).

Unlike gastrointestinal subjects, application of probiotics to metabolic syndrome–related disorders is a relatively new concept, expanding to treatment of hyperglycemia, dyslipidemia, and NAFLD (Burcelin et al., 2011). Studies demonstrating reduction in levels of total cholesterol, non-HDL cholesterol, triglycerides, and glucose have been published at the last years (Ejtahed et al., 2011; Moroti et al., 2012; Ataie-Jafari et al., 2009). The effect of probiotics on NAFLD is one of the areas of this research.

Thus, in NASH patients, a formula containing a mix of *Lactobacillus plantarum*, *L. delbrueckii*, *L. acidophilus*, *L. rhamnosus*, and *Bifidobacterium bifidum* has been shown to decrease IHTG content and induce significant reduction in serum aspartate aminotransferase (AST) (Wong et al., 2013b). Another study of fatty liver has found reduction in patients' liver aminotransferases after administration of 500 million/day of *L. bulgaricus* and *Streptococcus thermophilus* for 3 months (Aller et al., 2011). In an animal model of Apo E$^{-/-}$ mice with DSS-induced liver injury, VSL#3 has reversed insulin resistance and prevented development of histological features of steatohepatitis. Conditioned media obtained from cultured probiotics has caused the direct transactivation of peroxisome proliferator–activated receptor γ (PPAR-γ), farnesoid-X receptors and vitamin D receptor (Mencarelli et al., 2012).

Recently, an elegant mechanistic study shading light on pathways of probiotic functioning in NASH was published (Endo et al., 2013). Butyrate is a short-chain fatty acid (SCFA) produced by microbiota in the colon and distal small intestine by fermentation of resistant starch, dietary fibers, and low-digestible polysaccharides. MIYAIRI 588 strain of *Clostridium butyricum* is a butyrate-producing Gram-positive anaerobe which has been shown to slow a progression of steatosis to hepatocarcinogenesis in choline-depleted, L-amino acid–defined rat model (Endo et al., 2013). The mechanism of the prevention has involved an activation of AMP-activated protein kinase (AMPK) and Akt, induction of nuclear factor 2 (Nrf2), and PPAR-α, on the one hand, and suppression of SREBP, UCP-2, and PPAR-γ, on the other hand, in choline-deficient rats. Expression of tight junction proteins zonula occluden 1 and occludin has also been improved in probiotic versus choline-deficient group. All those molecular changes have resulted in decreased triglyceride accumulation and improved insulin sensitivity in MIYAIRI 588-supplemented group. An assumption made by the authors was that butyric acid is a key regulator of hepatic triacylglycerol distribution, which has been additionally reinforced by in vitro experiments with Caco-2 cells (Endo et al., 2013).

Despite promising results in treatment of NAFLD with probiotics, this branch remains an issue of a new investigation, where strains and dosages of probiotic microorganisms and length of treatment period have to be defined, and safety issues have to be related. Thus, one small, non-placebo-controlled study conducted on four patients has found an increase in hepatic lipid content following supplementation of NAFLD patients with 1 sachet of VSL#3 for 4 months (Solga et al., 2008), indicating a high importance of those unrelated issues.

ROLE OF PREBIOTICS IN FATTY LIVER DISEASE

The definition of a prebiotic given by the International Scientific Association for Probiotics and Prebiotics (ISAPP) in 2008 is "a selectively fermented ingredient that results in specific changes, in the composition and/or activity of the gastrointestinal microbiota, thus conferring benefit(s) upon host health" (Roberfroid et al., 2010). The criteria of classification of a compound as a prebiotic include fermentability in in vitro fecal culture simulating nature gastrointestinal medium, an ability to constitute substrate for at least one beneficial microorganism, and selectivity in stimulation of growth and/or activity of limited number of beneficial genera of microorganisms. Classical compounds found to match those criteria are fructo-oligosaccharides (FOS), galacto-oligosaccharides (GOS), inulin, oligofructose, and their mixtures (Roberfroid et al., 2010). Polydextrose, isolated gums, resistant starch, lactulose, and lactitol have also been included to this group of nutrients (Slavin, 2013). The major contribution of a prebiotic to the host health is conditioned by its ability to improve beneficial intestinal microbiota. Nowadays studies elucidate prebiotic compounds that are appropriate to be candidates to supplemental treatment of wide spectrum of metabolic disorders.

Research works have demonstrated that nondigestible fructan oligofructose, mostly obtained from chicory root inulin, selectively increases bifidobacteria numbers in the large intestine and is a promising nutrient for controlling of metabolic alterations associated with obesity, including steatosis and dyslipidemia (Cani et al., 2007; Daubioul et al., 2000). Oligofructose and inulin have been found to decrease weight gain and hepatic triglycerides in rodent models of obesity, atherosclerosis, and high-fat diet (Daubioul et al., 2000; Correia-Sa et al., 2013; Anastasovska et al., 2012; Rault-Nania et al., 2006), although this decrease has not always been accompanied with plasma triglyceride reduction (Daubioul et al., 2000).

Trials to elucidate a mechanism of prebiotic action on liver metabolism have been resulted in a constant accumulation of new mechanistic evidence. Thus, supplementation of a regular animal diet with a commercial formulation, constituting a source of dextrin, an additional carbohydrate that has been suggested to have prebiotic characteristics, has resulted in the attenuation of the oxidative marker protein carbonyl and increase in GSH/GSSG ratio in rat liver homogenate. In the same study, oligofructose (in contrast to dextrin) has shown a moderate, if any, effect on liver redox status, demonstrating a meaningfulness of a specific type and dosage of prebiotic related to each condition (Kozmus et al., 2011). In another study, oligofructose has ameliorated a pro-oxidative effect of subcutaneous administration of D-galactose on BL/6J mice liver. Whereas D-galactose decreased the activity of hepatic superoxide dismutase and glutathione peroxidase, oligofructose has prevented this attenuation (Chen et al., 2011).

Apparently, activity of glucagon-like peptide (GLP) 1 is needed to enable metabolic modifications by prebiotics, at least oligofructose, in the liver (Cani et al., 2006). Canceling of activity of GLP-1 receptor by its antagonist exendin 9-39 prevents oligofructose-induced normalization of hepatic glucose production as well as improvement in insulin receptor substrate (IRS) and Akt phosphorylation in livers of diabetic mice. However, it seems that the reduction in phosphorylation of inflammatory factors nuclear factor κB (NF-κB) and inhibitor of κB kinase (IKK) β by oligofructose takes place by a GLP-1–independent manner. Inhibition of GLP-1 receptor by exedin 9-39 does not prevent the phosphorylation of these factors (Cani et al., 2006). Two independent studies of different types of prebiotics (a combination of chitin and β-glucan derived from *Aspergillus niger* (Neyrinck et al., 2012) and a mix of inulin and oligofructose (Parnell and Reimer, 2010) have demonstrated that prebiotics attenuate elevation in hepatic triglycerides in animal models of obesity and high-fat diet in a mechanism that is independent of fatty acid synthase and SREBP-1; although in one of those studies, the inulin-oligofructose mix has induced an elevation of both factors in lean mice (Parnell and Reimer, 2010), thus emphasizing the difference in lipid metabolism in lean and obese animals.

Unfortunately, to date, only few double-blind placebo-controlled clinical trials searching the effect of prebiotics on liver metabolism in NAFLD have been published. One of them demonstrates a lack of change in liver glucose production in type 2 diabetics as a result of supplementation of 20 g/day FOS for 4 weeks (Luo et al., 2000). Another trial compares ingestion of 16 g/day of oligofructose with maltodextrine (placebo) in NASH patients. It has been found that oligofructose is a potent agent to decrease significantly serum aminotransferases and AST after 8 weeks, and insulin levels after 4 weeks (Daubioul et al., 2005). Supplementation of 10 g/day of inulin for 3 weeks accompanied with dietary changes has resulted in decrease in hepatic lipogenesis and plasma triglycerides, without changes in plasma cholesterol, liver acetyl-CoA carboxylase, and SREBP-1 (Letexier et al., 2003). Several trials of prebiotics and synbiotics have been conducted on cirrhotic or liver transplant patients (Eguchi et al., 2011; Rayes et al., 2002; Malaguarnera et al., 2010) or individuals after liver resection (Rayes et al., 2012).

Today's research of prebiotics is focused on their effect as a microbiota-modulating component; the issue of elucidation of a prebiotic's role separate of probiotics remains unclear and probably irrelevant to a regular biosystem and functioning of gastrointestinal tract.

METHYL DONORS: CHOLINE, BETAINE, AND FOLIC ACID IN FATTY LIVER DISEASE

ROLE OF S-ADENOSYLMETHIONINE IN LIVER HEALTH AND DISEASE

Although S-adenosylmethionine (SAMe, Figure 14.1) is produced in all mammalian cells, liver is the major tissue of SAMe synthesis, where 50% of methionine metabolisms and 85% of transmethylation reactions take place. In fact, SAMe competes with ATP as the most widely used enzyme substrate (Lu and Mato, 2012).

The enzyme catalizing the biosynthesis of SAMe from methionine and ATP is methionine adenosyltransferase (also referred SAMe synthase). The synthesis of SAMe is regulated by hypoxia, glutathione, and availability of methionine, and modified by oxidant injury and redox state of the cell (Kalhan et al., 2011; Avila et al., 1998; Pajares et al., 1992; Martinez-Chantar et al., 2003; Sanchez-Gongora et al., 1996; Lu et al., 2000). SAMe mediates a variety of metabolic pathways, several of which are listed below:

a. Transmethylation pathway where SAMe donates its methyl group to a large variety of acceptor molecules (Lu and Mato, 2012).
b. Transsulfuration pathway, utilizing SAMe in cysteine biosynthesis through its conversion to homocysteine, followed by homocysteine's transformation to cysteine by a vitamin B_6-requiring process. The transsulfuration pathway is particularly active in the liver, making SAMe important precursor of GSH (Lu, 2009).
c. Polyamine synthesis. Polyamines are low-molecular-weight, positively charged molecules that are ubiquitous in all living cells. Polyamines play a crucial role in many biochemical processes including regulation of transcription and translation, cell growth, and apoptosis (Perez-Leal and Merali, 2012; Lu and Mato, 2012).

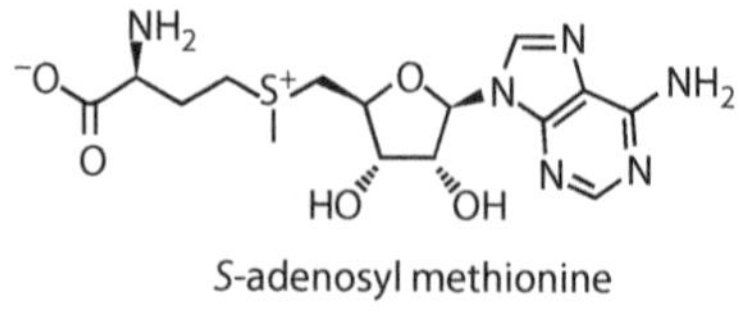

S-adenosyl methionine

FIGURE 14.1   Structure of SAMe.

Supplementary SAMe has been tried in liver diseases of different etiology with promising results. Although the results of clinical studies of SAMe supplementation in alcoholic liver disease are controversial (Medici et al., 2011; Mato et al., 1999), in rat models, it has been able to prevent ethanol-induced liver damage by inhibiting the TLR-mediated pathway (Khachatoorian et al., 2013). There were also encouraging findings following SAMe supplementation in hepatitis C (HCV) patients. Thus, an improvement has been found in SAMe-supplemented (1600 mg/day), previously nonresponsive patients in their reaction to peginterferon-ribavirin therapy; 48% of patients have had undetectable levels of viral RNA by week 24 of the therapy (Feld et al., 2011). In another study, supplementation of the peginterferon-ribavirin treatment with SAMe and betaine led to 58% of previously nonresponsive patients to achieve early viral response; however, only 3% have achieved sustained viral response (Filipowicz et al., 2010).

ROLE OF METHYL DONORS IN FATTY LIVER DISEASE

In an animal model of fatty liver following high-fat sucrose diet, an effect of supplementation of methyl donors on diet-induced gene expression, epigenetic, somatic, and biochemical changes have been studied (Cordero et al., 2013). The methyl donors, which have included choline, betaine, folic acid, and vitamin B_{12}, have been supplemented to male and female Wistar rats for 8 weeks. First, the supplementation with methyl donors has prevented liver fat accumulation. Second, the obesogenic diet has decreased methylation of CpG islands of fatty acid synthase promoter in males, whereas in females, it has led to hypermethylation. In the female group, but not the male group, methyl donor supplementation has increased methylation of specific CpGs. At the level of mRNA expression, methyl donors have increased acetyl CoA carboxylase α and decreased proinflammatory chemokine ligand CCL2. Interestingly, the obesogenic diet by itself has not significantly changed the expression of these genes as compared with a control group (Cordero et al., 2013).

Supplementation with betaine (Figure 14.2), a normal component of the methionine cycle and an important liver osmotic regulator, is an alternative way to increase methionine levels and to prevent fatty liver damage. Clinical studies demonstrate successful reduction of hepatic steatosis (Abdelmalek et al., 2009; Miglio et al., 2000), liver fibrosis, and plasma levels of liver enzymes (Abdelmalek et al., 2001) by betaine treatment.

Choline (Figure 14.2) is probably one of the most intriguing agents in methyl donor group. It is a precursor of several compounds as betaine and acetylcholine; the most relevant for proper liver functioning is phosphatidylcholine required for synthesis of

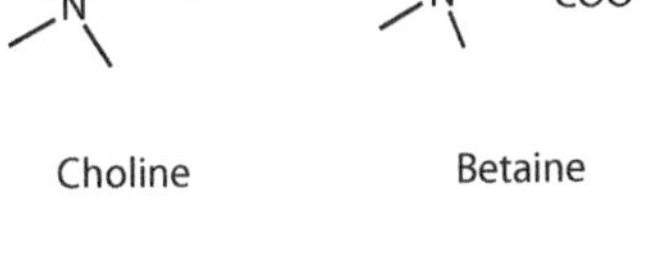

Choline   Betaine

FIGURE 14.2   Structure of choline and betaine.

VLDL followed by export of triacylglycerols from the liver. A prominent feature of choline-deficient diet, the development of liver dysfunction, is reflected in liver fat accumulation and leakage of liver enzymes (AST) to plasma (Fischer et al., 2007). Animal studies demonstrate reversibility of damage caused by choline-deficient diet by choline supplementation, resolving both steatosis and inflammation, and decreasing plasma AST and ALT levels (Takeuchi-Yorimoto et al., 2013).

Because it is synthesized in vertebrates from methionine, choline's nutritional essentiality in human is arguable; however, in several conditions, as in long-term total parenteral nutrition (TPN), choline deficiency has been found to be one of the major factors for development of liver steatosis (Buchman et al., 2001). The only source of choline other than diet is from the *de novo* biosynthesis of phosphatidylcholine, which is catalyzed by phosphatidylethanolamine-*N*-methyltransferase (PEMT) (Fischer et al., 2010; Zeisel, 2006). The PEMT gene has several estrogen response elements in its promoter region, and the gene is induced by estrogen, contributing to the reason of difference between premenopausal and postmenopausal women in their reaction to a choline-deficient diet (Fischer et al., 2010; Resseguie et al., 2007). Indeed, among general population, postmenopausal women are more susceptible to choline-deficient diet, whereas treatment with estrogen reduces this susceptibility (Fischer et al., 2007).

One of the requirements of endogenous choline synthesis is an obligatory requirement for one-carbon groups derived from donors such as folate and vitamin B_{12} metabolism (Kohlmeier et al., 2005). Individuals who are carriers of the 5,10-methylenetetrahydrofolate dehydrogenase-1958A gene allele are more likely than noncarriers to develop signs of choline deficiency on a low-choline diet, unless they are treated with a folic acid supplement (Kohlmeier et al., 2005).

There is a recommendation for adequate intake of dietary choline, standing by 550 mg/day for men and 425 mg/day for women. The recommendation has been established for prevention of choline depletion–induced liver dysfunction. However, high doses of choline (>6 g) have been associated with excessive cholinergic stimulation, such as vomiting, salivation, sweating, and gastrointestinal effects and fishy body odor. The tolerable upper limit for choline has been set at 3 g/day (Zeisel, 2010).

MILK THISTLE

Milk thistle (*Silybum marianum*) is a plant of Asteracea family, which has been used medicinally for more than 2000 years, primarily as a treatment for liver dysfunction. The major active components of milk thistle are flavonolignans with a general name "silymarin," consisting of eight compounds, the most prominent of which is silibinin (silibin). Additionally, a flavonoid taxifolin is an ingredient of the plant (Hackett et al., 2013). As non–water-soluble compounds, flavonolignans demonstrate low bioavailability; however, in capsules they are bound to phosphatidylcholine increasing their absorption. One of the characteristics of milk thistle extracts is a rapid glucoronidation and a fast excretion into the bile and urine (Ladas et al., 2010). Commercial extracts differ of their bioavailability and activity, and pharmacokinetic data have to be presented regarding each product (Hackett et al., 2013). This paragraph is discussing clinical findings associated with milk thistle components and liver diseases of different etiology.

For the last decade, the components of milk thistle have been clinically studied for their protective role in liver disease, especially in hepatitis C (HCV) patients. According to estimations, 8%–33% of the patients in the United States use silymarin for treatment of chronic HCV (Seeff et al., 2008), although the results of clinical studies are controversial.

Interestingly, the effect of milk thistle extract on liver diseases of differentiated etiology is reflected by different effects. Loguercio et al. (2012) tried a commercial silibin extract combined with phosphatidylcholine and vitamin E on 138 NAFLD patients, 30 of them with HCV. The combination has increased the proportion of patients with normal plasma levels of liver enzymes: AST and ALT in general NAFLD and γ-glutamyltranspeptidase in HCV-positive patients. In HCV-positive patients, levels of TNF-β and matrix metalloproteinases have been significantly reduced following the combination treatment, a result that has not been observed in general NAFLD patients. Levels of hepatic steatosis according to the ultrasonographic analysis have not differed between the treatment and the placebo groups; however, among the patients who had agreed to liver biopsy after the treatment (mostly NAFLD patients), the mean severity score for liver steatosis has significantly decreased from the baseline up to month 12 with the combination treatment, but not with the placebo; the data have not been achieved from HCV patients (Loguercio et al., 2012).

One of the reasons of difference in the reaction to the milk thistle extract by NAFLD and HCV patients may be related to separate kinetics of its conjugation and disposition in two conditions. Thus, one study (Schrieber et al., 2011) comparing disposition of silymarin between those two groups has found that plasma levels of silibin B had been higher, whereas its conjugates had been lower in the NAFLD rather than in chronic HCV patients. Moreover, enterohepatic cycling of flavono-lignins has been observed only in NAFLD and not in chronic HCV patients, thus contributing even more to higher plasma levels in NAFLD. The authors conclude that the effect of milk thistle is expected to be more intensive in NAFLD than in HCV (Schrieber et al., 2011). The low availability and lack of enterohepatic cycling in HCV patients, are probably able to be overcome by increasing concentrations of oral silymarin to 700 mg/day, which is higher than a standard dosage, but still well tolerable and safe (Hawke et al., 2010). However, when HCV, NAFLD, and HCV-cirrhotic patients were compared, the highest exposure to the flavonolignans has been observed in cirrhotic patient; cirrhotic patients have also achieved the highest caspase 3/7 activity following the exposure to silymarin indicating its pro-apoptotic role (Schrieber et al., 2008).

An effect of ingestion of 140 mg silymarin three times daily (a final dosage of 420 mg/day) has been studied in acute hepatitis patients for 4 weeks with additional 4 weeks of follow-up. Such symptoms as dark urine, scleral icterus, and jaundice have recovered at more rapid rate in patients randomized to silymarin than a placebo group; however, the direct measurements of liver function including direct bilirubin, AST, and ALT have not differed between the silymarin and the placebo groups (El-Kamary et al., 2009).

Despite the high expectations on the effect of silymarin on reducing of HCV RNA replication, clinical studies of oral silymarin supplementation have failed to demonstrate it (Hawke et al., 2010; Fried et al., 2012; Tanamly et al., 2004). Intravenous injections of silibinin have succeeded to reduce viral RNA replication in previous peginterferon-ribavirin nonresponders; however, this effect has not been maintained after the end of infusions by oral silibinin supplementation, even though the PegIFN/ribavirin therapy has been combined with the oral mode. This result probably explains the difference in pharmacokinetics of intravenous and oral supplementation between the antiviral effect of silibinin in vitro compared with lack of the one in clinical studies (Ferenci et al., 2008).

Hepatitis B is another condition popular for silymarin supplementation. A recent meta-analysis of the effect of simylarin on chronic hepatitis B patients undertaken by Chinese study group has demonstrated encouraging results for combining of silymarin with antiviral drug therapy. Silymarin was equivalent to antiviral drugs or protection liver drugs in serum transaminases, viral load, and hepatic fibrosis markers. Additionally, silymarin combined with antiviral drugs or antiviral and protection liver drugs significantly reduced levels of serum transaminases, hepatic fibrosis markers, and serum TGF-β1, TNF-α, IL-6 versus antiviral or protection liver drugs alone. However, the authors point at serious limitations in studies chosen for their meta-analysis: not all studies were double-blinded; no reasons for withdrawal have been noted; Chinese studies have been more condensed than typical Western ones (Wei et al., 2013).

In alcoholic cirrhosis, no significant silymarin-related findings have been demonstrated in English-language literature at the last decade, besides small increase in GSH (Lucena et al., 2002). In 1989, a randomized, double-blind, placebo-controlled trial was published demonstrating a significant reduction in mortality of alcoholic cirrhosis patients in silymarin-treated patients as compared with a placebo group (Ferenci et al., 1989); however, there are no later reports confirming this result.

Silymarin has been reported to attenuate oxidative stress and liver toxicity in workers of natural gas industry chronically exposed to hydrogen sulfide (H_2S) gas. Silymarin has reduced the levels of ALT, AST, and ALP proteins in workers' plasma. TNF-α G-308A polymorphism has been significantly associated with decreasing in AST (p = 0.04) and ALT (p = 0.003). These results suggest that decrease in the enzyme levels is less effective in subjects with high production of TNF-α (Mandegary et al., 2013).

In conclusion, oral silymarin can be used as a protective agent in NAFLD and in cirrhotic patients, whereas in HCV and HCB patients, more effective dosages and ways of administration have to be considered and investigated.

GREEN TEA

Green tea is produced from unfermented leafs of *Camellia sinensis*. Green tea flavonoids contain mostly catechins (Figure 14.3): epicatechin (EC), epigallocatechin (EGC), epicatechin gallate (ECG), and epigallocatechin gallate (EGCG) (Masterjohn and Bruno, 2012). In a process of tea fermentation to black tea, catechins are condensed to theaflavin dimers and thearubigin polymers (Mulder et al., 2005). Antioxidant, anti-inflammatory, hypolipidemic, and absorption-reducing activity of green tea have been studied in animal models and partly strengthened by

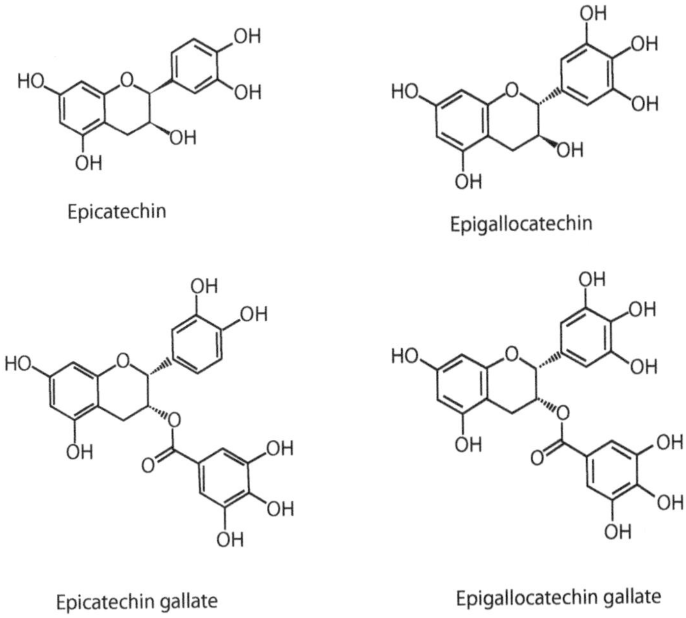

FIGURE 14.3   Structure of green tea flavonoids.

human studies. Animal models of NAFLD have demonstrated NF-κB inactivation, TLR downregulation, decrease in lipid and glucose absorption, reduction in ROS generation and increase in enzymatic antioxidant activities (Masterjohn and Bruno, 2012). Despite findings from animal models, evidence of protective effect on liver disease from human trials are limited; randomized, double-blinded trials are needed to prove them.

Catechins and theaflavins are absorbed in the small intestine, whereas larger thearubigins are metabolized by the intestinal flora to hydroxyphenyl-γ-valerolactones and phenolic acids, which undergo absorption from the large intestine. A study on nine healthy volunteers revealed lower levels of catechins following black tea consumption as compared with green tea; meanwhile, there was no difference between the two types of tea in excretion of hippuric acid, which might be a major metabolite produced from catechins (Mulder et al., 2005).

ROS attack on DNA and its further metabolism produce 8-hydroxy-2′-deoxyguanosine (8-OHdG), which is excreted in urine and constitutes a biomarker for DNA damage. Chemopreventive effect of green tea polyphenols (GTP) has been studied in randomized, double-blinded, placebo-controlled phase IIa chemoprevention trial in 124 individuals who have been seropositive for both hepatitis B surface antigen (HBsAg) and aflatoxin–albumin adducts. The participants have been taking GTP capsules daily at doses of 500 mg, 1000 mg, or a placebo for 3 months (Luo et al., 2006). Levels of urine 8-OHdG have been reduced by 3 months of GTP consumption at a dose-dependent manner (treatment for 1 month has not demonstrated a significant reduction in marker excretion).

In animal models of NAFLD, EGCG attenuates fibrosis and reduces levels of proinflammatory markers iNOS, COX-2, and TNF-α. At the level of signal transduction, EGCG downregulates an activation of TGF/SMAD, PI3 K/Akt/FoxO1, and NF-κB (Xiao et al., 2013).

Publications related to green tea toxicity reveal a need to consider safety issues. A study that has supplemented noncirrhotic and cirrhotic HCV participants with 400 mg of pure EGCG, has found that the effect of EGCG is higher in cirrhotic than in noncirrhotic patients. Plasma concentrations of EGCG have been up to 3-fold higher in cirrhotic patients, and an area under the curve (AUC) has been increased 2-fold (Halegoua-De Marzio et al., 2012). The Spanish Liver Toxicity Registry published in 2008 has reported that among 13 herbal-induced hepatotoxicity cases, *C. sinensis* was the main causative herb for liver damage; three of general 13 reported cases have been related to it (Garcia-Cortes et al., 2008). Clinical pharmacokinetic and animal toxicological information indicated that consumption of concentrated green tea extracts on an empty stomach is more likely to lead to adverse effects than its consumption in the fed state (Sarma et al., 2008). Although no changes in ALT, AST, GGT, bilirubin, urea, and uric acid have been observed in supplementation of green tea polyphenols at a dosage of 714 mg/day for 3 weeks in healthy men (Frank et al., 2009), the previously mentioned toxicity reports and case studies demonstrate the importance of regular follow-up in individuals using green tea extract supplements.

NONCLINICAL EVIDENCE OF A ROLE OF NUTRACEUTICALS IN PREVENTION AND TREATMENT OF FATTY LIVER DISEASE

There are a limited number of human trials studying the effect of nutraceuticals in fatty liver disease. A variety of natural compounds tried on animal models have been determined as candidates for prevention and treatment of the condition. Unfortunately, no single model system completely resembles the etiology of NAFLD. Moreover, those that most closely resemble human NAFLD also involve comorbidities such as obesity and diabetes, making it difficult to define the hepatoprotective activities of natural compounds (Masterjohn and Bruno, 2012). A wide variety of herbal and other nutraceuticals have been demonstrated as potentially hepatoprotective in animal models, including vitamin D (Eliades et al., 2013), *Opuntia ficus indica* (Moran-Ramos et al., 2012), *Cassia tora* seeds (Tzeng et al., 2013), caffeine (Sugiura et al., 2012), *Ginkgo biloba* (Wang et al., 2012), ginsenosides (Shen et al., 2013), etc.; however, this section is focusing only on several of potentially hepatoprotective nutraceuticals.

RESVERATROL

Resveratrol is a widely studied polyphenolic compound in a number of plants and their products such as grapes, wine, and berry fruits. It is considered to be a potential agent for treatment and prevention of diabetes, coronary heart disease, and cancer (Xu and Si, 2012). In obese rats, resveratrol decreases liver fat accumulation, probably by increasing carnitine palmitoyl transferase Ia (CPT-1a) and acyl-coenzyme A oxydase and decreasing acetyl-CoA activities. The polyphenol increases an activity of AMPK and PGC-1α (Alberdi et al., 2013). The increase in PGC-1α may explain a resveratrol-induced upregulation of mitochondrial biogenesis and increased expression of uncoupling protein 2 (UCP-2), which have been achieved in another study (Poulsen et al., 2012).

CURCUMIN

Curcuma longa, or turmeric, has been used for thousands of years in Eastern countries and traditional medicine. Modern research has revealed anti-inflammatory and chemopreventive properties of curcumin, an active component of *Cur. longa* rhizome, especially in attenuation of NF-κB pathway. Curcumin is not an exclusive, yet the most studied, component of turmeric possessing anti-inflammatory activities (Aggarwal et al., 2013).

Regarding fatty liver, experimental results have revealed that curcumin attenuates lipid accumulation in liver (Oner-Iyidogan et al., 2013; Yiu et al., 2011). Moreover, following supplementation of extract of *Curcuma longa*, reduction in activity of 3-hydroxy-3-methyl-glutaryl-CoA (HMG-CoA) reductase has been observed in livers of rats fed with high-cholesterol diet (Yiu et al., 2011). Liver SREBP-1c expression has been downregulated by curcumin in obese mice with hepatic steatosis (Kuo et al., 2012). Impaired functions of liver mitochondria in those mice have been improved by curcumin, demonstrating normalization in mitochondrial DNA, NRF1, and mitochondrial transcription factor A (TFAM) gene expression, reduced hepatic NF-κB activity, and levels of thiobarbituric acid reactive substances (TBARS). All those changes have resulted in restored mitochondrial oxidative metabolism and biogenesis (Kuo et al., 2012). As a potential hepatoprotective agent, curcumin has to be tried in randomized clinical studies to elucidate its effects on fatty liver.

α-LIPOIC ACID

α-Lipoic acid (thioctic acid, LA; Figure 14.4) is found naturally in mitochondria, where it is bound to the subunit E2 and acts as a coenzyme for pyruvate dehydrogenase and α-ketoglutarate dehydrogenase. Humans can synthesize LA de novo from fatty acids and cysteine, but only in very small amounts. Therefore, LA needs to be absorbed from exogenous sources (Goraca et al., 2011). Anticancer, antiaging, and antidiabetic activities have been related to this compound (Novotny et al., 2008; Rochette et al., 2013; Shay et al., 2009).

It has been found that LA is possible to prevent fatty liver damage in animals. In rats, LA administration has been shown to improve fructose diet-induced hepatic

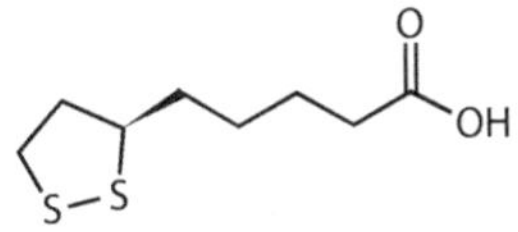

α-lipoic acid

FIGURE 14.4   Structure of α-lipoic acid.

insulin resistance and glucose intolerance. Liver oxidative stress has been attenuated, and antioxidant capacity and antioxidant enzymes expression have increased. PPAR-γ levels have been upregulated, whereas UCP-2 and PPAR-δ protein expression have decreased. The administration with LA has restored the basal gene expression of PPARδ, SREBP-1c, and lipogenic enzymes fatty acid synthase and glycerol-3-phosphate acyltransferase. Lipoic acid also has prevented fructose-mediated enhancement of glucokinase activity (Castro et al., 2013). In a model of methionine- and choline-deficient mice, supplementation with α-linoleic acid has decreased hepatic lipid accumulation and hepatic inflammation, including NF-κB activation. The levels of antioxidant markers TBARS and 4-hydroxynonenal have been decreased as well as plasma ALT and AST levels (Min et al., 2012).

BITTER MELON

Bitter melon (*Momordica charantia* L.) is a tropical vine that produces fruits traditionally used for treatment of diabetes. A hepatoprotective effect of bitter melon is now being demonstrated in animal models of fatty liver (Chen and Li, 2005; Senanayake et al., 2004a, b, 2012). Senanayake et al. published several reports related to liver triglyceride and a cholesterol-lowering effect of freeze-dried bitter melon powder and its methanol fraction in rats fed diet with or without cholesterol supplementation (Senanayake et al., 2004a,b, 2012). In a series of mechanistic experiments, the same group has prepared either liver slices or hepatocytes from rat livers and demonstrated that supplementation with bitter melon extract has summarized in decreased incorporation of [1(2)-^{14}C] acetate and [1-^{14}C] oleic acid into triglycerides of liver slices and hepatocytes. Bitter melon–supplemented rats have also shown an enhanced mRNA expression of CPT-IA, which is the rate-limiting enzyme for fatty acid oxidation. Thus, a proposed mechanism for reduction of hepatic steatosis by bitter melon is decreased synthesis of hepatic triclycerides and enhanced fatty acid oxidation (Senanayake et al., 2012).

BLACK RICE EXTRACT

Black rice (*Oryza sativa* L., Japonica) is a cyanidin-3-glucoside–rich cultivar regarded as a health-promoting food and widely consumed in Eastern Asia. Anthocyanin extract from black rice (BRE) can decrease serum TGs levels and protect the liver from alcohol-induced injury (Um et al., 2013).

A high-fat diet–induced hepatic steatosis is accompanied by a significant increase in serum levels of free fatty acids, triglyceride (TG), total cholesterol, and insulin. Supplementary black rice extract is potent to alleviate hepatic steatosis and to decrease serum TG and total cholesterol levels. Dietary BRE also increases expression of fatty acid metabolism–related genes, including CPT-1A, acyl-CoA oxidase, cytochrome P450, and PPAR-α (Jang et al., 2012).

In a model of alcoholic liver disease, administration of BRE along with alcohol decreases levels of serum AST, ALT, and GGT, the MDA, and concentrations of serum and hepatic TG and total cholesterol. Rats treated with RBE have shown a better profile of the antioxidant system, including normalized glutathione peroxidase, superoxide dismutase and glutathione *S*-transferase activities (Hou et al., 2010). Up to date, no clinical studies regarding BRE hepatoprotective effect have been conducted.

CONCLUDING REMARKS

Although nutraceuticals have been used for thousands of years in traditional medicine, their scientific research is a relatively novel area. Integration of nutraceuticals in the conventional therapies needs more evidence form clinical trials. The last two decades have accelerated the rate of this study, resulting in our knowledge of potential nutraceutical therapeutic agents.

Regarding fatty liver disease, an improvement of gut microbiota demonstrates very promising effects on preventing and treatment of this condition. Other potential agents such as milk thistle, methyl donors, and, when correct dosages are used, green tea polyphenols have been revealed. A variety of other nutraceuticals have been studied, and mechanisms of their action have been elucidated in vitro and in vivo. Insufficiency or lack of randomized, placebo-controlled clinical studies, and meta-analyses do not allow us to conclude about the clinical meaning of those agents. Their involvement in anti-inflammatory, anti-lipogenic, and antioxidative pathways propose a good beginning for executing clinical trials and defining safety issues and effective dosages for each nutraceutical. Matching of each nutraceutical to a specific liver condition is an important challenge in their research.

REFERENCES

Abdelmalek, M. F., P. Angulo, R. A. Jorgensen, P. B. Sylvestre, and K. D. Lindor. 2001. Betaine, a promising new agent for patients with nonalcoholic steatohepatitis: results of a pilot study. *Am J Gastroenterol* 96:2711–7.

Abdelmalek, M. F., S. O. Sanderson, P. Angulo et al. 2009. Betaine for nonalcoholic fatty liver disease: results of a randomized placebo-controlled trial. *Hepatology* 50:1818–26.

Aggarwal, B. B., W. Yuan, S. Li, and S. C. Gupta. 2013. Curcumin-free turmeric exhibits anti-inflammatory and anticancer activities: identification of novel components of turmeric. *Mol Nutr Food Res* 57:1529–42.

Alberdi, G., V. M. Rodriguez, M. T. Macarulla, J. Miranda, I. Churruca, and M. P. Portillo. 2013. Hepatic lipid metabolic pathways modified by resveratrol in rats fed an obesogenic diet. *Nutrition* 29:562–7.

Aller, R., D. A. De Luis, O. Izaola et al. 2011. Effect of a probiotic on liver aminotransferases in nonalcoholic fatty liver disease patients: a double blind randomized clinical trial. *Eur Rev Med Pharmacol Sci* 15:1090–5.

Anastasovska, J., T. Arora, G. J. Sanchez Canon et al. 2012. Fermentable carbohydrate alters hypothalamic neuronal activity and protects against the obesogenic environment. *Obesity (Silver Spring)* 20:1016–23.

Asrih, M., and F. Jornayvaz. 2013. Inflammation as a link between nonalcoholic fatty liver disease and insulin resistance. *J Endocrinol* 218:R25–36.

Ataie-Jafari, A., B. Larijani, H. Alavi Majd, and F. Tahbaz. 2009. Cholesterol-lowering effect of probiotic yogurt in comparison with ordinary yogurt in mildly to moderately hypercholesterolemic subjects. *Ann Nutr Metab* 54:22–7.

Avila, M. A., M. V. Carretero, E. N. Rodriguez, and J. M. Mato. 1998. Regulation by hypoxia of methionine adenosyltransferase activity and gene expression in rat hepatocytes. *Gastroenterology* 114:364–71.

Buchman, A. L., M. E. Ament, M. Sohel et al. 2001. Choline deficiency causes reversible hepatic abnormalities in patients receiving parenteral nutrition: proof of a human choline requirement: a placebo-controlled trial. *JPEN J Parenter Enteral Nutr* 25:260–8.

Burcelin, R., M. Serino, C. Chabo, V. Blasco-Baque, and J. Amar. 2011. Gut microbiota and diabetes: from pathogenesis to therapeutic perspective. *Acta Diabetol* 48:257–73.

Cani, P. D., C. Knauf, M. A. Iglesias, D. J. Drucker, N. M. Delzenne, and R. Burcelin. 2006. Improvement of glucose tolerance and hepatic insulin sensitivity by oligofructose requires a functional glucagon-like peptide 1 receptor. *Diabetes* 55:1484–90.

Cani, P. D., A. M. Neyrinck, F. Fava et al. 2007. Selective increases of bifidobacteria in gut microflora improve high-fat-diet-induced diabetes in mice through a mechanism associated with endotoxaemia. *Diabetologia* 50:2374–83.

Caselli, M., F. Cassol, G. Calo, J. Holton, G. Zuliani, and A. Gasbarrini. 2013. Actual concept of "probiotics": is it more functional to science or business? *World J Gastroenterol* 19:1527–40.

Castro, M. C., M. L. Massa, G. Schinella, J. J. Gagliardino, and F. Francini. 2013. Lipoic acid prevents liver metabolic changes induced by administration of a fructose-rich diet. *Biochim Biophys Acta* 1830:2226–32.

Chauhan, B., G. Kumar, N. Kalam, and S. H. Ansari. 2013. Current concepts and prospects of herbal nutraceutical: a review. *J Adv Pharm Technol Res* 4:4–8.

Chen, H. L., C. H. Wang, Y. W. Kuo, and C. H. Tsai. 2011. Antioxidative and hepatoprotective effects of fructo-oligosaccharide in D-galactose-treated Balb/cJ mice. *Br J Nutr* 105:805–9.

Chen, Q., and E. T. Li. 2005. Reduced adiposity in bitter melon (Momordica charantia) fed rats is associated with lower tissue triglyceride and higher plasma catecholamines. *Br J Nutr* 93:747–54.

Cordero, P., A. M. Gomez-Uriz, J. Campion, F. I. Milagro, and J. A. Martinez. 2013. Dietary supplementation with methyl donors reduces fatty liver and modifies the fatty acid synthase DNA methylation profile in rats fed an obesogenic diet. *Genes Nutr* 8:105–13.

Correia-Sa, I., H. de-Sousa-Lopes, M. J. Martins, I. Azevedo, E. Moura, and M. A. Vieira-Coelho. 2013. Effects of raftilose on serum biochemistry and liver morphology in rats fed with normal or high-fat diet. *Mol Nutr Food Res*.

Crawford, J. M. 2012. Histologic findings in alcoholic liver disease. *Clin Liver Dis* 16:699–716.

Daubioul, C. A., Y. Horsmans, P. Lambert, E. Danse, and N. M. Delzenne. 2005. Effects of oligofructose on glucose and lipid metabolism in patients with nonalcoholic steatohepatitis: results of a pilot study. *Eur J Clin Nutr* 59:723–6.

Daubioul, C. A., H. S. Taper, L. D. De Wispelaere, and N. M. Delzenne. 2000. Dietary oligofructose lessens hepatic steatosis, but does not prevent hypertriglyceridemia in obese zucker rats. *J Nutr* 130:1314–9.

de Wit, N., M. Derrien, H. Bosch-Vermeulen et al. 2012. Saturated fat stimulates obesity and hepatic steatosis and affects gut microbiota composition by an enhanced overflow of dietary fat to the distal intestine. *Am J Physiol Gastrointest Liver Physiol* 303:G589–99.

Eguchi, S., M. Takatsuki, M. Hidaka, A. Soyama, T. Ichikawa, and T. Kanematsu. 2011. Perioperative synbiotic treatment to prevent infectious complications in patients after elective living donor liver transplantation: a prospective randomized study. *Am J Surg* 201:498–502.

Ejtahed, H. S., J. Mohtadi-Nia, A. Homayouni-Rad et al. 2011. Effect of probiotic yogurt containing Lactobacillus acidophilus and Bifidobacterium lactis on lipid profile in individuals with type 2 diabetes mellitus. *J Dairy Sci* 94:3288–94.

El-Kamary, S. S., M. D. Shardell, M. Abdel-Hamid et al. 2009. A randomized controlled trial to assess the safety and efficacy of silymarin on symptoms, signs and biomarkers of acute hepatitis. *Phytomedicine* 16:391–400.

Eliades, M., E. Spyrou, N. Agrawal et al. 2013. Meta-analysis: vitamin D and non-alcoholic fatty liver disease. *Aliment Pharmacol Ther* 38:246–54.

Endo, H., M. Niioka, N. Kobayashi, M. Tanaka, and T. Watanabe. 2013. Butyrate-producing probiotics reduce nonalcoholic fatty liver disease progression in rats: new insight into the probiotics for the gut-liver axis. *PLoS One* 8:e63388.

Feld, J. J., A. A. Modi, R. El-Diwany et al. 2011. *S*-Adenosyl methionine improves early viral responses and interferon-stimulated gene induction in hepatitis C nonresponders. *Gastroenterology* 140:830–9.

Ferenci, P., B. Dragosics, H. Dittrich et al. 1989. Randomized controlled trial of silymarin treatment in patients with cirrhosis of the liver. *J Hepatol* 9:105–13.

Ferenci, P., T. M. Scherzer, H. Kerschner et al. 2008. Silibinin is a potent antiviral agent in patients with chronic hepatitis C not responding to pegylated interferon/ribavirin therapy. *Gastroenterology* 135:1561–7.

Filipowicz, M., C. Bernsmeier, L. Terracciano, F. H. Duong, and M. H. Heim. 2010. *S*-Adenosyl-methionine and betaine improve early virological response in chronic hepatitis C patients with previous nonresponse. *PLoS One* 5:e15492.

Fischer, L. M., K. A. da Costa, L. Kwock, J. Galanko, and S. H. Zeisel. 2010. Dietary choline requirements of women: effects of estrogen and genetic variation. *Am J Clin Nutr* 92:1113–9.

Fischer, L. M., K. A. da Costa, L. Kwock et al. 2007. Sex and menopausal status influence human dietary requirements for the nutrient choline. *Am J Clin Nutr* 85:1275–85.

Frank, J., T. W. George, J. K. Lodge et al. 2009. Daily consumption of an aqueous green tea extract supplement does not impair liver function or alter cardiovascular disease risk biomarkers in healthy men. *J Nutr* 139:58–62.

Fried, M. W., V. J. Navarro, N. Afdhal et al. 2012. Effect of silymarin (milk thistle) on liver disease in patients with chronic hepatitis C unsuccessfully treated with interferon therapy: a randomized controlled trial. *JAMA* 308:274–82.

Garcia-Cortes, M., Y. Borraz, M. I. Lucena et al. 2008. [Liver injury induced by "natural remedies": an analysis of cases submitted to the Spanish Liver Toxicity Registry]. *Rev Esp Enferm Dig* 100:688–95.

Goraca, A., H. Huk-Kolega, A. Piechota, P. Kleniewska, E. Ciejka, and B. Skibska. 2011. Lipoic acid—biological activity and therapeutic potential. *Pharmacol Rep* 63:849–58.

Guandalini, S. 2011. Probiotics for prevention and treatment of diarrhea. *J Clin Gastroenterol* 45 Suppl:S149–53.

Hackett, E. S., D. C. Twedt, and D. L. Gustafson. 2013. Milk thistle and its derivative compounds: a review of opportunities for treatment of liver disease. *J Vet Intern Med* 27:10–6.

Halegoua-De Marzio, D., W. K. Kraft, C. Daskalakis, X. Ying, R. L. Hawke, and V. J. Navarro. 2012. Limited sampling estimates of epigallocatechin gallate exposures in cirrhotic and noncirrhotic patients with hepatitis C after single oral doses of green tea extract. *Clin Ther* 34:2279–2285 e1.

Hawke, R. L., S. J. Schrieber, T. A. Soule et al. 2010. Silymarin ascending multiple oral dosing phase I study in noncirrhotic patients with chronic hepatitis C. *J Clin Pharmacol* 50:434–49.

Henao-Mejia, J., E. Elinav, C. Jin et al. 2012. Inflammasome-mediated dysbiosis regulates progression of NAFLD and obesity. *Nature* 482:179–85.

Hou, Z., P. Qin, and G. Ren. 2010. Effect of anthocyanin-rich extract from black rice (*Oryza sativa* L. Japonica) on chronically alcohol-induced liver damage in rats. *J Agric Food Chem* 58:3191–6.

Jang, H. H., M. Y. Park, H. W. Kim et al. 2012. Black rice (*Oryza sativa* L.) extract attenuates hepatic steatosis in C57BL/6 J mice fed a high-fat diet via fatty acid oxidation. *Nutr Metab (Lond)* 9:27.

Johnston, B. C., J. Z. Goldenberg, P. O. Vandvik, X. Sun, and G. H. Guyatt. 2011. Probiotics for the prevention of pediatric antibiotic-associated diarrhea. *Cochrane Database Syst Rev*:CD004827.

Kalhan, S. C., J. Edmison, S. Marczewski et al. 2011. Methionine and protein metabolism in non-alcoholic steatohepatitis: evidence for lower rate of transmethylation of methionine. *Clin Sci (Lond)* 121:179–89.

Karoli, R., J. Fatima, A. Chandra, U. Gupta, F. U. Islam, and G. Singh. 2013. Prevalence of hepatic steatosis in women with polycystic ovary syndrome. *J Hum Reprod Sci* 6:9–14.

Khachatoorian, R., D. Dawson, E. M. Maloney, J. Wang, B. A. French, and S. W. French. 2013. SAMe treatment prevents the ethanol-induced epigenetic alterations of genes in the Toll-like receptor pathway. *Exp Mol Pathol* 94:243–6.

Kohlmeier, M., K. A. da Costa, L. M. Fischer, and S. H. Zeisel. 2005. Genetic variation of folate-mediated one-carbon transfer pathway predicts susceptibility to choline deficiency in humans. *Proc Natl Acad Sci USA* 102:16025–30.

Kozmus, C. E., E. Moura, M. P. Serrao et al. 2011. Influence of dietary supplementation with dextrin or oligofructose on the hepatic redox balance in rats. *Mol Nutr Food Res* 55:1735–9.

Kuo, J. J., H. H. Chang, T. H. Tsai, and T. Y. Lee. 2012. Curcumin ameliorates mitochondrial dysfunction associated with inhibition of gluconeogenesis in free fatty acid-mediated hepatic lipoapoptosis. *Int J Mol Med* 30:643–9.

Ladas, E., D. J. Kroll, and K. M. Kelly. 2010. Milk thistle. In *Encyclopedia of dietary science*, edited by P. M. Coates. New York: Informa Healthcare.

Letexier, D., F. Diraison, and M. Beylot. 2003. Addition of inulin to a moderately high-carbohydrate diet reduces hepatic lipogenesis and plasma triacylglycerol concentrations in humans. *Am J Clin Nutr* 77:559–64.

Li, D. Y., M. Yang, S. Edwards, and S. Q. Ye. 2013. Nonalcoholic fatty liver disease: for better or worse, blame the gut microbiota? *JPEN J Parenter Enteral Nutr* 37:787–93.

Loguercio, C., P. Andreone, C. Brisc et al. 2012. Silybin combined with phosphatidylcholine and vitamin E in patients with nonalcoholic fatty liver disease: a randomized controlled trial. *Free Radic Biol Med* 52:1658–65.

Lu, S. C. 2009. Regulation of glutathione synthesis. *Mol Aspects Med* 30:42–59.

Lu, S. C., Z. Z. Huang, H. Yang, J. M. Mato, M. A. Avila, and H. Tsukamoto. 2000. Changes in methionine adenosyltransferase and *S*-adenosylmethionine homeostasis in alcoholic rat liver. *Am J Physiol Gastrointest Liver Physiol* 279:G178–85.

Lu, S. C., and J. M. Mato. 2012. *S*-Adenosylmethionine in liver health, injury, and cancer. *Physiol Rev* 92:1515–42.

Lucena, M. I., R. J. Andrade, J. P. de la Cruz, M. Rodriguez-Mendizabal, E. Blanco, and F. Sanchez de la Cuesta. 2002. Effects of silymarin MZ-80 on oxidative stress in patients with alcoholic cirrhosis. Results of a randomized, double-blind, placebo-controlled clinical study. *Int J Clin Pharmacol Ther* 40:2–8.

Luo, H., L. Tang, M. Tang et al. 2006. Phase IIa chemoprevention trial of green tea polyphenols in high-risk individuals of liver cancer: modulation of urinary excretion of green tea polyphenols and 8-hydroxydeoxyguanosine. *Carcinogenesis* 27:262–8.

Luo, J., M. Van Yperselle, S. W. Rizkalla, F. Rossi, F. R. Bornet, and G. Slama. 2000. Chronic consumption of short-chain fructooligosaccharides does not affect basal hepatic glucose production or insulin resistance in type 2 diabetics. *J Nutr* 130:1572–7.

Machado, M. V., and H. Cortez-Pinto. 2012. Gut microbiota and nonalcoholic fatty liver disease. *Ann Hepatol* 11:440–9.

Malaguarnera, M., M. P. Gargante, G. Malaguarnera et al. 2010. Bifidobacterium combined with fructo-oligosaccharide versus lactulose in the treatment of patients with hepatic encephalopathy. *Eur J Gastroenterol Hepatol* 22:199–206.

Mandegary, A., A. Saeedi, A. Eftekhari, V. Montazeri, and E. Sharif. 2013. Hepatoprotective effect of silyamarin in individuals chronically exposed to hydrogen sulfide; modulating influence of TNF-alpha cytokine genetic polymorphism. *Daru* 21:28.

Martinez-Chantar, M. L., M. U. Latasa, M. Varela-Rey et al. 2003. L-methionine availability regulates expression of the methionine adenosyltransferase 2A gene in human hepatocarcinoma cells: role of S-adenosylmethionine. *J Biol Chem* 278:19885–90.

Masterjohn, C., and R. S. Bruno. 2012. Therapeutic potential of green tea in nonalcoholic fatty liver disease. *Nutr Rev* 70:41–56.

Mato, J. M., J. Camara, J. Fernandez de Paz et al. 1999. *S*-Adenosylmethionine in alcoholic liver cirrhosis: a randomized, placebo-controlled, double-blind, multicenter clinical trial. *J Hepatol* 30:1081–9.

Medici, V., M. C. Virata, J. M. Peerson et al. 2011. *S*-Adenosyl-L-methionine treatment for alcoholic liver disease: a double-blinded, randomized, placebo-controlled trial. *Alcohol Clin Exp Res* 35:1960–5.

Mencarelli, A., S. Cipriani, B. Renga et al. 2012. VSL#3 resets insulin signaling and protects against NASH and atherosclerosis in a model of genetic dyslipidemia and intestinal inflammation. *PLoS One* 7:e45425.

Miglio, F., L. C. Rovati, A. Santoro, and I. Setnikar. 2000. Efficacy and safety of oral betaine glucuronate in non-alcoholic steatohepatitis. A double-blind, randomized, parallel-group, placebo-controlled prospective clinical study. *Arzneimittelforschung* 50:722–7.

Min, A. K., M. K. Kim, H. S. Kim et al. 2012. Alpha-lipoic acid attenuates methionine choline deficient diet-induced steatohepatitis in C57BL/6 mice. *Life Sci* 90:200–5.

Moran-Ramos, S., A. Avila-Nava, A. R. Tovar, J. Pedraza-Chaverri, P. Lopez-Romero, and N. Torres. 2012. Opuntia ficus indica (nopal) attenuates hepatic steatosis and oxidative stress in obese Zucker (*fa/fa*) rats. *J Nutr* 142:1956–63.

Morelli, L., and L. Capurso. 2012. FAO/WHO guidelines on probiotics: 10 years later. *J Clin Gastroenterol* 46 Suppl:S1–2.

Moroti, C., L. F. Souza Magri, M. de Rezende Costa, D. C. Cavallini, and K. Sivieri. 2012. Effect of the consumption of a new symbiotic shake on glycemia and cholesterol levels in elderly people with type 2 diabetes mellitus. *Lipids Health Dis* 11:29.

Mulder, T. P., A. G. Rietveld, and J. M. van Amelsvoort. 2005. Consumption of both black tea and green tea results in an increase in the excretion of hippuric acid into urine. *Am J Clin Nutr* 81:256S–260S.

Neyrinck, A. M., S. Possemiers, W. Verstraete, F. De Backer, P. D. Cani, and N. M. Delzenne. 2012. Dietary modulation of clostridial cluster XIVa gut bacteria (Roseburia spp.) by chitin-glucan fiber improves host metabolic alterations induced by high-fat diet in mice. *J Nutr Biochem* 23:51–9.

Novotny, L., P. Rauko, and C. Cojocel. 2008. Alpha-Lipoic acid: the potential for use in cancer therapy. *Neoplasma* 55:81–6.

Oner-Iyidogan, Y., H. Kocak, M. Seyidhanoglu et al. 2013. Curcumin prevents liver fat accumulation and serum fetuin-A increase in rats fed a high-fat diet. *J Physiol Biochem* 69:677–86.

Pajares, M. A., C. Duran, F. Corrales, M. M. Pliego, and J. M. Mato. 1992. Modulation of rat liver S-adenosylmethionine synthetase activity by glutathione. *J Biol Chem* 267:17598–605.

Parnell, J. A., and R. A. Reimer. 2010. Effect of prebiotic fibre supplementation on hepatic gene expression and serum lipids: a dose-response study in JCR:LA-cp rats. *Br J Nutr* 103:1577–84.

Perez-Leal, O., and S. Merali. 2012. Regulation of polyamine metabolism by translational control. *Amino Acids* 42:611–7.

Poulsen, M. M., J. O. Larsen, S. Hamilton-Dutoit et al. 2012. Resveratrol up-regulates hepatic uncoupling protein 2 and prevents development of nonalcoholic fatty liver disease in rats fed a high-fat diet. *Nutr Res* 32:701–8.

Prakash, S., C. Tomaro-Duchesneau, S. Saha, and A. Cantor. 2011. The gut microbiota and human health with an emphasis on the use of microencapsulated bacterial cells. *J Biomed Biotechnol* 2011:981214.

Raman, M., I. Ahmed, P. M. Gillevet et al. 2013. Fecal microbiome and volatile organic compound metabolome in obese humans with nonalcoholic fatty liver disease. *Clin Gastroenterol Hepatol* 11:868–75.

Rault-Nania, M. H., E. Gueux, C. Demougeot, C. Demigne, E. Rock, and A. Mazur. 2006. Inulin attenuates atherosclerosis in apolipoprotein E-deficient mice. *Br J Nutr* 96:840–4.

Rayes, N., T. Pilarski, M. Stockmann, S. Bengmark, P. Neuhaus, and D. Seehofer. 2012. Effect of pre- and probiotics on liver regeneration after resection: a randomised, double-blind pilot study. *Benef Microbes* 3:237–44.

Rayes, N., D. Seehofer, S. Hansen et al. 2002. Early enteral supply of lactobacillus and fiber versus selective bowel decontamination: a controlled trial in liver transplant recipients. *Transplantation* 74:123–7.

Resseguie, M., J. Song, M. D. Niculescu, K. A. da Costa, T. A. Randall, and S. H. Zeisel. 2007. Phosphatidylethanolamine N-methyltransferase (PEMT) gene expression is induced by estrogen in human and mouse primary hepatocytes. *FASEB J* 21:2622–32.

Roberfroid, M., G. R. Gibson, L. Hoyles et al. 2010. Prebiotic effects: metabolic and health benefits. *Br J Nutr* 104:S1–63.

Rochette, L., S. Ghibu, C. Richard, M. Zeller, Y. Cottin, and C. Vergely. 2013. Direct and indirect antioxidant properties of alpha-lipoic acid and therapeutic potential. *Mol Nutr Food Res* 57:114–25.

Roingeard, P. 2013. Hepatitis C virus diversity and hepatic steatosis. *J Viral Hepat* 20:77–84.

Salari, P., S. Nikfar, and M. Abdollahi. 2012. A meta-analysis and systematic review on the effect of probiotics in acute diarrhea. *Inflamm Allergy Drug Targets* 11:3–14.

Sanchez-Gongora, E., J. G. Pastorino, L. Alvarez et al. 1996. Increased sensitivity to oxidative injury in chinese hamster ovary cells stably transfected with rat liver S-adenosylmethionine synthetase cDNA. *Biochem J* 319:767–73.

Sarma, D. N., M. L. Barrett, M. L. Chavez et al. 2008. Safety of green tea extracts: a systematic review by the US Pharmacopeia. *Drug Saf* 31:469–84.

Schrieber, S. J., R. L. Hawke, Z. Wen et al. 2011. Differences in the disposition of silymarin between patients with nonalcoholic fatty liver disease and chronic hepatitis C. *Drug Metab Dispos* 39:2182–90.

Schrieber, S. J., Z. Wen, M. Vourvahis et al. 2008. The pharmacokinetics of silymarin is altered in patients with hepatitis C virus and nonalcoholic Fatty liver disease and correlates with plasma caspase-3/7 activity. *Drug Metab Dispos* 36:1909–16.

Schuppan, D., and J. M. Schattenberg. 2013. Non-alcoholic steatohepatitis: pathogenesis and novel therapeutic approaches. *J Gastroenterol Hepatol* 28 Suppl 1:68–76.

Seeff, L. B., T. M. Curto, G. Szabo et al. 2008. Herbal product use by persons enrolled in the hepatitis C Antiviral Long-Term Treatment Against Cirrhosis (HALT-C) Trial. *Hepatology* 47:605–12.

Senanayake, G. V., N. Fukuda, S. Nshizono et al. 2012. Mechanisms underlying decreased hepatic triacylglycerol and cholesterol by dietary bitter melon extract in the rat. *Lipids* 47:495–503.

Senanayake, G. V., M. Maruyama, M. Sakono et al. 2004a. The effects of bitter melon (Momordica charantia) extracts on serum and liver lipid parameters in hamsters fed cholesterol-free and cholesterol-enriched diets. *J Nutr Sci Vitaminol (Tokyo)* 50:253–7.

Senanayake, G. V., M. Maruyama, K. Shibuya et al. 2004b. The effects of bitter melon (Momordica charantia) on serum and liver triglyceride levels in rats. *J Ethnopharmacol* 91:257–62.

Shay, K. P., R. F. Moreau, E. J. Smith, A. R. Smith, and T. M. Hagen. 2009. Alpha-lipoic acid as a dietary supplement: molecular mechanisms and therapeutic potential. *Biochim Biophys Acta* 1790:1149–60.

Shen, L., Y. Xiong, D. Q. Wang et al. 2013. Ginsenoside Rb1 reduces fatty liver by activating AMP-activated protein kinase in obese rats. *J Lipid Res* 54:1430–8.

Slavin, J. 2013. Fiber and prebiotics: mechanisms and health benefits. *Nutrients* 5:1417–35.

Solga, S. F., G. Buckley, J. M. Clark, A. Horska, and A. M. Diehl. 2008. The effect of a probiotic on hepatic steatosis. *J Clin Gastroenterol* 42:1117–9.

Spencer, M. D., T. J. Hamp, R. W. Reid, L. M. Fischer, S. H. Zeisel, and A. A. Fodor. 2011. Association between composition of the human gastrointestinal microbiome and development of fatty liver with choline deficiency. *Gastroenterology* 140:976–86.

Sugiura, C., S. Nishimatsu, T. Moriyama, S. Ozasa, T. Kawada, and K. Sayama. 2012. Catechins and caffeine inhibit fat accumulation in mice through the improvement of hepatic lipid metabolism. *J Obes* 2012:520510.

Sweeney, T. E., and J. M. Morton. 2013. The human gut microbiome: a review of the effect of obesity and surgically induced weight loss. *JAMA Surg* 148:563–9.

Takeuchi-Yorimoto, A., T. Noto, A. Yamada, Y. Miyamae, Y. Oishi, and M. Matsumoto. 2013. Persistent fibrosis in the liver of choline-deficient and iron-supplemented L-amino acid–defined diet-induced nonalcoholic steatohepatitis rat due to continuing oxidative stress after choline supplementation. *Toxicol Appl Pharmacol* 268:264–77.

Tanamly, M. D., F. Tadros, S. Labeeb et al. 2004. Randomised double-blinded trial evaluating silymarin for chronic hepatitis C in an Egyptian village: study description and 12-month results. *Dig Liver Dis* 36:752–9.

Tzeng, T. F., H. J. Lu, S. S. Liou, C. J. Chang, and I. M. Liu. 2013. Cassia tora (Leguminosae) seed extract alleviates high-fat diet-induced nonalcoholic fatty liver. *Food Chem Toxicol* 51:194–201.

Um, M. Y., J. Ahn, and T. Y. Ha. 2013. Hypolipidaemic effects of cyanidin 3-glucoside rich extract from black rice through regulating hepatic lipogenic enzyme activities. *J Sci Food Agric.*

Vrieze, A., P. F. de Groot, R. S. Kootte, M. Knaapen, E. van Nood, and M. Nieuwdorp. 2013. Fecal transplant: a safe and sustainable clinical therapy for restoring intestinal microbial balance in human disease? *Best Pract Res Clin Gastroenterol* 27:127–37.

Vrieze, A., E. Van Nood, F. Holleman et al. 2012. Transfer of intestinal microbiota from lean donors increases insulin sensitivity in individuals with metabolic syndrome. *Gastroenterology* 143:913–6 e7.

Wang, S. D., Z. Q. Xie, J. Chen et al. 2012. Inhibitory effect of Ginkgo biloba extract on fatty liver: regulation of carnitine palmitoyltransferase 1a and fatty acid metabolism. *J Dig Dis* 13:525–35.

Wei, F., S. K. Liu, X. Y. Liu et al. 2013. Meta-analysis: silymarin and its combination therapy for the treatment of chronic hepatitis B. *Eur J Clin Microbiol Infect Dis* 32:657–69.

Wong, V. W., C. H. Tse, T. T. Lam et al. 2013a. Molecular characterization of the fecal microbiota in patients with nonalcoholic steatohepatitis—a longitudinal study. *PLoS One* 8:e62885.

Wong, V. W., G. L. Won, A. M. Chim et al. 2013b. Treatment of nonalcoholic steatohepatitis with probiotics. A proof-of-concept study. *Ann Hepatol* 12:256–62.

Xiao, J., C. T. Ho, E. C. Liong et al. 2013. Epigallocatechin gallate attenuates fibrosis, oxidative stress, and inflammation in non-alcoholic fatty liver disease rat model through TGF/SMAD, PI3 K/Akt/FoxO1, and NF-kappa B pathways. *Eur J Nutr.*

Xu, Q., and L. Y. Si. 2012. Resveratrol role in cardiovascular and metabolic health and potential mechanisms of action. *Nutr Res* 32:648–58.

Yiu, W. F., P. L. Kwan, C. Y. Wong et al. 2011. Attenuation of fatty liver and prevention of hypercholesterolemia by extract of Curcuma longa through regulating the expression of CYP7A1, LDL-receptor, HO-1, and HMG-CoA reductase. *J Food Sci* 76:H80–9.

Zeisel, S. H. 2006. Choline: critical role during fetal development and dietary requirements in adults. *Annu Rev Nutr* 26:229–50.

Zeisel, S. H. 2010. Choline. In *Encyclopedia of dietary supplements*, edited by P. M. Coates. New York: Informa Healthcare.

Index

Page numbers followed by f and t indicate figures and tables, respectively.

303